2006
YEAR BOOK OF
OBSTETRICS, GYNECOLOGY, AND WOMEN'S HEALTH®

The 2006 Year Book Series

Year Book of Allergy, Asthma, and Clinical Immunology™: Drs Rosenwasser, Boguniewicz, Milgrom, Routes, and Weber

Year Book of Anesthesiology and Pain Management™: Drs Chestnut, Abram, Black, Gravlee, Lee, Mathru, and Roizen

Year Book of Cardiology®: Drs Gersh, Cheitlin, Elliott, Graham, Sundt, and Waldo

Year Book of Critical Care Medicine®: Drs Dellinger, Parrillo, Balk, Bekes, Dorman, and Dries

Year Book of Dentistry®: Drs McIntyre, Belvedere, Buhite, Davis, Henderson, Johnson, Jureyda, Ohrbach, Olin, Scott, Spencer, and Zakariasen

Year Book of Dermatology and Dermatologic Surgery™: Drs Thiers and Lang

Year Book of Diagnostic Radiology®: Drs Osborn, Birdwell, Dalinka, Gardiner, Levy, Maynard, Oestreich, and Rosado de Christenson

Year Book of Emergency Medicine®: Drs Burdick, Hamilton, Handly, Quintana, and Werner

Year Book of Endocrinology®: Drs Mazzaferri, Bessesen, Clarke, Howard, Kennedy, Leahy, Meikle, Molitch, Rogol, and Schteingart

Year Book of Family Practice®: Drs Bowman, Apgar, Dexter, Miser, Neill, and Scherger

Year Book of Gastroenterology™: Drs Lichtenstein, Burke, Campbell, Dempsey, Drebin, Ginsberg, Katzka, Kochman, Morris, Rombeau, Shah, and Stein

Year Book of Hand Surgery and Upper Limb Surgery®: Drs Chang and Steinmann

Year Book of Medicine®: Drs Barkin, Frishman, Loehrer, Garrick, Phillips, Pillinger, and Snydman

Year Book of Neonatal and Perinatal Medicine®: Drs Fanaroff, Maisels, and Stevenson

Year Book of Neurology and Neurosurgery®: Drs Gibbs and Verma

Year Book of Nuclear Medicine®: Drs Coleman, Blaufox, Royal, Strauss, and Zubal

Year Book of Obstetrics, Gynecology, and Women's Health®: Dr Shulman

Year Book of Oncology®: Drs Loehrer, Arceci, Glatstein, Gordon, Hanna, Morrow, and Thigpen

Year Book of Ophthalmology®: Drs Rapuano, Cohen, Eagle, Flanders, Hammersmith, Myers, Nelson, Penne, Sergott, Shields, Tipperman, and Vander

Year Book of Orthopedics®: Drs Morrey, Beauchamp, Peterson, Swiontkowski, Trigg, and Yaszemski

Year Book of Otolaryngology-Head and Neck Surgery®: Drs Paparella, Gapany, and Keefe

Year Book of Pathology and Laboratory Medicine®: Drs Raab, Parwani, Bejarano, and Bissell

Year Book of Pediatrics®: Dr Stockman

Year Book of Plastic and Aesthetic Surgery™: Drs Miller, Bartlett, Garner, McKinney, Ruberg, Salisbury, and Smith

Year Book of Psychiatry and Applied Mental Health®: Drs Talbott, Ballenger, Buckley, Frances, Jensen, and Markowitz

Year Book of Pulmonary Disease®: Drs Phillips, Barker, Lewis, Maurer, Tanoue, and Willsie

Year Book of Rheumatology, Arthritis, and Musculoskeletal Disease™: Drs Panush, Furst, Hadler, Hochberg, Lahita, and Paget

Year Book of Sports Medicine®: Drs Shephard, Alexander, Cantu, Feldman, McCrory, Nieman, Rowland, Sanborn, and Shrier

Year Book of Surgery®: Drs Copeland, Bland, Cerfolio, Daly, Eberlein, Fahey, Mozingo, Pruett, and Seeger

Year Book of Urology®: Drs Andriole and Coplen

Year Book of Vascular Surgery®: Dr Moneta

2006

Year Book of OBSTETRICS, GYNECOLOGY, AND WOMEN'S HEALTH®

Editor-in-Chief

Lee P. Shulman, MD

Professor of Obstetrics and Gynecology; Chief, Division of Reproductive Genetics, Department of Obstetrics and Gynecology, Feinberg School of Medicine, Northwestern University, Chicago, Illinois

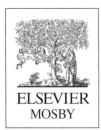

ELSEVIER
MOSBY

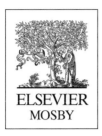

ELSEVIER
MOSBY

Vice President, Continuity Publishing: Timothy M. Griswold
Publishing Director, Continuity: J. Heather Cullen
Associate Developmental Editor: Timothy Maxwell
Senior Manager, Continuity Production: Idelle L. Winer
Senior Issue Manager: Donna M. Adamson
Illustrations and Permissions Coordinator: Dawn Vohsen

Printed in the United States of America
Composition by Thomas Technology Solutions, Inc.
Printing/binding by Sheridan Books, Inc.

Editorial Office:
Elsevier
Suite 1800
1600 John F. Kennedy Blvd.
Philadelphia, PA 19103-2899

International Standard Serial Number: 1090-798X
International Standard Book Number: 1-4160-3311-4
                                                       978-1-4160-3311-0

Editors

Raquel D. Arias, MD
Associate Professor, Obstetrics and Gynecology, Associate Dean for Women, Keck School of Medicine; Clinical Associate Professor, Gerontology, University of Southern California; Director, William H. Hindle Breast Diagnostic Center, Women's and Children's Hospital, Los Angeles, California

Randall Barnes, MD
Associate Professor, Feinberg School of Medicine, Northwestern University, Chicago, Illinois

Serdar E. Bulun, MD
Professor and Friends of Prentice Distinguished Physician Chief, Division of Reproductive Biology Research, Department of Obstetrics and Gynecology, Feinberg School of Medicine, Northwestern University, Chicago, Illinois

Sherman Elias, MD
John J. Sciarra Professor and Chair, Department of Obstetrics and Gynecology, Feinberg School of Medicine, Northwestern University, Chicago, Illinois

Jean A. Hurteau, MD
Director, Division of Gynecologic Oncology, University of Illinois at Chicago, Chicago, Illinois

Gary H. Lipscomb, MD
Professor and Associate Chair of Clinical Affairs, Director, Division of Gynecologic Specialties, Department of Obstetrics and Gynecology, University of Tennessee Health Science Center, Memphis, Tennessee

John M.G. van Vugt, MD, PhD
Professor of Fetal Medicine, VU University Medical Center, Amstelveen, The Netherlands

Contributing Editors

Megan E. App, MD, MPH
Assistant Professor of Clinical Obstetrics and Gynecology, University of Illinois at Chicago, Chicago, Illinois

Candace Susanne Brown, MSN, PharmD
Professor, Departments of Pharmacy, Obstetrics and Gynecology, and Psychiatry, University of Tennessee Health Science Center, Lakeland, Tennessee

Yvonne Collins, MD
Assistant Professor of Clinical Obstetrics and Gynecology, University of Illinois at Chicago, Chicago, Illinois

Michael R. Drews, MD
Associate Clinical Professor, Department of Obstetrics and Gynecology in Reproductive Sciences, University of Dentistry and Medicine of New Jersey, Robert Wood Johnson Medical School; Reproductive Medicine Associates of New Jersey, Morristown, New Jersey

Patricia M Garcia, MD, MPH
Associate Professor, Division of Maternal-Fetal Medicine, Feinberg School of Medicine, Northwestern University, Chicago, Illinois

Vanessa A. M. Givens, MD
Assistant Professor, Department of Obstetrics and Gynecology, University of Tennessee Health Science Center, Memphis, Tennessee

Stephen A. Grochmal, MD
Associate Clinical Professor of Obstetrics and Gynecology, Division of Operative Gynecology, Endoscopy and Laser Surgery, Howard University College of Medicine, New York, New York

Thomas J. Herzog, MD
Professor of Clinical Obstetrics and Gynecology, Director, Division of Gynecologic Oncology, Irving Comprehensive Cancer Center, College of Physicians and Surgeons, Columbia University, New York, New York

Elba A. Iglesias, MD
Assistant Professor of Pediatrics, North Shore-Long Island Jewish Health System; Division of Adolescent Medicine, Schneider Children's Hospital, New Hyde Park, New York

H.N. Lafeber, MD, PhD
Professor of Neonatology, VU University Medical Center, Amsterdam, The Netherlands

F.K. Lotgering, MD, PhD
Professor of Obstetrics, Head, Division of Obstetrics, University Medical Centre Nijmegen, Nijmegen, The Netherlands

David Scott Miller, MD
Director and Dallas Foundation Chair in Gynecologic Oncology, Professor of Obstetrics and Gynecology, University of Texas Southwestern Medical Center, Dallas, Texas

Bradley J. Monk, MD
Associate Professor, University of California, Irvine Medical Center, Orange, California

Owen P. Phillips, MD
Professor, Department of Obstetrics and Gynecology, University of Tennessee Health Science Center, Memphis, Tennessee

Gustavo Rodriguez, MD
Associate Professor, Feinberg School of Medicine, Northwestern University, Chicago, Illinois

E.A.P. Steegers, MD, PhD
Professor and Head, Division of Obstetrics and Prenatal Medicine, Department of Obstetrics and Gynecology, Erasmus University Medical Center, Rotterdam, The Netherlands

Mary D. Stephenson, MD, MSc
Professor of Obstetrics and Gynecology, Section of Reproductive Endocrinology & Infertility, Director, Recurrent Pregnancy Loss Program, University of Chicago, Chicago, Illinois

Stephen Thung, MD
Assistant Professor, Department of Obstetrics and Gynecology, Yale University School of Medicine, New Haven, Connecticut

Serdar H. Ural, MD
Assistant Professor of Obstetrics and Gynecology, Director, High Risk Obstetrics Clinic, Division of Maternal Fetal Medicine, University of Pennsylvania School of Medicine, Philadelphia, Pennsylvania

Paul Pierre van den Berg, MD, PhD
Professor of Obstetrics, Department of Obstetrics and Gynecology, University Medical Center Groningen, Groningen, The Netherlands

H.P. van Geijn, MD, PhD
Professor of Obstetrics and Gynecology, Head, Department of Obstetrics and Gynecology, VU University Medical Center, Amsterdam, The Netherlands

George D. Wendel, Jr., MD
Professor, Residency Program Director, Vice-Chair for Education, Obstetrics and Gynecology Department, University of Texas Southwestern Medical School, Dallas, Texas

S. Diane Yamada, MD
Assistant Professor, Section of Gynecologic Oncology, Department of Obstetrics and Gynecology, University of Chicago, Chicago, Illinois

Nikki B. Zite, MD, MPH
Assistant Professor, Department of Obstetrics and Gynecology, University of Tennessee Medical Center, Knoxville, Tennessee

Table of Contents

Journals Represented

Journals represented in this YEAR BOOK are listed below.

Acta Obstetricia et Gynecologica Scandinavica
Acta Paediatrica
American Journal of Clinical Nutrition
American Journal of Clinical Pathology
American Journal of Epidemiology
American Journal of Human Genetics
American Journal of Obstetrics and Gynecology
American Journal of Pathology
American Journal of Perinatology
American Journal of Public Health
Annals of Oncology
Annals of Plastic Surgery
Archives of Disease in Childhood, Fetal and Neonatal Edition
Archives of Neurology
Archives of Pathology and Laboratory Medicine
Archives of Pediatrics and Adolescent Medicine
Australian and New Zealand Journal of Obstetrics and Gynaecology
Brain Research
Breast Journal
British Journal of Anaesthesia
British Journal of General Practice
British Journal of Obstetrics and Gynaecology
British Journal of Urology International
British Medical Journal
Cancer Epidemiology, Biomarkers and Prevention
Circulation
Clinical Infectious Diseases
Contraception
Endocrinology
Epidemiology
European Journal of Obstetrics, Gynecology and Reproductive Biology
European Urology
Fertility and Sterility
Gastroenterology
Gynecologic Oncology
Human Reproduction
International Journal of Cancer
International Journal of Gynaecology and Obstetrics
International Journal of Gynecological Cancer
International Journal of Gynecology & Obstetrics
Journal of Acquired Immune Deficiency Syndromes
Journal of Adolescent Health
Journal of Applied Physiology
Journal of Bone and Joint Surgery (American Volume)
Journal of Clinical Endocrinology and Metabolism
Journal of Clinical Microbiology
Journal of Clinical Oncology
Journal of Computer Assisted Tomography
Journal of Heart and Lung Transplantation

Journal of Lower Genital Tract Disease
Journal of Medical Genetics
Journal of Obstetrics and Gynaecology
Journal of Pediatric Adolescent Gynecology
Journal of Pediatrics
Journal of Public Health Dentistry
Journal of Reproductive Medicine
Journal of Ultrasound in Medicine
Journal of Urology
Journal of Women's Health
Journal of the American Medical Association
Lancet
Lancet Oncology
Maturitas
Medicine and Science in Sports and Exercise
Menopause: The Journal of The American Menopause Society
Metabolism: Clinical and Experimental
Modern Pathology
Molecular and Cellular Biology
New England Journal of Medicine
Obstetrics and Gynecology
Pediatric Research
Pediatrics
Placenta
Proceedings of the National Academy of Sciences
Radiology
Science
Southern Medical Journal
Surgery
The Oncologist
Ultrasound in Obstetrics and Gynecology
Urology

STANDARD ABBREVIATIONS

The following terms are abbreviated in this edition: acquired immunodeficiency syndrome (AIDS), cardiopulmonary resuscitation (CPR), central nervous system (CNS), cerebrospinal fluid (CSF), computed tomography (CT), deoxyribonucleic acid (DNA), electrocardiography (ECG), health maintenance organization (HMO), human immunodeficiency virus (HIV), intensive care unit (ICU), intramuscular (IM), intravenous (IV), magnetic resonance (MR) imaging (MRI), ribonucleic acid (RNA), and ultrasound (US).

NOTE

To facilitate the use of the YEAR BOOK OF OBSTETRICS, GYNECOLOGY, AND WOMEN'S HEALTH as a reference tool, all illustrations and tables included in this publication are now identified as they appear in the original article. This change is meant to help the reader recognize that any illustration or table appearing in the YEAR BOOK OF OBSTETRICS, GYNECOLOGY, AND WOMEN'S HEALTH may be only one of many in the original article. For this reason, figure and table numbers will often appear to be out of sequence within the YEAR BOOK OF OBSTETRICS, GYNECOLOGY, AND WOMEN'S HEALTH.

Introduction

I continue to be amazed at the changes in women's health care, especially when I compare current medical practice with clinical care at the completion of my residency in 1987. From the application of genomic advances to almost all aspects of women's health care to the development of robotic and minimally invasive surgical techniques to the improvements in assisted reproductive technologies, our improved understanding of the pathophysiology of obstetrical and gynecological conditions has truly improved our ability to provide effective diagnosis and treatment to an increasing number of women.

What cannot be lost in this changing and expanding understanding of the scientific and clinical basis of obstetrical and gynecological conditions is that effective medicine requires the clinician to be a caring and empathetic caregiver. Our compassion and humanity remain central to the provision of effective health care regardless of the scientific and technological advances that characterize current and future clinical paradigms. Indeed, the desire and ability to apply these advances to the widest possible community of women who may require such care could be the definitive expression of compassion and humanity as it pertains to medicine.

This is the second edition of the YEAR BOOK OF OBSTETRICS, GYNECOLOGY, AND WOMEN'S HEALTH that has been edited by the current board of editors and contributing editors. Our goal remains simple: to provide you with an encompassing review of the important clinical and scientific advances in obstetrics, gynecology, and women's health gathered from published articles in well-recognized peer-reviewed journals. Our decision to expand our editorial board to include recognized experts from around the world is one that was made to create a YEAR BOOK that is more likely to present a more accurate view of the important scientific and clinical advances in women's health care. From the feedback that we have thus far received, we believe that this new formula has worked and we will thus continue to utilize this system for future editions.

Readers of the YEAR BOOK series will recognize some minor changes to the overall content of this year's edition that will hopefully serve to better present the changing milieu of women's health care. Several new categories have been added, including fecal incontinence, botanicals, preimplantation diagnosis, and cancer genetics. In addition, sections relating to the more personal aspects of women's health care have been expanded. In this way, we hope to "practice what we preach" by presenting an updated review of the scientific, clinical, *and* interpersonal and emotive aspects of women's health care and thus better present the entirety of women's health care worldwide.

I am indebted to the editors and contributing editors for their hard work, dedication, patience, and friendship throughout this process. I would also like to thank and recognize our editorial assistants, David Strosnider and Rebecca Shulman, for their invaluable contributions to the composition of this edition of the YEAR BOOK. And finally, on behalf of all of the editors, contributing editors, and editorial assistants, I would like to thank you, the reader, for your interest in women's health and your dedication to improving the care of women throughout the world. We want to provide you with the best possible review of current scientific and clinical advancements so that you can continue to provide the most effective care and best serve the interests of women. In this way, this edition of the YEAR BOOK is dedicated to the clinicians who provide obstetrical and gynecological care, who teach students, residents, and colleagues, who provide vital emotional support at the worst of times and share in the joy of the best of times. We hope that this YEAR BOOK will be of some assistance to your pursuit of professional and personal goals.

The editorial board welcome your comments and opinions about this edition of the YEAR BOOK. Please feel free to contact us by email at shulmandoc@hotmail.com. Many thanks again and best wishes.

Lee P. Shulman MD

MEDICAL EDUCATION, PRACTICE ISSUES, GENERAL

WOMEN'S HEALTH

1 General Issues

Teaching Students to Question
Loy GL, Gelula MH, Vontver L (Univ of Illinois at Chicago; Univ of Washington, Seattle)
Am J Obstet Gynecol 191:1752-1756, 2004   1–1

Background.—The ability to ask the "right" questions is fundamental to critical thinking, an essential component of medical education. Interaction between students and instructors can create learning opportunities for the student, and this interaction is accomplished through students' questions. Knowing how to ask a critical question would enable students to engage the attending faculty. The purpose of this study was to teach the strategies of critical questioning to medical students to determine the effects of this instruction on students' critical thinking skills, confidence in their ability to ask questions, and interaction between student and instructor.

Methods.—A series of workshops was designed to teach students to systematically ask critical questions in a nonconfrontational way. Eight workshop modules were presented in two 90-minute sessions held 1 week apart. The study group was composed of 62 consenting adults in their third-year obstetrics and gynecology clerkship. The students were divided according to alternate rotations to either attend the workshops (28 students) or not attend (41 students).

Results.—The medical students who attended the workshops scored higher than the non-attending group on the California Critical Thinking Skills Test mean total score (study group 25.1 [±0.7 SEM] vs control group 22.9 [±0.6 SEM]), subscales of interference (12.6 [±0.3 SEM] vs 11.2 [±0.3 SEM]), and deductive reasoning (12.7 [±0.3 SEM]).

Conclusions.—Critical thinking in medical students is improved by teaching students to ask critical questions as measured by the California Critical Thinking Skills Test.

▶ The authors report on the results of a series of 8 workshop modules presented during two 90-minute sessions held 1 week apart, titled "How to Ask the Right Question," in which third-year medical students on their core clerkship in obstetrics and gynecology participated. A control group was comprised of students on alternate periods during which no workshops were given. The hypotheses were that teaching students the strategies of critical questioning would improve critical thinking skills, improve student confidence in their own ability to ask questions, and increase interactions between student and instructor. Medical students who attended the workshops scored higher on the California Critical Thinking Skills Tests, a survey instrument that measures the predisposition toward thinking critically, as compared to controls.

The authors conclude the following:

1. If questions are conceived during attending rounds and discussed as a group, that improved knowledge building occurs.
2. By creating a learning opportunity within a clinical situation and applying reasoning skills, the learner improves retention of those skills.
3. Increasing student-initiated contact with instructors during clinical rotations remains an important goal to counter the pressures of time constraints and the variations in instructor attentiveness. Frequent and interactive contact with instructors improves the probability of acquisition of knowledge and skills. Critical questioning skills are an important part of lifelong learning.

These skills may ultimately be shown to correlate with clinical performance and outcomes and therefore warrant further evaluation.

S. Elias, MD

Factors Detracting Students From Applying for an Obstetrics and Gynecology Residency

Gariti DL, Zollinger TW, Look KY (Indiana Univ, Indianapolis)
Am J Obstet Gynecol 193:289-293, 2005   1–2

Objective.—This study compares perception about the characteristics of obstetrics-gynecology (OG) of medical students who choose to pursue a residency in OG and those students who choose to enter another specialty.

Study Design.—Fourth-year medical students were asked to complete a survey addressing their perceptions about OG. Responses were compared of (1) those entering OG to those entering other specialties, (2) those entering OG to those who seriously considered entering OG but chose another discipline, and (3) males to females. Chi-square tests were used for the comparisons.

Results.—Of the 267 eligible students, 137 (51.1%) completed the survey. Clerkship satisfaction was rated as high by 88.9% of students choosing OG vs 10.2% ($P < .0005$) of those who chose another discipline. The emerging predominance of female providers detracted 38.5% of males vs 10.2% of females ($P < .0005$).

Conclusion.—Student perception of an OG clerkship may detract them from pursuing OG as a career.

▶ The authors report the results of a survey study of fourth-year medical students to examine differences in their perceptions about obstetrics and gynecology regarding the clerkship, lifestyle, gender issues, and practice economics. Students choosing obstetrics and gynecology and those choosing other specialties were surveyed. Students entering obstetrics and gynecology were more satisfied with their obstetrics and gynecology clerkship than were students pursuing other specialties. The authors suggest that the quality of interactions between obstetrics and gynecology faculty and residents during their clerkship experience is an important factor for recruitment into the specialty. Lifestyle issues, such as a lack of control over work hour distributions, appear to make obstetrics and gynecology an unattractive choice. Exposing students to various career opportunities in obstetrics and gynecology may help with recruitment. Options that should be cited include subspecialization, alternative modes of practice (eg, gynecology-only practice), part-time practices, group practices, and the new trend toward the laborist model of practice. Finally, many male students do not see a place for themselves in the future of the obstetrics and gynecology workforce. Thus, it is important for male medical students to interact with male obstetrician-gynecologist practitioners as role models, who can assure them that there is indeed a place for them in the specialty. Increasing the number of male applicants for obstetrics and gynecology residencies could significantly improve the overall recruitment into the specialty. We must make obstetrics and gynecology attractive to the best and brightest medical students to ensure the highest quality of health care to women.

S. Elias, MD

Teaching Residents How to Teach Improves Quality of Clerkship
Hammoud MM, Haefner HK, Schigelone A, et al (Univ of Michigan, Ann Arbor)
Am J Obstet Gynecol 191:1741-1745, 2004   1–3

Objective.—To evaluate the impact of a resident's teaching skills workshop on the ratings of the obstetrics and gynecology clerkship by third-year medical students.

Study Design.—The 6-week obstetrics and gynecology clerkship at the University of Michigan is provided at 4 different sites including the University of Michigan Hospital. At the end of each rotation, medical students complete an evaluation form assessing various aspects of their learning experience, including the overall quality of clerkship. A workshop, "Teaching Residents How to Teach," was conducted at the University of Michigan Hospital, whereas the other 3 sites served as the control. Clerkship evaluations were compared before and after the workshop using Student t test.

Results.—Students at the University of Michigan Hospital rated all items on the evaluation form higher after the teaching workshop. The overall quality of the clerkship at the University of Michigan Hospital improved ($P = .05$), whereas the other sites remained stable.

Conclusions.—A "Teaching the Residents How to Teach" workshop improves the overall quality of the clerkship.

▶ Obstetrics and gynecology has been one of the lowest rated clerkships by medical students nationally. This may be one of the factors in the decline of medical students choosing careers in obstetrics and gynecology, although other factors such as lifestyle and perceived reduced practice opportunities for male medical students also appear to be important. Residents play a major role in teaching medical students. The authors of this study sought to determine whether a 1-day teaching skills workshop for residents would affect medical student clerkship evaluations. Specifically, they looked at items on the clerkship evaluations that they would expect to improve based on the teaching curriculum, including the quality of resident teaching and the overall quality of the clerkship. The workshop was conducted at the University of Michigan Hospital; 3 other clerkship sites served as controls. Clerkship evaluations were compared before and after the workshop. They found that students' evaluations for the 3 months after the retreat were significantly higher with respect to the clarity of the goals and objectives of the clerkship, expectations of student performance, and quality of feedback compared with students' evaluations from the control clerkships sites. The authors considered one of the most important observations from the study was that 14 of the 16 residents who filled out evaluations of the retreat agreed or strongly agreed that their commitment to teaching medical students had increased on the basis of the teaching workshop. Overall, the quality of the clerkship was believed to be improved by the "Teaching the Residents How to Teach" workshop. However, the authors observed that there is a time factor after which the residents' enthusiasm in teaching decreases; therefore, residents' teaching skills must constantly be reinforced to continue the desired effect of improving the quality of the clerkship. Teaching workshops for faculty should also be studied to determine whether they, too, would further improve the clerkship experience for medical students.

S. Elias, MD

Impact of Work Hour Restrictions on Resident Case Experience in an Obstetrics and Gynecology Residency Program
Blanchard MH, Amini SB, Frank TM (Case Western Reserve Univ, Cleveland, Ohio)
Am J Obstet Gynecol 191:1746-1751, 2004   1–4

Objective.—The purpose of this study was to evaluate senior resident case experience before and after enactment of work hour restrictions.

Study Design.—Obstetrics and gynecology experience from 2 postgraduate year 4 classes were evaluated before and after adoption of work hour restrictions. Data were limited to experience obtained during the fourth year of residency. Data were analyzed with the 2-sample t test and Wilcoxon rank sum test, and adjusted for changes in institutional procedural volume.

Results.—There were significant decreases in resident experience in total abdominal hysterectomy ($P = .018$), procedures for genuine stress urinary incontinence ($P = .004$), and hysteroscopy ($P = .006$). Decreases were seen in resident experience in vaginal birth after cesarean section ($P = .011$), primary cesarean section ($P = .31$), and vacuum delivery ($P = 007$), despite increase in institutional volume.

Conclusion.—Work hour restrictions have had impact on resident case experience in obstetrics and gynecology. Variance in institutional case numbers account for only some of these changes.

▶ Historically, physicians in training have worked long duty hours, often in excess of 100 hours per week. There has been considerable concern about the effects of these long work hours on patient safety as well as the adverse personal health consequences on residents. In response to these concerns, the Accreditation Council on Graduate Medical Education set the standard of limiting resident work hours to 80 hours per week. In this study, the authors evaluated the impact of restricting work hours on senior resident case experience by comparing 2 cohorts. Cohort 1 consisted of those postgraduate year 4 residents graduating in June 2002 (before duty hour limitations), and cohort 2 consisting of postgraduate year 4 residents graduating in June 2003 (after work restrictions were enacted). They found significant decreases in resident experience for the following procedures: total abdominal hysterectomy, general stress urinary incontinence, hysteroscopy, vaginal birth after cesarean section, primary cesarean section, and vacuum delivery. This brings into question the number of cases necessary for a resident to become proficient in performing a given procedure. The authors cite studies that indicate hospital quality improvement data showing that for certain types of procedures (amniocentesis, coronary arterial bypass surgery), morbidity and mortality rates are lower when performed by physicians who do the procedures frequently. However, these data come from postresidency practice settings. Whether they are applicable to residency training must still be evaluated. Priorities may have to be realigned for residency training within the 80-hour work week to ensure that time is best utilized for education and that opportunities for surgical experiences are optimized.

S. Elias, MD

Laparoscopic Training and Practice in Gynecologic Oncology Among Society of Gynecologic Oncologists Members and Fellows-in-Training
Frumovitz M, Ramirez PT, Greer M, et al (Univ of Texas, Houston)
Gynecol Oncol 94:746-753, 2004   1–5

Background.—Laparoscopy has become an important surgical tool in the current clinical era. The uses of this technique and the training required for excellence have not been well studied in the field of gynecologic oncology. The objective of this study was to gain information regarding the opinion of indications for laparoscopy and the adequacy of training in laparoscopy within the discipline of gynecologic oncology.

Methods.—A survey was mailed to the Society of Gynecologic Oncologists (SGO) and fellows-in-training in December 2002. Anonymous responses were analyzed, and statistics including frequency distributions and nonparametric tests were applied to analyze the results.

TABLE 1.

Variable	SGO Members	Fellows-in-Training
Responded to survey	336 (45%)	57 (49%)
Perform laparoscopy	272 (84%)	57 (100%)
Most common procedure:	69%	N/A
Adnexal mass management		
Perform >50% cases via scope	3%	N/A
Rate skills "very good" or "good"	78%	N/A
Rate training "very good" or "good"	N/A	25%
Believe scope indicated for prophylactic BSO	81%	97%
Believe scope indicated for	56%	83%
uterine cancer (LAVH/staging)		
Believe scope indicated for	52%	74%
ovarian cancer—second look		
Believe scope indicated for	4%	0%
ovarian cancer—debulking		
Believe scope indicated for	16%	19%
cervical cancer—trachelectomy/staging		
Belong to a laparoscopic society	13%	N/A

Abbreviations: SGO, Society of Gynecologic Oncologists; *N/A*, not applicable; *BSO*, bilateral salpingo-oophorectomy; *LAVH*, laparoscopically assisted radical hysterectomy.

Findings.—A total of 336 SGO members and 57 fellows-in-training responded to the survey. Table 1 reports the major findings from the survey. The vast majority of SGO members (84%) currently perform laparoscopic surgeries with the cited goal of decreasing length of stay, improving quality of life, and improving cosmetic results. For those who do not perform laparoscopy, the concern of increased operative time was the most significant barrier cited. Interestingly, 78% of SGO members rated their skills as "very good" or "good," while only 25% of fellows thought that their training was "very good" or "good."

Conclusions.—Most members of the SGO who responded do perform laparoscopy for selected indications, and most actually developed their skills after fellowship training. Interestingly, most current fellows do not perceive their present training to be adequate.

▶ Many of the early developments that advanced the field of laparoscopy occurred within the discipline of gynecology, first in Western Europe then in the United States. Other surgical specialties now enthusiastically embrace these methods widely after initially often expressing derision for those who performed laparoscopic surgery. Within the field of gynecologic oncology, the role of laparoscopy has been debated. Advocates cite its ability to decrease length of stay and enhance recovery, while others counter that randomized studies have not adequately demonstrated equivalency to laparotomy for cancer resection and staging, and that the laparoscopic approach takes more time while being potentially associated with a higher complication rate.

Obviously, the shortcomings of this analysis are that these data were collected via survey, which can have a number of associated biases. One concern is that those who returned their surveys were not necessarily representative of the greater societal membership. An additional concern is that the accuracy and veracity of the responses cannot be confirmed in an objective manner.

These criticisms notwithstanding, this article is an important contribution in that it highlights the marked disparity in laparoscopic indications and training. In terms of future implications, the most important issue is fellowship education. This is highlighted by the fact that 39% of the respondents have received no laparoscopic training and 46% received limited training (<5 cases per month). In addition, the fellows-in-training thought they received good training during residency, but only 25% thought they were currently receiving good laparoscopic training during fellowship. Hopefully, this disparity will be corrected as fellowships need to make laparoscopic training a high priority and incorporate a formalized laparoscopic curriculum that will facilitate core skill learning in training our next generation of gynecologic oncologists.

T. J. Herzog, MD

The Effects of the Women, Infants, and Children's Supplemental Food Program on Dentally Related Medicaid Expenditures
Lee JY, Rosier RG, Norton EC, et al (Univ of North Carolina, Chapel Hill)
J Public Health Dent 64:76-81, 2004   1–6

Objective.—This study estimates the effects of the Special Supplemental Nutrition Program for Women, Infants, and Children (WIC) on dentally related Medicaid expenditures for young children.

Methods.—We used a five-year cohort study design to compare dentally related Medicaid expenditures for children enrolled in WIC versus those not enrolled for each year of life up to age 5 years. There were 49,795 children born in North Carolina in 1992 who met the inclusion criteria for the study. Their birth records were linked to Medicaid enrollment and claims files, WIC master files, and the Area Resource File. Our analysis strategy included a logit and OLS two-part model with CPI dollar adjustments.

Results.—Children who participated in WIC at ages 1 and 2 years had significantly less dentally related expenditures than those who did not participate. WIC participation at age 3 years did not have a significant effect. Fewer WIC children received dental care under general anesthesia than non-WIC children.

Conclusions.—The WIC program has the potential for decreasing dentally related costs to the Medicaid program, while increasing use of dental services.

▶ This study was performed to assess the Special Supplemental Nutrition Program for Women, Infants, and Children (WIC) and related dental expenses. A total of 49,795 children from North Carolina were analyzed. Logit and an ordinary least squares (OLS) 2-part model with Consumer Price Index (CPI) dollar adjustments were used for analysis. It was interestingly and clearly seen that when the earlier children were participating in WIC, their dental expenditures were significantly decreasing. Because dental care is as important as physical and mental health, it is imperative to strongly consider this information in prevention and better use of dental health resources. In addition, early-age participation can lead to economic savings in the long run.

S. H. Ural, MD

Female Patients' Sex Preferences in Selection of Gynecologists and Surgeons
Childs AJ, Friedman WH, Schwartz MP, et al (Mercer Univ, Savannah, Ga; Med College of Georgia, Augusta)
South Med J 98:405-408, 2005   1–7

Objectives.—In this study, the authors investigated sex preferences for gynecologists and surgeons among female patients, and explored potential contributing factors.

Methods.—One hundred forty-six female patients were surveyed in a private practice office concerning their sex preferences and past obstetric/gynecologic care. For data comparisons, χ^2 or Fisher exact tests were used.

Results.—Gynecologist sex preferences were similar between male (30%), female (35%), and no sex preferences (35%). Patients who had a female obstetrician at their first delivery or began their gynecologic care with a female were more likely to prefer a female gynecologist. Multiparous patients were more likely to state no preference for a gynecologist. There were no statistical differences in sex preferences when patients were stratified by age, race, educational background, age of first gynecologist visit, or the age at their first delivery. About half of the patients (51%) stated that they preferred a male surgeon; only 3% preferred a female surgeon, and 46% stated they had no preference.

Conclusions.—Our investigation demonstrated that women's preferences for a gynecologist were divided equally between preferring a male, a female, and having no preference. Our study did find, however, that about half of the female patients preferred a male surgeon.

▶ The authors report a survey study of 146 female patients in a male single-physician private family practice office setting. Their data showed that female patients are approximately equally divided between their preference for a male gynecologist (30%), female gynecologist (35%), or no gender preference (35%). Of note, approximately 50% of women preferred a male surgeon, whereas only 3% preferred a female surgeon. A major potential bias in this study, which the authors acknowledge, was that the survey was performed in a male physician's office. Even though the patients in the study group did not receive any obstetric or gynecologic care from the provider, they chose a male physician for other medical needs. The authors go on to recommend that further investigations are required. In the discussion of their report, the authors point to other studies suggesting that patients are searching for physicians they emotionally connect with and who spend time listening intently to them rather than focusing on sex alone. This is an important message for male medical students who may be reluctant to enter obstetrics and gynecology because they perceive that they will be disadvantaged in attracting patients compared with female gynecologists. We must make obstetrics and gynecology an attractive career choice for both female and male medical students to provide the best physicians possible for the care of women.

S. Elias, MD

The Development of a Computer-Assisted Curriculum in Reproductive Endocrinology and Infertility for Residents
Alvero R, Lund K, Armstrong A, et al (Univ of Colorado, Aurora; Natl Insts of Child Health and Human Development, Bethesda, Md; Univ of Washington, Seattle)
Am J Obstet Gynecol 191:1777-1781, 2004   1–8

Objective.—This study was undertaken to determine the features of an effective computer-based residency curriculum in reproductive endocrinology and infertility.

Study Design.—A review of the literature to determine those features that have been used by training programs in medicine. Reproductive endocrinology and infertility division directors, current obstetrics and gynecology residents, and obstetrics and gynecology practitioners in the community were surveyed to evaluate critical subjects for study.

Results.—Programs most successful in using computers in training health care providers use a case-based approach that prioritizes important subjects. Areas of greatest importance to the 3 groups surveyed include infertility, dysfunctional uterine bleeding, and management of the climacteric, and several other areas were also deemed critical.

Conclusion.—Benefits of computer-based learning include consistency, the ability to develop problem solving skills for life-long learning, and a self-paced approach, but its validity as a teaching tool will require rigorous appraisal.

▶ Computer-based learning (CBL) is increasingly used in many educational settings, including residency training. CBL allows consistency in content, self-paced learning, learning exposure time in light of reduced resident work hours, and opportunities for problem-based learning. In this survey study, the authors evaluated the Council on Resident Education in Obstetrics and Gynecology Educational Objectives in Reproductive Endocrinology and Infertility. The educational objectives were collapsed into 18 topics and evaluated on a 5-point Likert scale ranging from "not important" to "critical." The survey included faculty members of a reproductive endocrinology and infertility division, practicing obstetrician-gynecologists, and obstetrics and gynecology residents. There was a consensus that the most important topics were infertility, dysfunctional uterine bleeding, and amenorrhea. The most disagreement among the groups was in pediatric gynecology and developmental anomalies of the urogenital tract. The authors suggested that the process of lifelong learning may be one of the advantages of problem-based learning, and instruments such as the Self-Directed Learning Readiness Scale can be used to assess this skill. However, although CBL is increasingly available, that is not sufficient justification for its use. The case must still be made as to whether it is an important improvement over traditional educational methods such as didactic lectures. CBL will never replace the dynamic interactions between new residents and faculty, especially in the clinical setting.

S. Elias, MD

Limitations of the Pelvic Examination for Evaluation of the Female Pelvic Organs
Padilla LA, Radosevich DM, Milad MP (Univ of New Mexico, Albuquerque; Univ of Minnesota; Northwestern Univ, Chicago)
Int J Gynaecol Obstet 88:84-88, 2005   1–9

Objective.—To assess factors influencing an accurate pelvic examination under the best possible circumstances.

Methods.—Before undergoing laparoscopy or laparotomy, 84 women under general anesthesia underwent pelvic examinations by an attending gynecologist, a gynecology resident, and a medical student blinded to the indication for surgery. Surgical findings were compared with the examiners' findings. Dependent variables (uterine size, uterine contour, and presence of adnexal masses) and effect modifiers (examiner experience and body mass index) were analyzed.

Results.—The overall pelvic examination was accurate 70.2% of the time for attending gynecologists, 64.0% for residents, and 57.3% for medical students. The sensitivity to detect adnexal masses was much lower than the sensitivity to assess uterine size or uterine contour. Obesity noticeably reduced detection of adnexal masses.

Conclusion.—The bimanual examination appears to be a limited screening test for the female upper genital tract even under the best possible circumstances. Uterine assessment appears to be more accurate than adnexal assessment.

▶ The bimanual pelvic examination has long been considered as an essential part of the female physical examination. However, the sensitivity, specificity, and predictive values of such a screening examination have never been well evaluated. In this study, 84 women underwent pelvic examination under anesthesia immediately before either laparotomy or laparoscopy by an attending gynecologist, a gynecology resident, and a medical student, each blinded to the indication for surgery. Examiners recorded their pelvic examination findings, including adnexal size and presence of adnexal masses, as well as uterine position, size, mobility, and contour. The results showed that the overall pelvic examination was accurate in 70.2% of the time for attending gynecologists, 64.0% for residents, and 57.3% for medical students. The sensitivity of detecting an adnexal mass was clearly poorer than uterine assessment. Obesity, as expected, was an independent factor decreasing the pelvic examination's accuracy. The authors recommend that programs be designed to standardize performance of pelvic examinations and establish quality control similar to other diagnostic tests such as ultrasonography. Until proficiency can be demonstrated, supervision of those performing pelvic examinations is warranted.

S. Elias, MD

Racial/Ethnic Differences in the Prevalence of Depressive Symptoms Among Middle-Aged Women: The Study of Women's Health Across the Nation (SWAN)
Bromberger JT, Harlow S, Avis N, et al (Univ of Pittsburgh, Pa; Univ of Michigan, Ann Arbor; Wake Forest Univ, Winston-Salem, NC; et al)
Am J Public Health 94:1378-1385, 2004   1–10

Objectives.—We examined racial/ethnic differences in significant depressive symptoms among middle-aged women before and after adjustment for socioeconomic, health-related, and psychosocial characteristics.

Methods.—Racial/ethnic differences in unadjusted and adjusted prevalence of significant depressive symptoms (score ≥ 16 on the Center for Epidemiologic Studies Depression [CES-D] Scale) were assessed with univariate and multiple logistic regressions.

Results.—Twenty-four percent of the sample had a CES-D score of 16 or higher. Unadjusted prevalence varied by race/ethnicity ($P < .0001$). After adjustment for covariates, racial/ethnic differences overall were no longer significant.

Conclusions.—Hispanic and African American women had the highest odds, and Chinese and Japanese women had the lowest odds, for a CES-D score of 16 or higher. This variation is in part because of health-related and psychosocial factors that are linked to socioeconomic status.

▶ Increasing study of menopause and associated health-related outcomes of the onset of menopause has considerably improved our knowledge of the effects of estrogen deprivation as well as our abilities to provide effective evaluation and treatment for menopausal women. This study by Bromberger et al reviews the racial and ethnic differences in the prevalence of depressive symptoms among middle-aged women. The authors found that Hispanic and African American women have the highest odds of developing depressive symptoms, whereas Chinese and Japanese women have the lowest odds of developing such symptomatology. The role of the obstetrician/gynecologist continues to encompass unconventional aspects of women's health care; in this regard, recognizing signs and symptoms of depression and being able to provide therapeutic interventions is an important aspect of effective women's health care.

L. P. Shulman, MD

Pesticide Use and Menstrual Cycle Characteristics Among Premenopausal Women in the Agricultural Health Study

Farr SL, Cooper GS, Cai J, et al (Univ of North Carolina at Chapel Hill; Natl Inst of Environmental Health Sciences, Research Triangle Park, NC)
Am J Epidemiol 160:1194-1204, 2004   1-11

Abstract.—Menstrual cycle characteristics may have implications for women's fecundability and risk of hormonally related diseases. Certain pesticides disrupt the estrous cycle in animals. The authors investigated the cross-sectional association between pesticide use and menstrual function among 3,103 women living on farms in Iowa and North Carolina. Women were aged 21–40 years, premenopausal, not pregnant or breastfeeding, and not taking oral contraceptives. At study enrollment (1993–1997), women completed two self-administered questionnaires on pesticide use and reproductive health. Exposures of interest were lifetime use of any pesticide and hormonally active pesticides. Menstrual cycle characteristics of interest included cycle length, missed periods, and intermenstrual bleeding. The authors used generalized estimating equations to assess the association between pesticide use and menstrual cycle characteristics, controlling for age, body mass index, and current smoking status. Women who used pesticides experienced longer menstrual cycles and increased odds of missed periods (odds ratio = 1.5, 95% confidence interval: 1.2, 1.9) compared with women who never used pesticides. Women who used probable hormonally active pesticides had a 60–100% increased odds of experiencing long cycles, missed periods, and intermenstrual bleeding compared with women who had never used pesticides. Associations remained after control for occupational physical activity.

▶ This is a very important study emphasizing the association of pesticides and reproductive function in terms of menstrual cycle characteristics. These data are highly suggestive that some of the currently used pesticides may cause significant reproductive toxicity.

S. E. Bulun, MD

2 Molecular Biology

NOBOX Deficiency Disrupts Early Folliculogenesis and Oocyte-Specific Gene Expression

Rajkovic A, Pangas SA, Ballow D, et al (Baylor College of Medicine, Houston)
Science 305:1157-1159, 2004   2–1

Background.—In mice, primordial ovarian follicles form when individual oocytes are surrounded by somatic cells. Growing oocytes transcribe genes important for folliculogenesis and those needed for early embryonic development. *Figla* is a recognized oocyte-specific regulator of zona pellucida genes, but the transcriptional control of nearly all oocyte-specific genes is poorly understood. Transcription factors that regulate oocyte gene expression will be key mediators of fertility because stage-specific expression of the genes is a requisite for proper oocyte growth and subsequent embryogenesis. *Nobox* is an oocyte-specific homeobox gene that is expressed in germ cell cysts and in primordial and growing oocytes. The purpose of this study was to determine whether *Nobox* is critical in folliculogenesis.

Methods.—The *Nobox* locus was disrupted in murine embryonic stem cells. Ninety percent of the coding region was deleted, including exons that encode the homeodomain. Female and male heterozygote matings produced expected Mendelian ratios. $Nobox^{-/-}$ and $Nobox^{-/-}$ ovarian histology during early postnatal folliculogenesis were examined with 2 germ cell markers, GCNA1 and MSY2.

Results.—Lack of *Nobox* was found to accelerate the postnatal loss of oocytes and to abolish the transition from primordial to growing follicles. Follicles were replaced by fibrous tissue in female mice lacking *Nobox* in a manner similar to nonsyndromic ovarian failure in women. Genes preferentially expressed in oocytes, including *Oct4* and *Gdf9* were downregulated in $Nobox^{-/-}$ mice, whereas ubiquitous genes such as *Bmp4*, *Kit*, and *Bax* were unaffected.

Conclusions.—*Nobox* is crucial for specifying an oocyte-restricted gene expression pattern that is essential for postnatal follicle development.

▶ *Nobox* is an oocyte-specific homeobox gene. It plays a critical role in early folliculogenesis. The disruption of this gene causes accelerated oocyte death. Understanding the functions of the product of this gene may increase our understanding of premature ovarian failure and provide important information concerning the evaluation and treatment of infertility.

S. E. Bulun, MD

Comparison of Fine-Scale Recombination Rates in Humans and Chimpanzees

Winckler W, Myers SR, Richter DJ, et al (Massachusetts Gen Hosp, Boston; Harvard Med School, Boston; Broad Inst of Harvard and MIT, Cambridge, Mass; et al)
Science 308:107-111, 2005   2–2

Background.—Recombination in the human genome, as in yeast, occurs mainly at the so-called "hot spots" of recombination, such as the β-globin and human leukocyte antigen regions. Direct observation of recombination hot spots is laborious, and only recently has it become practical to study fine-scale recombination rates on a genomic scale. Hot spot activity can be disrupted by directed mutagenesis of single nucleotides, and different alleles of the same locus can show differences in recombination, indicating strong sequence specificity. However, no sequence motif has been identified as causing recombination hot spots. The observation that meiotic drive at hot spots has prompted the hypothesis that hot spots may be short lived because of evolutionary selection against sites that initiate double-strand breaks. This study compared fine-scale recombination patterns inferred from polymorphism data at orthologous loci in western chimpanzees and in 2 human population samples.

Methods.—Single-nucleotide polymorphisms (SNPs) were ascertained by resequencing in both species and by querying public databases. SNPs were validated and the sample expanded by genotyping SNPs in a larger panel of human beings and chimpanzees. Patterns of LD among SNPs were expressed by using the pairwise metric [D'], representing the extent of historic recombination among alleles. Statistical evidence for hot spots of recombination, and quantitative estimates of local rates of recombination, were calculated.

Results.—Strong statistical evidence for hot spots of recombination was obtained in both species. However, despite approximately 99% identity at the level of DNA sequence, recombination hot spots were found rarely in the positions in the 2 species. There was no observable correlation in the estimates of fine-scale recombination rates.

Conclusions.—Local patterns of recombination rate have evolved rapidly in a way that is disproportionate to the change in DNA sequence.

▶ These authors found an important explanation for phenotypic differences between closely related species. Although there is an approximately 99% identity at the level of DNA sequence between human beings and chimpanzees, they have demonstrated that the sites of recombination within the genomes of these 2 species were almost entirely different. Genetic recombination during meiosis through crossing over of genes between homologous chromosomes maintains genetic diversity. Therefore, differences in the patterns of recombination determined by epigenetic factors but not the DNA sequence itself may determine the major phenotypic differences between closely related species.

S. E. Bulun, MD

Growth Retardation and Abnormal Maternal Behavior in Mice Lacking Testicular Orphan Nuclear Receptor 4

Collins LL, Lee Y-F, Heinlein CA, et al (Univ of Rochester, NY; Oregon Health & Science Univ, Portland; Univ of Wisconsin, Madison; et al)
Proc Natl Acad Sci U S A 101:15058-15063, 2004   2–3

Abstract.—Testicular orphan nuclear receptor 4 (TR4) is a member of the nuclear receptor superfamily for which a ligand has not yet been found. *In vitro* data obtained from various cell lines suggest that TR4 functions as a master regulator to modulate many signaling pathways, yet the *in vivo* physiological roles of TR4 remain unclear. Here, we report the generation of mice lacking TR4 by means of targeted gene disruption (TR4$^{-/-}$). The number of TR4$^{-/-}$ pups generated by the mating of TR4$^{+/-}$ mice is well under that predicted by the normal Mendelian ratio, and TR4$^{-/-}$ mice demonstrate high rates of early postnatal mortality, as well as significant growth retardation. Additionally, TR4$^{-/-}$ females show defects in reproduction and maternal behavior, with pups of TR4$^{-/-}$ dams dying soon after birth with no indication of milk intake. These results provide *in vivo* evidence that TR4 plays important roles in growth, embryonic and early postnatal pup survival, female reproductive function, and maternal behavior.

▶ The orphan nuclear receptor TR4 is critical for maternal behavior. Although TR4-deficient mothers secreted milk into their breast ducts, these mice did not build nests or nurse their offspring. This gave rise to early growth retardation and death of the offspring with no milk in their stomachs. This is an important example of a critical role of a nuclear receptor in determining reproductive behavior.

S. E. Bulun, MD

Role of *K-ras* and *Pten* in the Development of Mouse Models of Endometriosis and Endometrioid Ovarian Cancer

Dinulescu DM, Ince TA, Quade BJ, et al (Massachusetts Inst of Technology, Cambridge; Whitehead Inst, Cambridge, Mass; Harvard Med School, Boston)
Nature Med 11:63-70, 2005   2–4

Abstract.—Epithelial ovarian tumors present a complex clinical, diagnostic and therapeutic challenge because of the difficulty of early detection, lack of known precursor lesions and high mortality rates. Endometrioid ovarian carcinomas are frequently associated with endometriosis, but the mechanism for this association remains unknown. Here we present the first genetic models of peritoneal endometriosis and endometrioid ovarian adenocarcinoma in mice, both based on the activation of an oncogenic *K-ras* allele. In addition, we find that expression of oncogenic *K-ras* or conditional *Pten* deletion within the ovarian surface epithelium gives rise to preneoplastic ovarian lesions with an endometrioid glandular morphology. Furthermore, the combination of the two mutations in the ovary leads to the induction of invasive and widely metastatic endometrioid ovarian adenocarcinomas with complete penetrance and a disease latency of only 7 weeks. The ovarian cancer model described in this study recapitulates the specific tumor histomorphology and metastatic potential of the human disease.

▶ This landmark study provides a proof of principle that overexpression or disruption of critical genes in a cell-specific manner can give rise to a common chronic disorder such as endometriosis. These data are also suggestive that activation or disruption of only a single critical gene is all that is required for the development of ovarian cancer in a focus of endometriosis.

S. E. Bulun, MD

Aryl Hydrocarbon Receptor-Mediated Transcription: Ligand-Dependent Recruitment of Estrogen Receptor α to 2,3,7,8-Tetrachlorodibenzo-*p*-Dioxin-Responsive Promoters
Matthews J, Wihlén B, Thomsen J, et al (Karolinska Institutet, Huddinge, Sweden)
Mol Cell Biol 25:5317-5328, 2005   2–5

Abstract.—Using chromatin immunoprecipitation assays, we studied the 2,3,7,8-tetrachlorodibenzo-*p*-dioxin (TCDD)-mediated recruitment of the aryl hydrocarbon receptor (AhR) and several co-regulators to the CYP1A1 promoter. AhR displayed a time-dependent recruitment, reaching a peak at 75 min and maintaining promoter occupancy for the remainder of the time course. Recruitment of AhR was followed by TIF2/SRC2, which preceded CBP, histone H3 acetylation, and RNA polymerase II (RNAPII). Simultaneous recruitment to the enhancer and the TATA box region suggests the formation of a large multiprotein complex bridging the two promoter regions. Interestingly, estrogen receptor α (ERα) displayed a TCDD- and time-dependent recruitment to the CYP1A1 promoter, which was increased by co-treatment with estradiol. Transfection in HuH7 human liver cells confirmed previously reported ERα enhancement of AhR activity. In contrast, TCDD did not induce the recruitment of ERα to the estrogen-responsive pS2 promoter, and after 120 min of co-treatment with estradiol, ERα is still present on the CYP1A1 promoter but no longer at pS2. RNA interference studies with T47D cells support a role for ERα in TCDD-dependent CYP1A1 expression. Our data suggest that ERα acts as a coregulator of AhR-mediated transcriptional activation and that the recruitment of ERα by AhR represents a novel mechanism AhR-ERα cross talk.

▶ These authors found a novel mechanism as to how ER and the dioxin receptor AhR can interact to regulate genes with critical function. These findings lend further credence to the concept that dioxin may interact with estrogen at many different levels to regulate various genes in a tissue- and gene-specific fashion. Such findings provide important insights into the mechanisms of estrogen metabolism and its impact on a variety of clinical outcomes.

S. E. Bulun, MD

Gene Expression Profiling of Leiomyoma and Myometrial Smooth Muscle Cells in Response to Transforming Growth Factor-β

Luo X, Ding L, Xu J, et al (Univ of Florida, Gainesville)
Endocrinology 146:1097-1118, 2005   2–6

Abstract.—Altered expression of the TGF-β system is recognized to play a central role in various fibrotic disorders, including leiomyoma. In this study we performed microarray analysis to characterize the gene expression profile of leiomyoma and matched myometrial smooth muscle cells (LSMC and MSMC, respectively) in response to the time-dependent action of TGF-β and, after pretreatment with TGF-β type II receptor (TGF-βRII) antisense oligomer-blocking/reducing TGF-β autocrine/paracrine actions. Unsupervised and supervised assessments of the gene expression values with a false discovery rate selected at $P \leq 0.001$ identified 310 genes as differentially expressed and regulated in LSMC and MSMC in a cell- and time-dependent manner by TGF-β. Pretreatment with TGF-βRII antisense resulted in changes in the expression of many of the 310 genes regulated by TGF-β, with 54 genes displaying a response to TGF-β treatment. Comparative analysis of the gene expression profile in TGF-βRII antisense- and GnRH analog-treated cells indicated that these treatments target the expression of 222 genes in a cell-specific manner. Gene ontology assigned these genes functions as cell cycle regulators, transcription factors, signal transducers, tissue turnover, and apoptosis. We validated the expression and TGF-β time-dependent regulation of IL-11, TGF-β-induced factor, TGF-β-inducible early gene response, early growth response 3, CITED2 (cAMP response element binding protein-binding protein/p300-interacting transactivator with ED-rich tail), Nur77, Runx1, Runx2, p27, p57, growth arrest-specific 1, and G protein-coupled receptor kinase 5 in LSMC and MSMC using real-time PCR. Together, the results provide the first comprehensive assessment of the LSMC and MSMC molecular environment targeted by autocrine/paracrine action of TGF-β, highlighting potential involvement of specific genes whose products may influence the outcome of leiomyoma growth and fibrotic characteristics by regulating inflammatory response, cell growth, apoptosis, and tissue remodeling.

▶ This highly informative study emphasizes that TGF-β is a major regulator of leiomyoma growth and associated fibrosis. Such information may be most valuable in the development of effective therapies for uterine fibroids.

S. E. Bulun, MD

Effect of Vaginal Distension on Blood Flow and Hypoxia of Urogenital Organs of the Female Rat

Damaser MS, Whitbeck C, Chichester P, et al (Hines Veterans Affairs Hosp, Ill; Loyola Univ, Maywood, Ill; Albany Med College, NY)
J Appl Physiol 98:1884-1890, 2005   2–7

Abstract.—Vaginal delivery of children causes traumatic injury to tissues of the pelvic floor and is correlated with stress urinary incontinence; however, the exact mechanism of organ and tissue injury leading to incontinence development is unknown. The purpose of this project was to test the hypothesis that vaginal distension results in decreased blood flow to, and hypoxia of, the urogenital organs responsible for continence, which would suggest an ischemic and/or reperfusion mechanism of injury. Thirteen female rats underwent vaginal distension for 1 h. Thirteen age-matched rats were sham-distended controls. Blood flow to the bladder, urethra, and vagina were determined using a microsphere technique. Hypoxia of these organs was determined by immunohistochemistry. Blood flow to all three organs was significantly decreased just before release of vaginal distension. Bladder blood flow decreased further immediately after release of vaginal distension and continued to be significantly decreased 15 min after the release. Blood flow to both the urethra and vagina tripled immediately after release, inducing a rapid return to normal values. Vaginal distension resulted in extensive smooth muscle hypoxia of the bladder, as well as extensive hypoxia of the vaginal epithelium and urethral hypoxia. Bladders from sham-distended rats demonstrated urothelial hypoxia as well as focal hypoxic areas of the detrusor muscle. We have clearly demonstrated that vaginal distension results in decreased blood flow to, and hypoxia of, the bladder, urethra, and vagina, supportive of hypoxic injury as a possible mechanism of injury leading to stress urinary incontinence.

▶ For a long time, it has been thought that the main etiology of pelvic floor dysfunction leading to prolapse and urinary incontinence has been from stretch injury of pelvic fascia, muscle, and nerves that occurs during labor and childbirth. Ischemic injuries from neglected labor and childbirth are well known to cause complete tissue necrosis and vaginal fistulas, particularly in developing countries. This study makes a compelling case for hypoxia as a mechanism of nerve and tissue injury that does not necessarily manifest as full tissue necrosis but could very well play a role in urogenital denervation and pelvic floor dysfunction.

D. S. Miller, MD

Circulating Endothelial Progenitor Cells During Human Pregnancy

Sugawara J, Mitsui-Saito M, Hoshiai T, et al (Tohoku Univ, Sendai, Japan)
J Clin Endocrinol Metab 90:1845-1848, 2005   2–8

Abstract.—The precise molecular and cellular mechanisms that regulate maternal vascular development during gestation are largely unknown. Endothelial progenitor cells (EPCs), which play an important role in vascular homeostasis, have been discovered in the circulation. We examined the level of circulating EPCs throughout uncomplicated pregnancies (n = 20) and assessed the correlation between serum estradiol levels and the number of EPCs. The number of circulating EPCs increased gradually and paralleled the progression of gestational age. In addition, the number of EPCs correlated significantly with the level of serum estradiol. The present study suggests that EPCs may play an important role in the regulation and maintenance of the placental development and vascular integrity during pregnancy.

▶ EPCs that play a role in vascular homeostasis have been detected in maternal circulation. The study demonstrates that EPCs increase in pregnancy as gestational age increases. Serum estradiol levels also appeared to increase with increasing EPC levels. These data may play an important role in future studies evaluating clinical pregnancy outcomes, including preeclampsia. However, determination of the origin of EPCs will likely be a critical finding in assessing the research and clinical value of EPCs.

S. H. Ural, MD

OBSTETRICS

3 Maternal/Fetal Physiology

Pregnancy-related Changes in Physical Activity, Fitness, and Strength
Treuth MS, Butte NF, Puyau M (Johns Hopkins Bloomberg School of Public Health, Baltimore, Md; Baylor College of Medicine, Houston)
Med Sci Sports Exerc 37:832-837, 2005   3–1

Purpose.—The objective was to examine the pregnancy-related changes in physical activity, fitness, and strength in women of varying body mass indices (BMI).

Methods.—Women ($N = 17$ low BMI, $N = 34$ normal BMI, and $N = 12$ high BMI, mean age ± SD = 30.7 ± 4.1 yr) were studied before pregnancy (0 wk) and postpartum (6 and 27 wk) for body composition and for physical activity, fitness, and strength. Physical activity was assessed by questionnaire, fitness by a maximal oxygen consumption ($\dot{V}O_2$) test on a cycle ergometer, and strength by the one-repetition maximum test. Data were analyzed by repeated measures ANOVA testing for time and BMI group.

Results.—Total physical activity differed qualitatively, but not quantitatively, with time. Significant time effects were observed for maximal workload, heart rate, respiration rate, ventilation, $\dot{V}O_2$, respiratory exchange ratio, and strength. $\dot{V}O_{2max}$, adjusted for weight, dropped by ~ 385 mL·min^{-1}) from 0 to 6 wk postpartum ($P < 0.0001$) and by ~ 234 mL·min^{-1} from 0 to 27 wk postpartum ($P < 0.01$). The high-BMI group had a lower $\dot{V}O_{2max}$ (adjusted for weight or fat-free mass) than the normal-BMI group ($P < 0.05$). Strength decreased for the leg press by 24% ($P < 0.02$) and for the latissimus pull down by 8% ($P < 0.01$) from 0 to 6 wk postpartum, and then increased by 44 and 12%, respectively (both $P < 0.05$), by 27 wk postpartum.

Conclusion.—Relative to prepregnancy performance, fitness and strength declined in the early postpartum period but improved by 27 wk postpartum.

▶ Pregnant women can and should exercise. This study's objective was to assess physiologic changes that can take place. The results demonstrated that especially in the near postpartum period, performance, fitness, and strength were decreased. A total of 124 women from the Houston area were included in the research project, and 63 completed the study with a term delivery without complications. Additional significant findings were that maximal oxygen consumption and leg strength were also decreased. Social and psychological factors may play a role in this decrease, but the effect of these findings on a woman's health needs to be determined.

S. H. Ural, MD

Systematic Micro-Array Based Identification of Placental mRNA in Maternal Plasma: Towards Non-invasive Prenatal Gene Expression Profiling
Tsui NBY, Chim SSC, Chiu RWK, et al (Chinese Univ of Hong Kong, Shatin)
J Med Genet 41:461-467, 2004   3–2

Background.—The discovery of fetal DNA in the plasma of pregnant women has spurred the development of several promising approaches to noninvasive prenatal diagnosis. However, fetal and maternal DNA species coexist in maternal plasma, so these DNA-based diagnostic tools depend mainly on the use of genetic markers that would allow discrimination between fetal and maternal DNA. The feasibility of noninvasive gene expression profiling was determined by an approach based on an oligonucleotide microarray for the efficient development of new placental-specific mRNA markers that could be detected in maternal plasma. In addition, direct empirical evidence that maternal plasma RNA analysis did allow noninvasive prenatal gene expression profiling was sought.

Methods.—Gene expression profiles between placental tissues and corresponding peripheral blood from pregnant women in their first and third trimesters were compared by oligonucleotide microarray analysis. Panels of potentially fetal-specific mRNA markers in maternal plasma were identified, and 6 transcripts were selected for additional evaluation by real-time quantitative reverse transcriptase polymerase chain reaction assays.

Results.—A direct relation was found between the detectability of transcripts in maternal plasma and their respective expression levels in placental tissues. In addition, correlations were found between the relative abundance of these 6 transcripts in maternal plasma and their abundance in the placental tissues.

Conclusions.—Circulating placental mRNA in maternal plasma could be used for noninvasive prenatal gene expression profiling. A microarray approach for rapid and systematic identification of new placental mRNA markers for use in such profiling was also presented.

▶ The discovery of fetal RNA in maternal plasma offers exciting new possibilities for noninvasive prenatal testing. Such work has built on the extensive earlier work of many centers looking for fetal cells and DNA in maternal blood. In this study, the group from the Chinese University of Hong Kong led by Dennis Lo report on the use of microarrays to identify specific fetal mRNA in maternal plasma and present potential applications of this new technology. Such advancements will likely lead to effective prenatal screening and diagnostic protocols and provide important information concerning embryonic and fetal development.

P. P. van den Berg, MD, PhD

Relationship of Intracellular Magnesium of Cord Blood Platelets to Birth Weight
Takaya J, Yamato F, Higashino H, et al (Kansai Med Univ, Osaka, Japan)
Metabolism 53:1544-1547, 2004   3–3

Abstract.—Magnesium (Mg^{2+}) has an important role in insulin action, and insulin stimulates Mg^{2+} uptake in insulin-sensitive tissues. Impaired biologic responses to insulin are referred to as insulin resistance. Diabetic patients and obese subjects are reported to have intracellular magnesium ($[Mg^{2+}]_i$) deficiency. Many epidemiologic studies have disclosed that restricted fetal growth has been associated with increased risk of insulin resistance in adult life. We studied the relationship of $[Mg^{2+}]_i$ in cord blood platelets to birth weight. The subjects were 19 infants who were small for gestational age (SGA) and 45 who were appropriate for gestational age (AGA). By using a fluorescent probe, mag-fura-2, we examined the basal and insulin-stimulated $[Mg^{2+}]_i$ of platelets in the cord blood. Cord plasma insulin-like growth factor-1 (IGF-1) and leptin levels were determined with the use of enzyme-linked immunosorbent assay (ELISA). Birth weight was correlated with cord plasma IGF-1 ($P < .001$) and leptin ($P < .005$). Mean basal $[Mg^{2+}]_i$, but not plasma $[Mg^{2+}]$ was lower in the SGA than in the AGA group (291 ± 149 µmol/L v 468 ± 132 µmol/L, $P < .001$). The basal $[Mg^{2+}]_i$

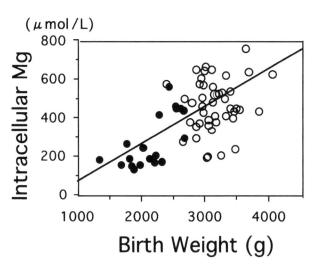

FIGURE 1.—The correlation of intracellular Mg^{2+} and birth weight. The basal level of intracellular $[Mg^{2+}]_i([Mg^{2+}]_i)$ of cord platelets is significantly correlated with birth weight ($P < .001$, $r = 0.60$). *open circles*, AGA; *filled circles*, SGA. *Abbreviations: AGA*, Appropriate for gestational age; *SGA*, small for gestational age. (Courtesy of Takaya J, Yamato F, Higashino H, et al: Relationship of intracellular magnesium of cord blood platelets to birth weight. *Metabolism* 53:1544-1547, 2004.)

was significantly correlated with the birth weight ($P < .001$) as well as birth length ($P < .001$). At 60 seconds after stimulation with insulin, there was no significant difference in stimulated $[Mg^{2+}]_i$ between the SGA and AGA groups. Although the SGA group had low $[Mg^{2+}]_i$, the platelets had good potentiality to compensate for low $[Mg^{2+}]_i$. $[Mg^{2+}]_i$ reflects the extent of fetal growth. Decreased $[Mg^{2+}]_i$ in SGA might underlie the initial pathophysiologic events leading to insulin resistance (Fig 1).

▶ This article from Japan focuses on a relationship between birth weight and cord blood platelet intracellular magnesium levels. Because of the known association between magnesium and insulin levels, it is unclear if Mg directly alters birth weight. It was seen that Mg inside cord blood platelets correlated with birth weight and length. It appeared that higher Mg was associated with higher weight. An association between Mg levels and adult insulin resistant diseases remains to be determined.

S. H. Ural, MD

Interluekin-6, Interleukin-8, and Soluble Tumor Necrosis Factor Receptor-I in the Cord Blood as Predictors of Chronic Lung Disease in Premature Infants

An H, Nishimaki S, Ohyama M, et al (Yokohama City Univ, Japan; Kanagawa Child Med Ctr, Japan)
Am J Obstet Gynecol 191:1649-1654, 2004   3–4

Objectives.—In order to predict the late-development of chronic lung disease of prematurity (CLD), cytokines in the cord blood were assessed in this study.

Study Design.—Eighteen premature infants with CLD were enrolled. Cord blood plasma levels of cytokines of these infants and 12 control infants without CLD were measured including interleukin (IL)-1β, IL-2, IL-4, IL-6, IL-8, IL-10, interferon (IFN)-γ, tumor necrosis factor (TNF)-α, soluble TNF receptor-I, and soluble IL-6 receptor using a cytometric bead array and an enzyme-linked immunosorbent assay.

Results.—The cord blood IL-6, IL-8, and sTNFR-I levels were significantly elevated in CLD infants compared with those in control ($P < .05$). IL-1β, IL-2, IL-4, IL-10, and IFN-γ were undetectable in both groups. CLD infants with maternal chorioamnionitis had higher IL-6 than those without chorioamnionitis ($P < .01$). In CLD infants, IL-6 was higher in the infants who required prolonged oxygen therapy ($P < .05$).

Conclusion.—Elevated inflammatory cytokines in the cord blood are associated with the progression to CLD (Fig 5).

▶ Can lung disease be predicted in premature infants? This important study was performed to assess this question. Certain factors were analyzed from blood obtained from the umbilical cord immediately after the delivery. It was clearly shown that inflammatory cytokines in the cord blood were associated

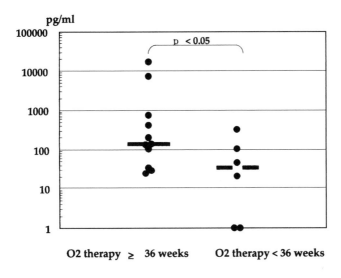

O2 therapy ≥ 36 weeks   O2 therapy < 36 weeks

Bars indicate median values

FIGURE 5.—Cord blood IL-6 and the duration of oxygen therapy in infants with CLD. In CLD infants, cord blood IL-6 levels were higher in the infants who required oxygen therapy over 36 weeks of corrected gestational age than those who did not need supplemental oxygen at this time. (138 vs 34.0 pg/mL, $P < .05$). *Abbreviation:* CLD, Chronic lung disease. (Courtesy of An H, Nishimaki S, Ohyama M, et al: Interluekin-6, interleukin-8, and soluble tumor necrosis factor receptor-I in the cord blood as predictors of chronic lung disease in premature infants.*Am J Obstet Gynecol* 191:1649-1654. Copyright 2004 by Elsevier.)

with CLD in infants that were born prematurely. With the results seen in the study, cytokines, particularly, can be used in assessing prediction of lung disease. This may further translate to prenatal assessment in future studies.

S. H. Ural, MD

Prenatal Environmental Tobacco Smoke Exposure Promotes Adult Atherogenesis and Mitochondrial Damage in Apolipoprotein E$^{-/-}$ Mice Fed a Chow Diet

Yang Z, Knight CA, Mamerow MM, et al (Univ of Alabama at Birmingham; Univ of Texas at Austin; Louisiana State Univ, Baton Rouge)
Circulation 110:3715-3720, 2004   3–5

Background.—Epidemiologic studies have suggested a relation between birth weights and adult cardiovascular disease development, which in turn suggests that a link may exist between the maternal-fetal environment and the development of adult cardiovascular disease. However, much more is known about the influence of the maternal-fetal environment on childhood vulnerability to reactive airway disease. Neonatal exposure to environmental tobacco smoke (ETS) has been linked to an increase in the incidence of childhood asthma and has been demonstrated in a variety of animal models.

A hypothesis was investigated that in utero ETS exposure promotes adult atherosclerotic lesion formation and mitochondrial damage.

Methods.—Atherosclerotic lesion formation, mitochondrial DNA damage, antioxidant activity, and oxidant load were determined in cardiovascular tissues obtained from adult apolipoprotein E$^{-/-}$ mice exposed to either filtered air or ETS in utero. The mice were fed a standard chow diet (4.5% fat) from weaning until euthanasia.

Results.—Male mice exposed in utero to ETS showed significant alterations in atherosclerotic lesion formation, mitochondrial DNA damage, antioxidant activity, and oxidant load.

Conclusions.—The hypothesis that prenatal exposure to environmental tobacco smoke is sufficient to promote the development of adult cardiovascular disease was supported by this study.

▶ This mouse model suggests that maternal cigarette smoking during pregnancy may give rise to significant adult cardiovascular disease, especially in vulnerable populations with various genetic backgrounds. Such findings may provide important information concerning the development of cardiovascular disease in adults.

S. E. Bulun, MD

Plasma Choline and Betaine and Their Relation to Plasma Homocysteine in Normal Pregnancy
Velzing-Aarts FV, Holm PI, Fokkema MR, et al (Groningen Univ, The Netherlands; Univ of Bergen, Norway; Med Ctr Haaglanden, The Hague, The Netherlands)
Am J Clin Nutr 81:1383-1389, 2005   3–6

Background.—Plasma concentrations of total homocysteine (tHcy) decrease during pregnancy. This reduction has been investigated in relation to folate status, but no study has addressed the possible role of betaine and its precursor choline.

Objective.—We investigated the courses of plasma choline and betaine during normal human pregnancy and their relations to plasma tHcy (Fig 1).

Design.—Blood samples were obtained monthly; the initial samples were taken at gestational week (GW) 9, and the last samples were taken ≈3 mo postpartum. The study population comprised 50 women of West African descent. Most of the subjects took folic acid irregularly.

Results.—Plasma choline (geometric mean; 95% reference interval) increased continuously during pregnancy, from 6.6 (4.5, 9.7) µmol/L at GW 9 to 10.8 (7.4, 15.6) µmol/L at GW 36. Plasma betaine decreased in the first half of pregnancy, from 16.3 (8.6, 30.8) µmol/L at GW 9 to 10.3 (6.6, 16.2) µmol/L at GW 20 and remained constant thereafter. We confirmed a reduction in plasma tHcy, and the lowest concentration was found in the second trimester. From GW 16 onward, an inverse relation between plasma tHcy

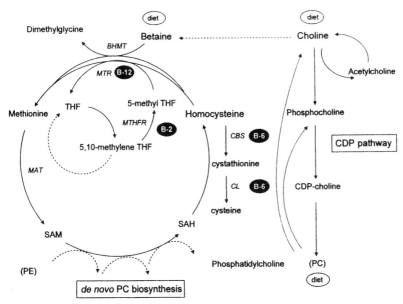

FIGURE 1.—Choline, betaine, and one-carbon metabolism. Choline is provided by food or can be formed de novo via sequential *S*-adenosylmethionine *(SAM)*-dependent methylation of phosphatidylethanolamine *(PE)* to form phosphatidylcholine *(PC)*, which in turn can be converted back to choline. Choline serves as a precursor in the synthesis of the neurotransmitter acetylcholine or is oxidized to betaine. The latter compound serves as a methyl donor in the betaine:homocysteine methyltransferase *(BHMT)* reaction, which converts homocysteine to methionine. This conversion is also catalyzed by methionine synthase *(MTR)*, which requires 5-methyltetrahydrofolate *(THF)* as methyl donor and couples the choline-betaine pathway to folate metabolism. The *solid arrows* represent single enzymatic reactions; the *dashed arrows* represent multiple enzyme reactions. *Abbreviations: CDP,* Cytidine 5′-diphosphate; *MTHFR,* 5,10-methylenetetrahydrofolate reductase; *MAT,* methionine adenosyltransferase; *SAH,* S-adenosylhomocysteine; *CBS,* cystathionine-β-synthase; *CL,* γ-cystathioninase. (Courtesy of Velzing-Aarts FV, Holm PI, Fokkema MR, et al: Plasma choline and betaine and their relation to plasma homocysteine in normal pregnancy. *Am J Clin Nutr* 81:1383-1389, 2005. Reproduced with permission by the *American Journal of Clinical Nutrition*. © *Am J Clin Nutr*, American Society for Clinical Nutrition.)

and betaine was observed. Multiple regression analysis showed that plasma betaine was a strong predictor of plasma tHcy from GW 20 onward.

Conclusions.—The steady increase in choline throughout gestation may ensure choline availability for placental transfer with subsequent use by the growing fetus. Betaine becomes a strong predictor of tHcy during the course of pregnancy. Both of these findings emphasize the importance of choline and betaine status during normal human pregnancy.

▶ The human diet is rich in choline, which serves as a precursor of betaine. Betaine remethylates homocysteine as an alternative for the remethylation by 5-methyltetrahydrofolate. The insight that prenatal choline availability is important for rat brain development with lifelong lasting effects also warrants special attention for this nutrient in human pregnancy. A longitudinal study on reference values of the metabolites choline, betaine, tHcy, and vitamins involved in one-carbon metabolism was conducted in 50 uneventful pregnancies of West African citizens of Curacao from 9 weeks gestational age until 15 weeks postpartum. The novel and most important result is finding a steady increase in maternal plasma choline throughout gestation. The increase in choline may be explained by the mobilization of maternal stores and enhanced de novo synthesis. This ensures choline availability for (active) placenta transfer to meet the fetal choline requirements, and emphasizes the importance of a higher dietary choline intake during pregnancy. Plasma betaine showed an inverse relation with tHcy with advancing gestation. Normally, there is only a weak relation to fasting plasma tHcy that is more pronounced in subjects with low folate concentrations. This finding emphasizes the importance of betaine during normal pregnancy and points to the possibility that a low betaine status may predispose to pregnancy complications associated with mild hyperhomocysteinemia. The importance of preconception choline and betaine status in relation with normal and adverse pregnancy outcome should be more extensively studied in future studies.

E. A. P. Steegers, MD, PhD

Congenital Heart Defects and Abnormal Maternal Biomarkers of Methionine and Homocysteine Metabolism

Hobbs CA, Cleves MA, Melnyk S, et al (Univ of Arkansas, Little Rock; Arkansas Children's Hosp Research Inst, Little Rock)
Am J Clin Nutr 81:147-153, 2005   3–7

Background.—It is well established that folic acid prevents neural tube defects. Although the mechanisms remain unclear, multivitamins containing folic acid may also protect against other birth defects, including congenital heart defects.

Objective.—Our goal was to establish a maternal metabolic risk profile for nonsyndromic congenital heart defects that would enhance current preventive strategies.

Design.—Using a case-control design, we measured biomarkers of the folate-dependent methionine and homocysteine pathway (Fig 1) among a population-based sample of women whose pregnancies were affected by congenital heart defects (224 case subjects) or unaffected by any birth defect (90 control subjects). Plasma concentrations of folic acid, homocysteine, methionine, S-adenosylmethionine (SAM), S-adenosylhomocysteine (SAH), vitamin B-12, and adenosine were compared, with control for lifestyle and sociodemographic variables.

Results.—After covariate adjustment, case subjects had higher mean concentrations of homocysteine ($P < 0.001$) and SAH ($P < 0.001$) and lower mean concentrations of methionine ($P = 0.019$) and SAM ($P = 0.014$) than did control subjects. Vitamin B-12, folic acid, and adenosine concentrations did not differ significantly between case and control subjects. Homocysteine, SAH, and methionine were identified as the most important biomarkers predictive of case or control status.

Conclusions.—The basis for the observed abnormal metabolic profile among women whose pregnancies were affected by congenital heart defects

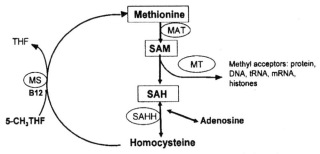

FIGURE 1.—The folate-dependent methionine and homocysteine metabolic pathway. Biomarkers indicated by *bold type* were measured in the present study. *Abbreviations: B12*, Vitamin B-12 (cobalamin); *MAT*, methionine adenosyltransferase; *mRNA*, messenger RNA; *MS*, methionine synthase; *MT*, methyltransferase; *SAH*, S-adenosylhomocysteine; *SAHH*, SAH hydrolase; *SAM*, S-adenosylmethionine; *THF*, tetrahydrofolate; *tRNA*, transfer RNA. (Courtesy of Hobbs CA, Cleves MA, Melnyk S, et al: Congenital heart defects and abnormal maternal biomarkers of methionine and homocysteine metabolism. *Am J Clin Nutr* 81:147-153, 2005. Reproduced with permission by the *American Journal of Clinical Nutrition.* © *Am J Clin Nutr*, American Society for Clinical Nutrition.)

cannot be defined without further analysis of relevant genetic and environmental factors. Nevertheless, a metabolic profile that is predictive of congenital heart defect risk would help to refine current nutritional intervention strategies to reduce risk and may provide mechanistic clues for further experimental studies.

▶ Congenital heart defects (CHDs) are the most prevalent congenital malformations worldwide. However, 85% of women with CHDs are now expected to reach adulthood. The origin of CHDs is highly heterogeneous, in which genetic factors of both parents are involved. During pregnancy, the mother serves as the environment of the developing child. Therefore, maternal endogenous (metabolic) and exogenous (environmental) influences are likely to play important roles. Evidence is increasing that periconceptional maternal folic acid treatment not only contributes to the prevention of neural tube defects but also of other birth defects, such as CHDs and orofacial clefts. Both increased plasma homocysteine and decreased folic acid may be detrimental to the developing embryo. Embryotoxic effects may include oxidative stress. A deranged maternal homocysteine metabolism resulting in hyperhomocysteinemia can be treated by folic acid and may explain a part of its beneficial effects.

In this case-control study of mothers of a child with CHD, some of the biomarkers of folate-related homocysteine metabolism have been investigated. The results showed a derangement in homocysteine metabolism resulting in hyperhomocysteinemia and hypomethionemia that was not caused by low folate or vitamin B_{12} levels. Hyperhomocysteinemia can be caused by genetic and several other health and lifestyle factors, such as a high protein intake, the use of alcohol, and smoking, as well as renal and liver dysfunctions and diabetes. This study emphasizes the importance of preconceptional screening of metabolic and nutritional risk factors and subsequent intervention programs aimed at the primary prevention of adverse pregnancy outcomes.

E. A. P. Steegers, MD, PhD

A New Model for Inflammation-Induced Preterm Birth: The Role of Platelet-Activating Factor and Toll-Like Receptor-4

Elovitz MA, Wang Z, Chien EK, et al (Univ of Pennsylvania, Philadelphia; Univ of Vermont, Burlington; Rhinehart Ctr for Reproductive Medicine, Evanston, Ill)
Am J Pathol 163:2103-2111, 2003   3–8

Abstract.—Preterm birth is a leading cause of neonatal morbidity and mortality. Despite a growing body of evidence correlating inflammation with preterm birth, the signal transduction pathways responsible for the emptying of the uterus in the setting of intrauterine inflammation has not been elucidated. We now report a unique, reproducible mouse model of localized intrauterine inflammation. This model results in 100% preterm delivery with no maternal mortality. Using our model, we also show that platelet-activating factor is a crucial mediator of both inflammation-induced preterm birth and fetal demise. Using C3H/HeJ mice, we demonstrate that toll-like receptor-4 (TLR-4) plays a role in lipopolysaccharide-induced preterm birth but not in inflammation-induced fetal death. Immunohistochemistry studies demonstrate the presence of the platelet-activating factor receptor in both endometrial glands and smooth muscle in uterine tissues. Molecular studies demonstrate the differential expression of platelet-activating factor receptor and TLR-4 in uterine and cervical tissue throughout gestation. Quantitative polymerase chain reaction revealed an up-regulation of TLR-4 in the fundal region of the uterus in response to intrauterine inflammation. The use of this model will increase our understanding of the significant clinical problem of inflammation-induced preterm birth and will elucidate signal transduction pathways involved in an inflammatory state.

▶ Because preterm birth remains a leading cause of neonatal morbidity and mortality, many groups are seeking to identify pathophysiologic processes that are associated with preterm labor. Inflammation has long been associated with preterm labor despite the lack of information concerning the specific pathways associated with adverse clinical outcomes. This group found that platelet-activating factor was a crucial mediator of inflammation-induced preterm birth and fetal demise and that a novel receptor played a role in preterm birth but not fetal death. Although such studies do not provide information of immediate clinical relevance, such studies will delineate the role(s) of inflammation in preterm birth and provide important clues for the development of effective therapies that will reduce the frequency of preterm birth.

P. P. van den Berg, MD, PhD

Implantation Site Intermediate Trophoblasts in Placenta Cretas

Kim K-R, Jun S-Y, Kim J-Y, et al (Univ of Ulsan, Seoul, Korea; Pochun Cha Univ, Seoul, Korea)

Mod Pathol 17:1483-1490, 2004   3–9

Abstract.—Placenta cretas are defined as abnormal adherences or in-growths of placental tissue, but their pathogenetic mechanism has not been fully explained. During histologic examination of postpartum uteri, we noticed that the number of implantation site intermediate trophoblasts was increased in the placental bed of placenta cretas. To validate our observation and to address the pathogenetic role of implantation site intermediate trophoblasts in placenta cretas, we examined postpartum uteri with placenta cretas ($n = 34$) and noncretas ($n = 22$), obtained from Cesarean or immediate postpartum hysterectomy specimens. Using antibody to CD146, a marker for implantation site intermediate trophoblasts, we found that placenta cretas had significantly thicker layer of implantation site intermediate trophoblasts (2300 ± 1200 µm) than noncretas (1500 ± 1200 µm, $P < 0.025$). We also observed that the confluent distribution of cells was more frequent in placenta cretas (97%) than noncretas samples (45%, $P < 0.001$), and that the total number of implantation site intermediate trophoblasts within the superficial myometrium of the placental bed was significantly higher in placenta cretas than noncretas (Fig 6). Using antibodies to Ki-67, Bcl-2 and cleaved caspase-3 to determine the proliferative index and apoptotic rates of implantation site intermediate trophoblasts, we found that they were close to zero in both groups and did not differ significantly. These findings suggest

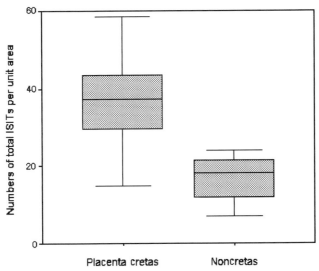

FIGURE 6.—Total number of implantation site intermediate trophoblasts (*ISITs*) per unit area within the superficial myometrium of placenta cretas and noncretas. (Courtesy of Kim K-R, Jun S-Y, Kim J-Y, et al: Implantation site intermediate trophoblasts in placenta cretas. *Mod Pathol* 17:1483-1490, 2004. Reprinted by Nature Publishing.)

that the increased number of implantation site intermediate trophoblasts observed in placenta cretas may be related to the pathogenesis of placental ingrowth, but the mechanism by which the increase in implantation site intermediate trophoblasts causes placenta cretas remains to be clarified.

▶ The study has demonstrated a larger number of implantation site intermediate trophoblasts, which suggests more intensive anchoring of placenta cretas than of control placentas. Several local factors have been implicated in the mechanism of excessive invasion. Among them are extracellular matrix-degrading proteinases, including plasminogen activators, metalloproteinases, and tissue inhibitors of matrix metalloproteinases (MMPs) that are secreted by the implantation site intermediate trophoblasts.[1] Immunologic factors are also likely to be involved in the sometimes excessive adherence of the placenta.

F. K. Lotgering, MD, PhD

Reference

1. Behrendtsen O, Alexander CM, Werb Z. Metalloproteinases mediate extracellular matrix degradation by cells from mouse blastocyst outgrowths. *Development* 114:447-456, 1992.

Polyol Concentrations in the Fluid Compartments of the Human Conceptus During the First Trimester of Pregnancy: Maintenance of Redox Potential in a Low Oxygen Environment

Jauniaux E, Hempstock J, Teng C, et al (Royal Free and Univ College, London; Univ of Colorado, Aurora; Univ of Cambridge, England)
J Clin Endocrinol Metab 90:1171-1175, 2005   3–10

Abstract.—Polyols are sugar alcohols formed by the reduction of aldoses and ketoses. Production is favored under conditions of low oxygenation, when it may provide an alternative means to production of lactate for regulating the oxidation-reduction balance of pyridine nucleotides. Polyols also act as important organic osmolytes and as precursors of cell membrane components. We measured free sugar and polyol concentrations in matched samples of maternal serum, intervillous fluid, coelomic fluid, and amniotic fluid from normal human pregnancies at 5-12 wk gestational age (Fig 2). The concentrations of fructose, inositol, sorbitol, erythritol, and ribitol were significantly higher in coelomic and amniotic fluids than in maternal serum, but the reverse was the case for glucose and glycerol. Intervillous fluid concentrations of inositol, mannitol, and sorbitol were also significantly higher than those in maternal serum. These results demonstrate that the polyol pathway, considered vestigial in adult tissues, is highly active in the human conceptus during early pregnancy. The pathway may serve to maintain ATP concentrations and cellular redox potential while the embryo develops in a low oxygen environment. Polyols may also play important physiological roles in development of the human conceptus, possibly drawing water and solutes across the placenta and expanding the gestational sac.

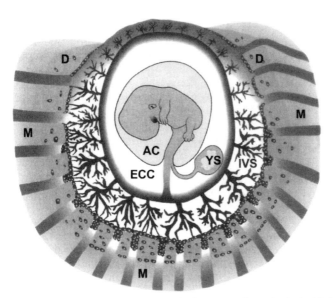

FIGURE 2.—Diagram of the gestational sac at 8–9 wk of pregnancy, illustrating the fetal fluid compartments. Amniotic fluid (AF) was withdrawn from the amniotic sac (AC), coelomic fluid (CF) was withdrawn from the exocoelomic cavity (ECC), and intervillous fluid (IF) was withdrawn from the intervillous space (IVS). Note that plugs of trophoblast block the tips of the spiral arteries throughout most of the placenta at this stage of development, preventing the inflow of maternal blood. *Abbreviations: D*, Decidua; *M*, myometrium; *YS*, yolk sac. (Modified from Janiaux E, Cindrova-Davies T, Johns J, et al: Distribution and transfer pathways of antioxidant molecules inside the first trimester human gestational sac. *J Clin Endocrinol Metab* 89:1452-1459, 2004. Courtesy of Jauniaux E, Hempstock J, Teng C, et al: Polyol concentrations in the fluid compartments of the human conceptus during the first trimester of pregnancy: Maintenance of redox potential in a low oxygen environment. *J Clin Endocrinol Metab* 90[2]:1171-1175, 2005. Copyright The Endocrine Society.)

▶ This group has previously shown that during the first trimester of human pregnancy, the human embryo and placenta develop in a low-oxygen environment.[1,2] Less is known about nutrition and the activity of metabolic pathways during this period. One of the obvious reasons for this is that it is difficult to obtain tissue samples during the first weeks of normal human pregnancy.

In the current study, the hypothesis investigated was that the polyol pathway, active under conditions of low oxygenation in embryonic tissues, may be important in the regulation of the oxidation-reduction balance of pyridine nucleotides. This may provide an alternative to the production of lactate and thus avoid excessive acidosis that may affect pregnancy outcome. Matched samples of maternal serum, intervillous fluid, coelomic fluid, and amniotic fluid were collected before surgical termination under general anesthesia, which may have affected the results. The authors found that several polyol pathway sugar metabolites were significantly higher in the extraembryonic fluids than in maternal serum; this seems to emphasize the importance of this pathway in the human fetoplacental unit during early normal pregnancy. This phylogenetically older system may be involved in the protection of the embryo from free radical–mediated teratogenesis, volume homeostasis of fetoplacental cells as well as fluid dynamics of pools of coelomic and amniotic fluid. The outcome of pregnancy depends largely on first-trimester embryonic and placental development. Understanding the physiology and pathophysiology of early embryonic and placental development will contribute to our knowledge of normal and abnormal pregnancy outcomes.

E. A. P. Steegers, MD, PhD

References

1. Rodesch F, Simon P, Donner C, et al: Oxygen measurements in endometrial and trophoblastic tissues during early pregnancy. *Obstet Gynecol* 80:283-285, 1992.
2. Jauniaux E, Watson AL, Hempstock J, et al: Onset of maternal arterial blood flow and placental oxidative stress: A possible factor in human early pregnancy failure. *Am J Pathol* 157:2111-2122, 2000.

The Openings of Uteroplacental Vessels With Villous Infiltration at Different Gestational Ages

Fujikura T (St Luke's Internatl Hosp, Tokyo)
Arch Pathol Lab Med 129:382-385, 2005   3–11

Context.—The number of uteroplacental vessels flowing into the intervillous space in mature placentas has been reported in some studies to increase and in others to decrease. Both villous infiltration and proliferation in the vessels have been neglected in histologic examinations and need to be studied.

Objective.—To clarify these conflicting findings regarding villous infiltration and proliferation in the uteroplacental vessels.

Design.—A retrospective study was done using placental sections of different gestational ages. The openings of the vessels in each section were counted, noting if they were with or without villous infiltration. The frequency of openings per section was calculated, and the findings were grouped by gestational age.

Results.—The frequency of total openings was significantly lower in the 41 to 37 weeks group (1.2) than in the 36 to 30 weeks group (2.0), the 29 to 20 weeks group (2.2), and the 19 to 13 weeks group (2.4) ($P < .001$). The frequency of openings with villous infiltration decreased similarly in mature placentas. Chorionic villi infiltrated the openings and proliferated in uteroplacental vessels. Differentiation between arteries and veins was difficult in the basal plate, because all vessels had veinlike structures.

Conclusions.—This decreasing frequency of openings in mature placentas suggests that the amount of intervillous blood flow is limited in full-term and postterm pregnancy. Villous infiltration into the vessels is considered a normal finding with gestation and can provide trophoblast for uteroplacental arteries. The relationship between placental development and villous proliferation in the vessels is presented.

▶ The study was performed to histologically evaluate villous infiltration and proliferation in the uteroplacental blood vessels. It was seen that term placentas had significantly lower openings when compared to placentas as early as 13 weeks of gestation. Differentiation between arterial and venous vessels was not possible upon histologic examination. Villous infiltration is a normal finding, and another interesting finding is that intervillous blood flow is possibly less in the term fetus. This brings up the question of how much this histologic/physiologic change factors into the onset of spontaneous labor. Future studies can use these findings as a precursor for clinical research.

S. H. Ural, MD

4 Prenatal Screening/ Diagnosis and Genetics

Prospective First-Trimester Screening for Trisomy 21 in 30,564 Pregnancies
Avgidou K, Papageorghiou A, Bindra R, et al (King's College, London; Harold Wood Hosp, Essex, England)
Am J Obstet Gynecol 192:1761-1767, 2005   4–1

Objective.—This study was undertaken to evaluate the performance of a 1-stop clinic for first-trimester assessment of risk (OSCAR) for trisomy 21 by a combination of maternal age, fetal nuchal translucency (NT) thickness,

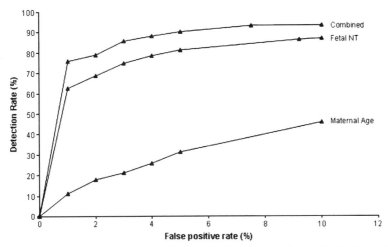

FIGURE 2.—Relationship between detection rates and false-positive rates in screening for trisomy 21 by maternal age alone, maternal age and fetal NT, and by the combination of maternal age, fetal NT, and maternal serum biochemistry. (Courtesy of Avgidou K, Papageorghiou A, Bindra R, et al: Prospective first-trimester screening for trisomy 21 in 30,564 pregnancies. *Am J Obstet Gynecol* 192:1761-1767. Copyright 2005 by Elsevier.)

TABLE 2.—Detection Rates for Different False-Positive Rates in Screening for Trisomy 21, by the Combination of Maternal Age, Fetal NT, and Maternal Serum-Free β-hCG and PAPP-A

Method of Screening	Trisomy 21	False-Positive Rate					
		1%	2%	3%	4%	5%	10%
Maternal age (MA)	196	22 (11.2%)	35 (17.9%)	42 (21.4%)	51 (26.0%)	61 (31.5%)	91 (46.4%)
MA and NT	196	123 (62.8%)	135 (68.9%)	167 (75.0%)	154 (78.6%)	160 (81.6%)	171 (87.2%)
MA, NT, β-hCG, and PAPP-A	196	149 (76.0%)	155 (79.1%)	168 (85.7%)	173 (88.3%)	177 (90.3%)	184 (93.9%)

(Courtesy of Avgidou K, Papageorghiou A, Bindra R, et al: Prospective first-trimester screening for trisomy 21 in 30,564 pregnancies. *Am J Obstet Gynecol* 192:1761-1767. Copyright 2005 by Elsevier.)

and maternal serum-free β-human chorionic gonadotrophin (hCG) and pregnancy-associated plasma protein-A (PAPP-A).

Study Design.—OSCAR was carried out in 30,564 pregnancies at 11 to 13+6 weeks. Patient-specific risks for trisomy 21 and detection and false-positive rates were calculated (Fig 2 and Table 2).

Results.—The median maternal age was 34 (range 15-49) years. Chromosomal abnormalities were identified in 330 pregnancies, including 196 cases of trisomy 21. The estimated risk for trisomy 21 was 1 in 300 or greater in 7.5% of the normal pregnancies, in 93.4% of those with trisomy 21 and in 88.8% of those with other chromosomal defects.

Conclusion.—The most effective method of screening for chromosomal defects is by first-trimester fetal NT and maternal serum biochemistry.

▶ Incorporation of first-trimester screening for fetal chromosome abnormalities is becoming a more common occurrence in the United States, Europe, and around the world. The primary reason for the increasing interest in first-trimester screening is the reported improved detection rates for fetal Down syndrome and trisomy 18 compared with the more conventional use of multi-marker serum analyte analysis in the second trimester. This current study comes from the Harris Birthright Research Center for Fetal Medicine in London and evaluates a first-trimester protocol utilizing maternal age, fetal NT, and maternal serum-free β-hCG and PAPP-A. The authors found that the most effective method of screening for chromosome defects is by combination of first-trimester measurement of fetal NT and maternal serum biochemistry. Of importance is that this article also provides an excellent review of the mathematic paradigms that go into the development of maternal screening protocols for fetal chromosome abnormalities. A challenge for clinicians who are considering the incorporation of such screening protocols into their obstetric practice is the use of novel ultrasonographic and serum markers for the delineation of risk for fetal chromosome abnormalities and the ability to counsel patients about this and other screening protocols that may be appropriate for them to consider during their pregnancies. Indeed, it may be the challenges of providing effective counseling for this and other screening protocols that may be the greatest barrier to effective incorporation of new and novel screening protocols for fetal chromosome abnormalities.

L. P. Shulman, MD

Evidence-Based Obstetric Ethics and Informed Decision-Making by Pregnant Women About Invasive Diagnosis After First-Trimester Assessment of Risk for Trisomy 21

Nicolaides KH, Chervenak FA, McCullough LB, et al (King's College, London; Cornell Univ, New York; Baylor College of Medicine, Houston)
Am J Obstet Gynecol 193:322-326, 2005   4–2

Objective.—The purpose of this study was to determine the ability of pregnant women to incorporate sophisticated screening information about risk assessment into their decisions about invasive testing in an appropriate way.

Study Design.—Assessment of risk for trisomy 21 was carried out by a combination of maternal age, fetal nuchal translucency (NT) thickness, and maternal serum free β-human chorionic gonadotrophin (hCG) and pregnancy-associated plasma protein-A (PAPP-A) at 11 to 13+6 weeks. The patients were counseled with regards to their estimated risk, and were informed that the only way to know for sure whether or not the fetus has a chromosomal abnormality is by having an invasive test, but these tests carry a risk of miscarriage of about 1%. They were also informed that although a risk of 1 in 300 or more was generally considered to be high, it was up to them to decide in favor or against invasive testing.

Results.—Assessment of risk was carried out in 30,564 singleton pregnancies with live fetuses at 11 to 13+6. The median maternal age was 34 (range 15-49) years and, in 14,816 (48.5%), the age was 35 years or greater. The rate of invasive testing increased exponentially with increasing estimated risk ($r = 0.917$, $P < .0001$). The estimated risk for trisomy 21 was 1 in 300 or more in 2565 (8.4%) women, and 1991 (77.6%) of these had invasive testing. The risk was less than 1 in 300 in 27,999 (91.6%) women, and 1286 (4.6%) of these had invasive testing.

Conclusion.—Pregnant women are able to use sophisticated screening information to make scientifically and ethically rational decisions about invasive testing for trisomy 21. These empiric data compliment the arguments of normative ethics to create evidence-based ethical standards for informed consent regarding invasive testing.

▶ In so far as the number and complexity of screening protocols for fetal chromosome abnormalities continues to expand, a seminal issue concerning obstetric care providers and their patients is the ability to provide effective counseling to women considering such screening protocols. Indeed, it is believed that the ability to provide effective counseling may be the main barrier to the effective incorporation of these screening protocols into obstetric care. One aspect of the counseling of such patients is the ability to effectively communicate assessment of risk after first-trimester screening so that patients can make truly informed decisions concerning the use of prenatal tests to further assess the increased risk detected by the first-trimester screening protocol. In this study from several well-recognized prenatal diagnostic centers around the world, the authors found that pregnant women were able to use sophisticated screening information to make scientific and ethically rational decisions about invasive testing for trisomy 21. Despite the findings of these renowned authors, clinicians should be concerned that in the absence of a large and well-trained cadre of counselors and maternal-fetal and genetics specialists, clinicians providing care to obstetric patients will nonetheless face considerable challenges in the counseling of patients who are not only considering screening protocols but are deciding whether to proceed with invasive testing after the detection of increased risk of fetal chromosome abnormalities. Clinicians should be aware that referral to counseling and genetics professionals maybe warranted to provide optimal care for their patients who are facing difficult diagnostic decisions in the face of novel screening outcomes.

L. P. Shulman, MD

Outcome of First-Trimester Pregnancies With Slow Embryonic Heart Rate at 6–7 Weeks Gestation and Normal Heart Rate by 8 Weeks at US
Doubilet PM, Benson CB (Harvard Med School, Boston)
Radiology 236:643-646, 2005   4–3

Purpose.—To determine retrospectively the outcome of pregnancies in which the embryo has a slow heart rate at 6.0–7.0 weeks gestation and a normal heart rate at follow-up ultrasonography (US) by 8.0 weeks gestation.

Materials and Methods.—Institutional review board approval was granted; informed consent was not required. The study was Health Insurance Portability and Accountability Act compliant. Singleton pregnancies with an embryonic heart rate measured on a 6.0–7.0-week US scan were identified. The heart rate was classified as slow if it was fewer than 90 beats per minute prior to 6.3 weeks or fewer than 110 beats/min at 6.3–7.0 weeks, normal if it was 100 or more beats/min at less than 6.3 weeks or 120 or more beats/min at 6.3–7.0 weeks, or borderline if it was 90–99 beats/min prior to 6.3 weeks or 110–119 beats/min at 6.3–7.0 weeks. Pregnancies were excluded from the analysis if they were lost to follow-up before the end of first trimester. The Fisher exact test was used for all statistical comparisons.

Results.—The rates of first-trimester demise were 60.6% for pregnancies with slow heart rates at 6.0–7.0 weeks (188 of 310), 17.4% for those with borderline heart rates (103 of 593), and 9.1% for those with normal heart rates (186 of 2034). There were 59 pregnancies with a slow heart rate at 6.0–7.0 weeks and a normal heart rate at follow-up US by 8.0 weeks; 15 (25.4%) resulted in first-trimester demise. This rate of demise was significantly higher than that of 7.2% (28 of 390) in pregnancies with a normal heart rate at 6.0–7.0 weeks and a normal heart rate by 8.0 weeks (*P* < .001, Fisher exact test). Pregnancies with a borderline heart rate early in pregnancy followed by a normal heart rate had a demise rate of 7.6% (nine of 118), which is similar to those with normal heart rates early in pregnancy followed by normal heart rates at follow-up (*P* = .84).

Conclusion.—When a slow embryonic heart rate is detected at 6.0–7.0 weeks, the likelihood of subsequent first-trimester demise remains elevated (approximately 25%) even if the heart rate is normal at follow-up. In such pregnancies, at least one follow-up scan in late first trimester is warranted.

▶ With the increasing utilization of first-trimester US for obstetric management, we have an expanding dataset concerning clinical outcomes with a variety of US findings. In particular, slow embryonic heartbeats are usually associated with poor perinatal outcomes. The authors of this study sought to determine whether pregnancies in which embryonic heartbeats were initially found to be slow and then subsequently found to be normal at follow-up US by

8 weeks' gestation had a different outcome than those with consistently slow embryonic heart rates. The authors found that regardless of increases in fetal heart rate after the initial measurement of a slow heart rate, first-trimester fetal demise rates remained considerably elevated. The finding of a slow first-trimester embryonic heart rate should lead to at least 1 follow-up scan in the first trimester. Although risk for fetal demise is considerably increased in such cases, there is still a good likelihood of a successful outcome, and patients should be appropriately counseled as to their risks as well as the appropriate management options available to them.

L. P. Shulman, MD

Quad Screen as a Predictor of Adverse Pregnancy Outcome
Dugoff L, for the FASTER Trial Research Consortium (Univ of Colorado, Denver; et al)
Obstet Gynecol 106:260-267, 2005   4–4

Objective.—To estimate the effect of second-trimester levels of maternal serum alpha-fetoprotein (AFP), human chorionic gonadotrophin (hCG), unconjugated estriol (uE$_3$), and inhibin A (the quad screen) on obstetric complications by using a large, prospectively collected database (the FASTER database).

Methods.—The FASTER trial was a multicenter study that evaluated first- and second-trimester screening programs for aneuploidy in women with singleton pregnancies. As part of this trial, patients had a quad screen drawn at 15-18 6/7 weeks. We analyzed the data to identify associations between the quad screen markers and preterm birth, intrauterine growth restriction, preeclampsia, and fetal loss. Our analysis was performed by evaluating the performance characteristics of quad screen markers individually and in combination. Crude and adjusted effects were estimated by multivariable logistic regression analysis. Patients with fetal anomalies were excluded from the analysis.

Results.—We analyzed data from 33,145 pregnancies. We identified numerous associations between the markers and the adverse outcomes. There was a relatively low, but often significant, risk of having an adverse pregnancy complication if a patient had a single abnormal marker. However, the risk of having an adverse outcome increased significantly if a patient had 2 or more abnormal markers. The sensitivity and positive predictive values using combinations of markers is relatively low, although superior to using individual markers.

Conclusion.—These data suggest that components of the quad screen may prove useful in predicting adverse obstetric outcomes. We also showed that the total number and specific combinations of abnormal markers are most useful in predicting the risk of adverse perinatal outcome.

▶ The combination of AFP, hCG, uE$_3$, and inhibin A has been called the quad screen. This combination of maternal serum markers has been shown to be the most effective screening test for Down syndrome in the second trimester. Based on data from the National Institute of Child Health and Human Development sponsored FASTER trial, the authors sought to determine whether a single marker or a combination of markers was associated with adverse obstetric outcomes in the absence of aneuploidy or neural tube defects. The data showed that the sensitivity and positive predictive values for the individual adverse outcomes are relatively low. However, the presence of 2 or more abnormal markers, although strongly associated with a number of adverse outcomes, was only a modest predictor of these outcomes and does not support the use of the quad screen as a screening test for adverse pregnancy outcomes in a general population. As the number of abnormal markers increased, the association with adverse outcomes became stronger. A major question is whether any single or multiple second-trimester maternal serum markers can be used for third-trimester interventions and prevent such adverse obstetric outcomes as preterm birth, intrauterine growth restriction, preeclampsia, or fetal loss. The authors suggest that the use of pregnancy-associated plasma protein-A, Doppler uterine artery studies, or other factors such as maternal demographic characteristics, might enhance the screening efficacy of the quad screen. These factors should be investigated.

S. Elias, MD

Cost-Effectiveness Analysis of Prenatal Population-Based Fragile X Carrier Screening
Musci TJ, Caughey AB (California Pacific Med Ctr, San Francisco; Univ of California–San Francisco; Univ of California–Berkeley)
Am J Obstet Gynecol 192:1905-1915, 2005   4–5

Objective.—To investigate the cost-effectiveness of a widespread prenatal population-based fragile X carrier screening program.

Study Design.—A decision tree was designed comparing screening versus not screening for the fragile X mental retardation protein 1 premutation in all pregnant women. Baseline values included a prevalence of fragile X mental retardation protein 1 premutations of 3.3 per 1000, a premutation expansion rate of 11.3%, and a 99% sensitivity of the screening test. The cost of the screening test was varied from $75 to $300. A sensitivity analysis of the probabilities, utilities, and costs was performed (Fig 2 and Table 3).

Results.—The screening strategy would lead to the identification of 80% of the fetuses affected by fragile X annually. Assuming the cost of $95 per test and only one child, the program would be cost effective at $14,858 per quality-adjusted life-year. The screening strategy remained cost effective up to $140 per test and 1 child per woman or for 2 children per woman up to a cost of $281 per test.

Conclusion.—Population-based screening for the fragile X premutation may be both clinically desirable and cost effective. Prospective pilot studies of this screening modality are needed in the prenatal setting.

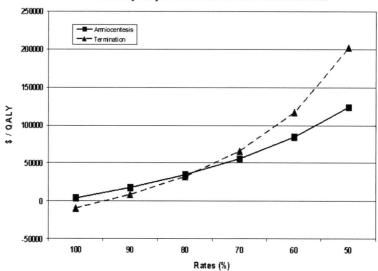

FIGURE 2.—Sensitivity analysis of fragile X screening program. Incremental CUA ratios (CUA ratio = dollars per QALY) varying the acceptance rates of amniocentesis, among women found to be screen positive, and termination rates among those patients whose fetus is found to have a full fragile X mutation. (Courtesy of Musci TJ, Caughey AB: Cost-effectiveness analysis of prenatal population-based fragile X carrier screening. *Am J Obstet Gynecol* 192:1905-1915. Copyright 2005 by Elsevier.)

▶ Fragile X is the most common cause of inherited mental retardation and is seen in approximately 1 in 4000 males and 1 in 6000 females. Males with fragile X exhibit unique physical features and behavioral characteristics and have moderate to severe developmental delay. Affected females usually have similar cognitive defects but usually present with less severe phenotypic abnormalities. Although the inheritance of fragile X is classically an X-linked mechanism, the molecular genetics of this condition are complex. The determination of whether a particular screening assay is appropriate for consideration of the general population requires a cost-effectiveness analysis to determine whether utilizing such a protocol would be cost effective for the population to be screened. To this end, the authors sought to determine the cost effectiveness

TABLE 3.—Sensitivity Analysis of Fragile X Carrier Prevalence and Expansion Rate

Fragile X Carrier Prevalence (60-200 CGG Repeats)	Expansion Rate	CUA Ratio ($/QALY)	No. Fragile X Identified/PRL	Amnios/1 Case of Fragile X Dx
0.001	0.375	$7748	20	11
0.002	0.1875	$10,502	13	17
0.003	0.125	$13,661	10	22
0.004	0.09375	$17,322	8	27
0.005	0.075	$21,613	6	33

PRL, Procedure-related loss.
(Courtesy of Musci TJ, Caughey AB: Cost-effectiveness analysis of prenatal population-based fragile X carrier screening. *Am J Obstet Gynecol* 192:1905-1915. Copyright 2005 by Elsevier.)

of a widespread prenatal population-based fragile X carrier screening program. The authors found that such a screening program could be both clinically desirable and cost effective. We have witnessed in the past several years the difficulties with incorporating cystic fibrosis screening into routine obstetric care. This incorporation occurred only after considerable studies looking into the ability of cystic fibrosis screening to be incorporated into obstetric care as well as the cost effectiveness of such screening. Although this study demonstrates a clear benefit for the consideration of fragile X screening in a general population, further studies will be needed to confirm and further delineate various medical, economic, and societal issues concerning the potential incorporation of fragile X screening for routine obstetric care. Until those studies have been accomplished, fragile X screening should be reserved for those individuals with personal or family histories of developmental delay and mental retardation.

L. P. Shulman, MD

High Levels of Fetal Cell-Free DNA in Maternal Serum: A Risk Factor for Spontaneous Preterm Delivery
Farina A, LeShane ES, Romero R, et al (Univ of Bologna, Italy; Tufts Univ, Boston; NIH, Bethesda, Md)
Am J Obstet Gynecol 193:421-425, 2005   4–6

Objective.—This study was conducted to determine whether there is a relationship between the concentration of fetal cell–free DNA in maternal serum and the duration of pregnancy in women who are at high risk for preterm delivery because of either preterm labor or preterm premature rupture of the membranes.

Study Design.—Sera were collected and frozen from 71 women with a male fetus. Maternal serum fetal cell–free DNA concentration was measured with the use of real-time polymerase chain reaction amplification of *DYS1*. Fetal cell–free DNA concentrations were converted to multiples of the median. The following groups were studied: group 1: women with preterm labor and intact membranes who were delivered at ≥ 36 weeks of gestation (n = 21); group 2: women with preterm labor who were delivered at <36 weeks of gestation (n = 29); and group 3: women with preterm premature rupture of the membranes in labor (n = 20) or not in labor (n = 1) who were delivered prematurely (<36 weeks of gestation). Kaplan-Meier and Cox regression analyses were used to analyze the relationship between fetal cell–free DNA concentrations and the likelihood of preterm delivery.

Results.—A cut-off value for fetal cell–free DNA of 1.82 multiples of the median was chosen for analysis. The cumulative rate of early preterm delivery (<30 weeks of gestation) was significantly higher for women with fetal cell–free DNA concentrations of ≥ 1.82 multiples of the median than those with fetal cell–free DNA concentrations below this cut-off (45% [95% CI, 36%-74%] vs 18% [95% CI, 11%-25%]; $P = .008$). The cumulative rate of preterm delivery (<36 weeks of gestation) was also significantly higher at

≥1.82 multiples of the median (73% [95% CI, 52%-93%] vs 66% [95% CI, 54%-79%]; $P = .02$). After adjustment for covariates, Cox analysis showed that fetal cell–free DNA at ≥1.82 multiples of the mechanisms of disease that are associated with a mean hazard rate of delivery of 1.57 ($P = .005$). *Conclusion.*—High concentrations of fetal cell–free DNA in maternal serum are associated with an increased risk of spontaneous preterm delivery. This observation may have implications for the understanding of the mechanisms of disease that is associated with preterm labor.

▶ The past decade has witnessed a veritable explosion of studies evaluating the potential of fetal cells and fetal DNA in maternal blood as a screening and diagnostic test for prenatal mendelian and chromosome abnormalities. Indeed, such technology is being used in Europe and some parts of the United States to provide noninvasive assessment of fetal RH status in isoimmunized women. However, studies over the past several years have demonstrated a potentially important impact of fetal DNA on maternal health and well-being. In this regard, the study by Farina et al shows that high concentrations of fetal cell–free DNA in maternal serum are associated with an increased risk of spontaneous preterm delivery. Although this study does not serve to provide information concerning potential therapeutic or preventative options based on these findings, it does provide important information as to the potential etiology if not of some cases of spontaneous preterm delivery. Our understanding of fetal DNA and its role in the maternal blood compartment remains a mystery and a topic of eager investigation.

L. P. Shulman, MD

Hypothyroidism Is Common in Turner Syndrome: Results of a Five-Year Follow-up
El-Mansoury M, Bryman I, Berntrop K, et al (Sahlgrenska Univ, Göteborg, Sweden; Lund Univ, Malmö, Sweden; Göteborg Univ, Sweden)
J Clin Endocrinol Metab 90:2131-2135, 2005   4–7

Abstract.—Turner syndrome (TS) is caused by a sex chromosome aberration. The aim was to study the prevalence and incidence of thyroid disease in adults with TS.

Women with TS (n = 91; mean age, 37.7 ± 11 yr) were compared with an age-matched female random population sample (n = 228). At baseline, 15 (16%) TS women were treated for hypothyroidism, and elevated serum TSH was found in another eight (9%). As a result, hypothyroidism was more common in women with TS (25%) than in controls (2%; $P < 0.0001$). Serum free T_4 was lower ($P = 0.02$), and serum TSH was higher ($P < 0.0001$) in TS women than in age-matched controls. Of all TS women with hypothyroidism, 10 (43%) had an elevated thyroid peroxidase antibody titer *vs.* 15 (22%) of those without hypothyroidism ($P < 0.05$), evenly distributed between the karyotype 45,X and mosaicism. A high body mass index, but not a family history or blood lipids, was associated with hypothyroidism in TS.

After the 5-yr follow-up, an additional 11 (16%) developed hypothyroidism, of whom four (36%) had elevated thyroid peroxidase. Altogether, 34 (37%) TS women had hypothyroidism after the 5-yr follow-up.

Autoimmune hypothyroidism was common, with an annual incidence of 3.2% in TS. Thyroid function should be checked regularly in TS.

▶ Hypothyroidism is common in adult women with TS. This study found an annual incidence of elevated thyrotropin (TSH) of 3%. Physicians caring for adults with TS should be aware of associated medical conditions including hypothyroidism, cardiovascular disease and dilatation of the aortic root, hyperlipidemia, hypertension, osteoporosis, and hearing loss. In addition to providing hormone replacement therapy, clinicians should also provide adequate surveillance of adults with TS that includes an annual medical history and physical exam; determination of hemoglobin, renal function, fasting blood glucose, lipid profile, liver enzymes, and TSH and free thyroxine (T_4) every 2 years; otologic evaluation at 10-year intervals; echocardiogram every 5 years; and measurements of bone mineral density at 3- to 5-year intervals.[1]

R. Barnes, MD

Reference

1. Saenger P, Wikland KA, Conway GS, et al: Recommendations for the diagnosis and management of Turner syndrome. *J Clin Endocrinol Metab* 86:3061-3069, 2001.

5 Maternal Complications

Prepregnancy Weight and Adverse Perinatal Outcomes in an Ethnically Diverse Population
Rosenberg TJ, Garbers S, Chavkin W, et al (Med and Health Research Association of NYC, Inc; Columbia Univ, New York)
Obstet Gynecol 102:1022-1027, 2003   5–1

Objective.—To examine the association between excessive prepregnancy weight and adverse outcomes, with a focus on women weighing over 200 lbs (91 kg) before pregnancy.

Methods.—Data were from the 1998-1999 New York City births file for 213,208 singletons with information on prepregnancy weight. Five categories of prepregnancy weight were constructed and used to predict gestational diabetes, preeclampsia, cesarean delivery, very low birthweight, macrosomia, and treatment in the neonatal intensive care unit (NICU). Statistical adjustments were made for mother's age, race or ethnicity, marital status, education, parity, social risk (eg, smoking), initiation of prenatal care, health insurance, and infant's sex.

Results.—Maternal prepregnancy weight was associated with several adverse outcomes. Women in the heaviest group (>300 lbs or >136 kg) had the highest adjusted odds ratios (OR) for gestational diabetes (OR 5.2), preeclampsia (OR 5.0), and cesarean delivery (OR 2.7) compared with women weighing 100-149 lbs (45-67 kg). Compared with the reference group, the heaviest women were more likely to have a macrosomic infant and an infant treated in the NICU (OR 4.2 and 1.9, respectively). Even among a subsample of women who did not have any diabetic or hypertensive diseases, excess weight significantly increased the likelihood of macrosomia and NICU treatment. Blacks were disproportionately represented in the two heaviest groups (49.8% of those weighing 200-299 lbs and 63.9% of those weighing over 300 lbs).

Conclusion.—In this population-based study of pregnant women, the adverse outcomes associated with excessive weight underline the urgency of weight loss interventions before pregnancy. The analysis also suggests that research is needed on rapidly growing racial or ethnic subgroups most at risk for obesity.

▶ The worldwide prevalence of obesity continues to increase rapidly. Associations have been made between obesity in pregnant women and pregnancy complications. There is some evidence that the obesity-related risks during pregnancy vary by race, with obese Hispanics and black women more likely to have adverse outcomes than obese white women. A large population-based dataset of New York City, including diverse populations and large numbers of prepregnant overweight or obese women, was used to study risks of subsequent pregnancy complications. Analysis was only performed on live births. Accordingly, possible associations between prepregnancy obesity and miscarriage or fetal demise could not be studied. The results of this study support previous findings of an increased risk of gestational diabetes, preeclampsia, cesarean delivery, having a macrosomic infant (both for diabetic and nondiabetic women), and having an infant treated in the NICU. Morbidly obese women showed a 40% risk of cesarean delivery. This gives rise to great concern, as maternal mortality and morbidity related to postoperative complications such as infection, operative injury, need for transfusion, thromboembolism, and hysterectomy are likely to be more frequent. With regard to ethnicity, it appeared that blacks were more often represented in the 2 heaviest categories and, therefore, may be at higher risk. This emphasizes the need for ongoing counseling by clinicians, emphasizing the importance of balanced nutrition and exercise, and the implementation of intervention programs to help reduce weight, especially before conception.

E. A. P. Steegers, MD, PhD

The Risk of Folate and Vitamin B_{12} Deficiencies Associated With Hyperhomocysteinemia Among Pregnant Women

Park H, Kim YJ, Ha EH, et al (Ewha Womans Univ, Seoul, South Korea)
Am J Perinatol 21:469-476, 2004   5–2

Abstract.—The purpose of this study was to compare the folate and vitamin B_{12} levels in pregnant and nonpregnant women to evaluate the risk for hyperhomocysteinemia and for folate and vitamin B_{12} deficiencies during pregnancy. Healthy pregnant women (n = 92; 24 to 28 gestational weeks; 18 to 39 years old) and nonpregnant women (n = 176; 18 to 39 years old) were sampled for serum levels of folate, vitamin B_{12}, and homocysteine. Pregnant women were less likely to have folate deficiency (8.0% versus 12.0%) but much more likely to have vitamin B_{12} deficiency (46.1% versus 0.6%) than nonpregnant women. Those with lower dietary vitamin intakes were more likely to have vitamin B_{12} deficiency. Serum folate and vitamin B_{12} were negatively correlated with homocysteine among pregnant women. Pregnant women with folate deficiency were more likely to have hyperhomocysteinemia than those without folate deficiency. The vitamin B_{12} level associated with hyperhomocysteinemia was lower in pregnant subjects than in nonpregnant subjects in this study, indicating that pregnant women require vitamin B_{12} supplementation.

▶ Pregnancy increases the requirements for vitamins; folate and vitamin B_{12} are 2 vitamins involved in critical metabolic pathways and, as such, are critical for maternal and fetal well-being. Folate and vitamin B_{12} deficiencies have been associated with adverse pregnancy outcomes, with folic acid supplementation now an integral part of preconception care. The authors found that pregnant women were more likely to be vitamin B_{12} deficient than nonpregnant women and that folate and vitamin B_{12} levels were negatively correlated with homocysteine levels in pregnant women. This study shows a clear need for appropriate vitamin B_{12} and folate supplementation for pregnant women, hopefully beginning before conception.

L. P. Shulman, MD

Impact of Prenatal Tobacco Smoke Exposure, as Measured by Midgestation Serum Cotinine Levels, on Fetal Biometry and Umbilical Flow Velocity Waveforms

Kalinka J, Hanke W, Sobala W (Med Univ of Lodz, Poland; Nofer Inst of Occupational Medicine, Lodz, Poland)
Am J Perinatol 22:41-47, 2005   5–3

Background.—Many studies have documented the association between maternal cigarette smoking during pregnancy and the elevated risk for low birth weight, preterm delivery, and intrauterine growth restriction. The constituents of sidestream smoke, which is the main component of environmental tobacco smoke, include carbon monoxide, carbon dioxide, and benzo(a)-pyrene, the same constituents of cigarette smoke inhaled by active smokers. In addition, the concentrations of chemicals found in sidestream smoke may greatly exceed those in the smoke from tobacco combustion (mainstream smoke). Many of these substances are known to pass through the placental barrier. The effect of tobacco smoke exposure, as measured by maternal serum concentration of cotinine, on fetal midgestation biometric parameters and umbilicial artery qualitative blood flow indices was evaluated in a prospective cohort study.

Methods.—The study cohort was composed of 114 healthy pregnant women at 20 to 24 weeks' gestation. The women were recruited from 2 antenatal care units in Lodz, Poland. These units were characterized by a high prevalence of smoking and exposure to environmental tobacco smoke. A standard questionnaire covering medical, socioeconomic, demographic, and constitutional aspects as well as tobacco smoking and environmental tobacco smoke exposure was administered, and every woman underwent routine US examination of fetal biometry and Doppler umbilical blood flow assessment as well as serum cotinine determination for assessment of tobacco smoke exposure.

TABLE 3.—Serum Cotinine Level Measured Between 20 and 24 Weeks of Pregnancy and the Mean Crude and Adjusted Values of Umbilical Artery Blood Flow Indices

| | | Umbilical Artery Blood Flow in 20-24 wk of Gestation | | | | | |
| Serum Cotinine Level (ng/mL) | n | Crude Values (Mean ± SD) | | | Adjusted Values* | | |
		S/D	RI	PI	S/D	RI	PI
< 2.0	8	2.86 ± 0.28	0.65 ± 0.04	1.07 ± 0.09	2.93	0.66	1.15
2.0-14	84	3.07 ± 0.54	0.67 ± 0.06	1.17 ± 0.17	3.18	0.67	1.20
> 14	22	3.53 ± 0.97	0.68 ± 0.11	1.25 ± 0.22	3.66	0.70	1.30
p		0.006	0.496	0.038	0.003	0.004	0.004

*Adjusted S/D, RI, and PI values were calculated for the mean serum cotinine level in each cotinine group, 20 weeks of gestation, male fetus gender, and femur length = 39.9, using linear regression model.
Abbreviations: SD, Standard deviation; *S/D*, systolic/diastolic index; *RI*, resistance index; *PI*, pulsatility index.
(Courtesy of Kalinka J, Hanke W, Sobala W: Impact of prenatal tobacco smoke exposure, as measured by midgestation serum cotinine levels, on fetal biometry and umbilical flow velocity waveforms. *Am J Perinatol* 22:41-47, 2005. Reprinted with permission from *American Journal of Perinatology*. Thieme Medical Publishers, Inc.)

Results.—Significant negative correlation was found between fetal biparietal diameter and serum cotinine concentration. Serum cotinine was found to be positively correlated with all the blood flow indices, after controlling for gestational age, gender, and femur length (Table 3). A midgestation umbilical artery systolic/diastolic index ratio of greater than 3 was found to be a significant risk factor for decreased birth weight.

Conclusions.—Exposure to tobacco smoke is a significant factor inducing increased resistance of umbilical blood flow as measured at 20 to 24 weeks' gestation. This could be one of the main mechanisms in decreased birth weight found among infants with prenatal exposure to tobacco smoke.

▶ This study analyzed the effects of tobacco smoke exposure on serum cotinine levels and umbilical artery Doppler waveform velocity. An increased resistance of umbilical blood flow was observed, and this may be a reason for lower birth weight in pregnant women who smoke. Future studies utilizing larger sample sizes are necessary to confirm these findings.

S. H. Ural, MD

Chorioamnionitis Increases Neonatal Morbidity in Pregnancies Complicated by Preterm Premature Rupture of Membranes

Ramsey PS, Lieman JM, Brumfield CG, et al (Univ of Alabama, Birmingham)
Am J Obstet Gynecol 192:1162-1166, 2005   5–4

Objective.—To compare morbidities of neonates born to women who developed chorioamnionitis after premature preterm rupture of membranes versus those who did not.

Study Design.—We reviewed outcomes in singleton pregnancies with confirmed premature preterm rupture of membranes at 24 weeks or beyond that resulted in delivery less than 37 weeks. Management of premature preterm rupture of membranes included the use of antibiotics, betamethasone if less than 32 weeks, and expectant management with induction at 34 weeks or greater. Composite neonatal major and minor morbidity rates were compared between pregnancies complicated by chorioamnionitis and those that were not.

Results.—From August 1998 to August 2000, 430 cases of premature preterm rupture of membranes were identified among 6003 deliveries (7.2%). Thirteen percent of women (56/430) with premature preterm rupture of membranes developed chorioamnionitis (Figure). The incidence of chorioamnionitis increased significantly with decreasing gestational age. The composite neonatal major morbidity rate was significantly higher in neonates whose mothers developed chorioamnionitis (55%) versus those who did not (18%, $P < .0001$). In a multiple logistic regression model, chorioamnionitis ($P < .0001$), infant gender ($P = 007$), latency ($P = .03$), and gestational age at delivery ($P < .0001$) were significantly associated with composite neonatal morbidity.

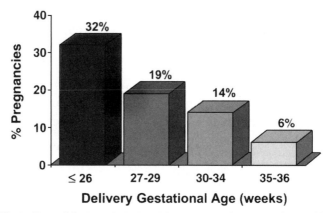

FIGURE.—Incidence of chorioamnionitis in PPROM pregnancies by gestational age at delivery. (Courtesy of Ramsey PS, Lieman JM, Brumfield CG, et al: Chorioamnionitis increases neonatal morbidity in pregnancies complicated by preterm premature rupture of membranes. *Am J Obstet Gynecol* 192:1162-1166. Copyright 2005 by Elsevier.)

Conclusion.—Neonatal morbidities are significantly higher among pregnancies with premature preterm rupture of membranes complicated by chorioamnionitis when compared with pregnancies that were not.

▶ The development of evidence-based paradigms for improving the health care of obstetric and gynecologic patients requires rigorous scientific evaluation of epidemiologic factors and how they affect clinical outcomes. To this end, Ramsey et al from the University of Alabama at Birmingham reviewed the outcomes in singleton pregnancies with confirmed premature preterm rupture of the membranes (PPROM) at 24 weeks or beyond that subsequently resulted in delivery at less than 37 weeks. What the authors found was that neonatal morbidity rates were significantly higher among those pregnancies with PPROM that were complicated by chorioamnionitis when compared with pregnancies that were not complicated by chorioamnionitis. The impact of this information can be profound, as management of pregnancies complicated by PPROM remains a topic of great controversy among obstetric providers. Essentially, the management of such patients requires a difficult decision between expected management and initiation of delivery. The information from this study addresses concerns regarding the expectant management of women with PPROM. Additional research will be needed to further evaluate potential risks and benefits of expectant management with PPROM and to better delineate effective treatment modalities for affected women.

L. P. Shulman, MD

Bacteria and Inflammatory Cells in Fetal Membranes Do Not Always Cause Preterm Labor

Steel JH, Malatos S, Kennea N, et al (Inst of Reproductive and Developmental Biology, London; Imperial College London; Vmax Ltd, Berkshire, England)
Pediatr Res 57:404-411, 2005   5–5

Abstract.—Intrauterine infection has been frequently linked with preterm labor before 30 wk of human pregnancy. Many different species of organisms have been detected, leading to the suggestion that infection-induced preterm labor is a generic inflammatory response to organisms rather than a specific response to a limited number of pathogens. The detection of organisms by microbiological culture is a laborious and unreliable process, so the aim of this study was to harness modern molecular techniques to detect organisms in tissues from human pregnancy. A DNA probe specific for conserved regions of bacterial 16S ribosomal RNA sequence was designed and labeled with fluorescein for fluorescence *in situ* hybridization. Organisms were detected in the great majority (>80%) of fetal membranes after prolonged premature rupture of the fetal membranes and after preterm labor, which was consistent with previous data. Organisms were also detected in fetal membranes after preterm delivery without labor and in term deliveries (with or without labour). Inflammatory cells were found frequently in the amnion or chorion of preterm fetal membranes but not in term tissues. Our primary finding is that fluorescence *in situ* hybridization is an appropriate method to detect organisms in human fetal membranes. In addition, our data show that bacteria may be present in fetal membranes without necessarily causing an inflammatory response, so the mere presence of bacteria may not be sufficient to cause preterm labor.

▶ The precise relationship between bacteria and inflammation remains unclear. Molecular detection techniques were used in this study, together with fluorescent in situ hybridization, to detect and identify bacteria. Surprisingly, bacteria were present in the majority of membrane samples, including those obtained from elective cesarean sections. From these data, bacteria alone or in conjunction with inflammatory cells does not cause preterm labor or premature preterm rupture of the membranes. Other processes must be involved, and further studies will be needed to delineate those pathophysiologic processes.

P. P. van den Berg, MD, PhD

6 Fetal Complications

A Review of Intrapartum Fetal Deaths, 1982 to 2002
Mattatall FM, O'Connell CM, Baskett TF (Dalhousie Univ, Halifax, NS, Canada)
Am J Obstet Gynecol 192:1475-1477, 2005   6–1

Background.—Among the known risk factors for intrapartum fetal deaths are malpresentation, abruptio placentae, and cord prolapse. One study has also reported that the risk of stillbirth related to intrapartum asphyxia is highest on weekends. Cases of unexpected intrapartum fetal death were identified and reviewed in 1 tertiary-level maternity hospital.

Methods.—The study included all deliveries at 1 Canadian hospital for 2 years. Live-in 24-hour consultant anesthesia and obstetric services were available during this period.

Results.—The period 1982 to 1992 generated 121,659 births at the study hospital. Of these, 835 were fetal deaths (6.9 per 1000). Of these deaths, 82 were reviewed, and 11 of these were identified as viable and not anomalous. Of the 11 deaths considered viable, 6 were deemed ideally preventable. Four of the deaths may have been prevented with improved fetal heart rate monitoring and interpretation because fetal distress would likely have been identified earlier had extended monitoring at admission or appropriate monitoring after admission been performed. However, insufficient evidence was available to show that fetal heart rate monitoring admission tests improve fetal outcomes.

Conclusions.—The use of electronic fetal heart rate monitoring and rapid operative delivery may further reduce the low rate of intrapartum fetal deaths.

▶ Our ability to provide epidemiologic information regarding intrapartum fetal death is an important part in developing more effective interventions to prevent adverse outcomes. In this study from Dalhousie University in Halifax, Nova Scotia, the authors reviewed more than 120,000 births finding the causes of intrapartum demises. Among these 82 fetal deaths were 20 fetuses with major anomalies; 51 were considered to be previable. Among the 6 deaths that were deemed to be ideally preventable, the authors felt that the use of electronic fetal monitoring and lack of operative delivery could reduce the already low rate of intrapartum fetal deaths. Although several studies in this year's YEAR BOOK attest to the poor positive predictive values for fetal heart rate monitoring and the prediction of adverse outcomes, it is clear that fetal heart rate monitoring is modern obstetric management. This well-done study by Mattatall et al confirms the important role of the fetal heart rate tracing in current obstetric care.

H. P. van Geijn, MD, PhD

Demographic Characteristics and Clinical Course in Infants With Moderate or Severe Neonatal Encephalopathy
West CR, Harding JE, Knight DB, et al (Liggins Inst, Auckland, New Zealand; Univ of Auckland, New Zealand, Natl Women's Hosp, Auckland, New Zealand)
Aust N Z J Obstet Gynaecol 45:151-154, 2005   6–2

Background.—Previous studies have reported the prevalence, contributing factors, demographics, and morbidity or neonatal encephalopathy. However, there are few published data on neonatal encephalopathy from New Zealand, which has a unique population and pattern of obstetric care provision. Only half of women of child-bearing age in Auckland, New Zealand, identify themselves as European, and most low-risk women are cared for during pregnancy by independently practicing midwives. The purpose of the present study was to determine the clinical course and outcomes and demographic characteristics of a cohort of term infants with moderate or severe neonatal encephalopathy in patients in a tertiary neonatal intensive care unit (NICU) in New Zealand.

Methods.—Infants admitted to NICU with neonatal encephalopathy were identified from the National Women's Hospital neonatal database from January 1997 to December 2000. The pool of potential study subjects during the review period included approximately 8000 inborn births and 4000 births in 2 level I hospitals in New Zealand. Clinical and demographic details were obtained. Ethnicity was self-identified by the mother. Trials of head cooling were ongoing during part of the period reviewed for this study, and data from cooled infants were included in the information on clinical course.

Results.—Seventy infants were identified, and 64 with moderate or severe neonatal encephalopathy were included in the analysis. Resuscitation was required for 61 patients (95%), respiratory support was needed for 53 patients (83%), and anticonvulsants were needed in 58 patients (91%). Death occurred in 2 infants (4%) with moderate encephalopathy and in 12 infants (86%) with severe encephalopathy. Subsequent neurodevelopment was abnormal in approximately 25% of infants who survived after a moderate to severe encephalopathy. There were no significant differences in inborn/outborn status, Apgar score, or cord pH between cooled and non-cooled infants.

Conclusions.—Important demographic characteristics and data regarding the clinical course of infants with neonatal encephalopathy are presented. Among infants with moderate or severe neonatal encephalopathy, the rate of subsequent neurodevelopmental abnormalities in survivors was nearly 25%.

▶ This paper presents important information concerning the characteristics of infants with moderate or severe neonatal encephalopathy. Neonatal resuscitation was associated with 95% of all affected newborns; death occurred in 4% of moderately affected newborns and 86% of severely affected infants. Of those infants that survived, abnormal neurodevelopment was observed in approximately 25% of infants with moderate or severe neonatal encephalopathy. Further studies are needed to better identify risk factors and effective interventions to prevent this dire neonatal complication.

H. N. Lafeber, MD, PhD

Do Hyperoxaemia and Hypocapnia Add to the Risk of Brain Injury After Intrapartum Asphyxia?
Klinger G, Beyene J, Shah P, et al (Hosp for Sick Children, Toronto; Mount Sinai Hosp, Toronto; Univ of Toronto)
Arch Dis Child Fetal Neonatal Ed 90:F49-F52, 2005   6–3

Background.—Episodes of hyperoxaemia and hypocapnia, which may contribute to brain injury, occur unintentionally in severely asphyxiated neonates in the first postnatal hours.

Objective.—To determine whether hyperoxaemia and/or hypocapnia during the first 2 hours of life add to the risk of brain injury after intrapartum asphyxia.

Methods.—Retrospective cohort study in term infants with post-asphyxial hypoxic ischaemic encephalopathy (HIE) born between 1985 and 1995. Severe and moderate hyperoxaemia were defined as PaO_2 >26.6 and PaO_2 >13.3 kPa (200 and 100 mm Hg). Severe and moderate hypocapnia were defined as $PaCO_2$ <2.6 and $PaCO_2$ <3.3 kPa (20 and 25 mm Hg). Adverse outcome ascertained by age 24 months was defined as death, severe cerebral palsy, or any cerebral palsy with blindness, deafness, or developmental delay. With outcome as the dependent variable, multivariate analyses were performed including hyperoxaemic and hypocapnic variables, and factors adjusted for initial disease severity.

Results.—Of 244 infants, 218 had known outcomes, 127 of which were adverse (64 deaths, 63 neurodevelopmental deficits). Multivariate analyses showed an association between adverse outcome and episodes of severe hyperoxaemia (odds ratio (OR) 3.85, 95% confidence interval (CI) 1.67 to 8.88, p = 0.002), and severe hypocapnia (OR 2.34, 95% CI 1.02 to 5.37, p = 0.044). The risk of adverse outcome was highest in infants who had both severe hyperoxaemia and severe hypocapnia (OR 4.56, 95% CI 1.4 to 14.9, p = 0.012).

Conclusions.—Severe hyperoxaemia and severe hypocapnia were associated with adverse outcome in infants with post-asphyxial HIE. During the first hours of life, oxygen supplementation and ventilation should be rigorously controlled.

▶ Resuscitation of the severely asphyxiated infant is challenging and requires attention be paid to the function of many organ systems. One of many difficulties encountered in this process is the balance between oxygen supplementation and carbon dioxide levels. To this end, the authors found that severe hyperoxemia and hypocapnia were associated with a marked increase risk for adverse outcomes. Although providing sufficient oxygen to the asphyxiated neonate is a central aspect of the resuscitation process, the balance between oxygen supplementation and ventilation must be rigorously controlled to maximize clinical outcomes.

H. N. Lafeber, MD, PhD

Behavioral Outcomes and Evidence of Psychopathology Among Very Low Birth Weight Infants at Age 20 Years
Hack M, Youngstrom EA, Cartar L, et al (Case Western Reserve Univ, Cleveland, Ohio; Kent State Univ, Ohio)
Pediatrics 114:932-940, 2004   6–4

Objective.—Information on the mental health of very low birth weight (VLBW; <1500 g) children in young adulthood is sparse. We thus sought to examine gender-specific behavioral outcomes and evidence of psychopathology in a cohort of VLBW young adults at 20 years of age.

Methods.—We compared a cohort of 241 survivors among VLBW infants who were born between 1977 and 1979 (mean birth weight: 1180 g; mean gestational age at birth: 29.7 weeks), 116 of whom were men and 125 of whom were women, with 233 control subjects from the same population in Cleveland who had normal birth weights (108 men and 124 women). Young adult behavior was assessed at 20 years of age with the Achenbach Young Adult Self-Report and the Young Adult Behavior Checklist for parents. In addition, the young adults and parents completed the ADHD Rating Scale for Adults. Gender-specific outcomes were adjusted for sociodemographic status.

Results.—VLBW men reported having significantly fewer delinquent behaviors than normal birth weight (NBW) control subjects, but there were no differences on the Internalizing, Externalizing, or Total Problem Behavior scales. Parents of VLBW men reported significantly more thought problems for their sons than did parents of control subjects. VLBW women reported significantly more withdrawn behaviors and fewer delinquent behavior problems than control subjects. Their rates of internalizing behaviors (which includes anxious/depressed and withdrawn behaviors) above the borderline clinical cutoff were 30% versus 16% (odds ratio: 2.2; 95% confidence interval [CI]: 1.2-4.1). Parents of VLBW women reported significantly higher scores for their daughters on the anxious/depressed, withdrawn, and attention problem subscales compared with control parents.

The odds ratios for parent-reported rates above the borderline-clinical cut-off among women for the anxious/depressed subscale was 4.4 (95% CI: 1.4-13.5), for thought problems was 3.7 (95% CI: 1.2-11.6), and for attention problems was 2.4 (95% CI: 1.0-5.5). There were no differences in the young adult self-report of attention-deficit/hyperactivity disorder (ADHD). Parents of VLBW men reported higher mean scores on the attention subtype of ADHD but not higher rates of ADHD.

Conclusion.—The increase in psychopathology among VLBW survivors in young adulthood indicates a need for anticipatory guidance and early intervention that might help to prevent or ameliorate potential psychopathology.

▶ Delineation of risks and outcomes for preterm delivery is an important process that allows for evidence-based counseling of families with preterm infants and the development of therapeutic interventions to improve clinical outcomes. Although many studies seek to evaluate short-term outcomes, this study compared a cohort of adolescents composed of VLBW infants born between 1977 and 1979 with a control group of adolescents who were term infants born in that same period. The authors found an increase in psychopathology among the adolescents who were VLBW infants. Such information can be critical for enabling clinicians to provide accurate prenatal counseling as well as facilitating early intervention to improve clinical outcomes in VLBW infants as they progress through childhood and early adulthood.

H. N. Lafeber, MD, PhD

7 Preeclampsia

Late First-Trimester Placental Disruption and Subsequent Gestational Hypertension/Preeclampsia
Silver RK, for the NICHD EATA Trial Group (Northwestern Univ, Evanston, Ill; et al)
Obstet Gynecol 105:587-592, 2005   7-1

Objective.—To evaluate the potential relationship between placental disruption in weeks 13 and 14 and the subsequent development of gestational hypertension or preeclampsia.

Methods.—Using subjects recruited during a randomized trial funded by the National Institute of Child Health and Human Development, which compared early amniocentesis and late transabdominal chorionic villus sampling (CVS) in weeks 13 and 14, rates of gestational hypertension and preeclampsia were compared between cases with varying degrees of placental disruption.

Results.—A total of 3,698 of 3,775 randomized subjects had cytogenetically normal pregnancies and were analyzed. A significantly higher rate of hypertension/preeclampsia was observed in the late CVS group (5.4%, n = 1,878) compared with the early amniocentesis cohort (3.5%, n = 1,820; P = .005). This difference persisted after controlling for maternal age, body mass index, parity, previous preterm delivery, smoking, and fetal gender. Early amniocentesis cases were further stratified on the basis of whether the placenta had been penetrated (n = 460) or not (n = 1,360). Risk of hypertensive complications was lowest if the placenta was not traversed (3.4%), greater with placental penetration (3.9%), and highest when the placenta was directly sampled during CVS (5.4%, P = .02).

Conclusion.—We hypothesize that focal disruption of the placenta at 13-14 weeks may increase the risk of hypertension/preeclampsia. These findings provide support for the theory that disturbances in early placentation lead subsequently to maternal hypertension.

► This is a secondary analysis from a larger randomized trial comparing late transabdominal CVS with early amniocentesis between 13 and 14 weeks of gestation. The authors identified an increased risk of nonspecific hypertensive disorders, including preeclampsia, in women who had chorionic villus sampling performed. The risks of hypertensive disorders were also stratified in the amniocentesis group to procedures that involved the placenta and those that did not, the former being associated with a higher risk. This study is of interest because it supports a potential and plausible relationship between early placenta disruption and subsequent gestational hypertensive disorders. It also identifies a potential increased risk of CVS and transplacental amniocentesis when compared with amniocentesis not involving the placenta. Unfortunately, the study was not initially designed to address hypertensive disorders and pregnancy, and the analysis did not stratify hypertensive disorders (severe preeclampsia, mild preeclampsia, gestational hypertension). Therefore, it remains unclear what the true impact of early placental disruption may have on maternal and neonatal outcomes.

S. Thung, MD

Long-Term Mortality After Preeclampsia
Funai EF, Friedlander Y, Paltiel O, et al (Yale Univ, New Haven, Conn; Hebrew Univ, Jerusalem; Hadassah Univ, Jerusalem; et al)
Epidemiology 16:206-215, 2005   7–2

Background.—Many believe that preeclampsia is not associated with future morbidity or mortality. We sought to investigate the long-term risk of mortality in women with preeclampsia, focusing on those known to be subsequently normotensive.

Study Design.—We ascertained deaths during 24–36 years' follow-up in a cohort of 37,061 women who delivered in Jerusalem in 1964–1976, including 1,070 women with preeclampsia. We used Cox proportional hazard models to estimate the risk of mortality associated with preeclampsia while controlling for the woman's age and education, history of diabetes, heart disease and low birth weight birth, the husband's social class, and the calendar year at the start of follow-up.

Results.—Compared with women who were not diagnosed with preeclampsia, the relative risk of death after preeclampsia was 2.1 (95% confidence interval = 1.8–2.5). Deaths from cardiovascular disease contributed most strongly to this increase. Among women with preeclampsia who had subsequent births without preeclampsia, the excess risk of mortality became manifest only after 20 years.

Conclusions.—These findings, together with other recent cohort studies, define preeclampsia as a risk marker for mortality from cardiovascular disease. They suggest that the observation of a normal blood pressure after preeclampsia should not discourage the search for other cardiovascular risk factors or abrogate the need for other preventive measures.

▶ Although the short-term morbidity and mortality rates associated with preeclampsia are well recognized, there is mounting evidence that preeclampsia is also associated with long-term medical disease and death. The authors of this study had the benefit of a uniquely large cohort of more than 37,000 women from Jerusalem who were followed up for a median of 30 years. They found a significant increased risk of death over the study period in women who had at least 1 episode of preeclampsia compared with women who had never had the disease (RR = 2.13). The authors also demonstrated that women who had subsequent pregnancies without recurrent preeclampsia, a group unlikely to have significant underlying chronic hypertension, also had an increased risk of death (RR = 1.95). The persistent long-term risk in women with normal subsequent pregnancies suggests that the adverse effects of preeclampsia may not be limited to commonly associated chronic medical conditions, such as diabetes and chronic hypertension, but caused by actual injury that occurs as a result of preeclampsia itself.

S. Thung, MD

Preeclampsia and Future Cardiovascular Disease: Potential Role of Altered Angiogenesis and Insulin Resistance

Wolf M, Hubel CA, Lam C, et al (Massachusetts Gen Hosp, Boston; Brigham and Women's Hosp, Boston; Beth Israel-Deaconess Med Ctr, Boston; et al)
J Clin Endocrinol Metab 89:6239-6243, 2004   7–3

Abstract.—Altered angiogenesis and insulin resistance are associated with preeclampsia and cardiovascular disease (CVD), and women with preeclampsia appear to be at increased risk of future CVD. We hypothesized that these factors are detectable in asymptomatic postpartum women with a history of preeclampsia and may represent pathophysiological mechanisms bridging preeclampsia and future CVD. We measured fasting insulin, glucose, vascular endothelial growth factor, and its circulating inhibitor, soluble fms-like tyrosine kinase (sFlt-1) in 29 normotensive women with a history of preeclampsia and 32 women with prior normotensive pregnancies at 18.0 ± 9.7 months postpartum. The homeostasis model of insulin resistance ($HOMA_{IR}$) [(insulin [microunits per milliliter] $\times$ glucose [millimoles per liter])/22.5] was calculated. Compared with women with normal pregnancies, women with prior preeclampsia had significantly increased levels of sFlt-1 (41.6 ± 6.7 vs. 30.4 ± 10.2; $P < 0.01$) and median $HOMA_{IR}$ (2.8 vs. 1.9; $P = 0.04$). Membership in the upper quartile of either sFlt-1 or $HOMA_{IR}$ was associated with prior preeclampsia (odds ratio 5.7; 95% confidence interval 1.7, 20.0; $P < 0.01$), and all five women in the upper quartiles of both sFlt-1 and $HOMA_{IR}$ had a history of preeclampsia. Women with a history of preeclampsia demonstrate altered expression of angiogenesis-related proteins and increased $HOMA_{IR}$ more than 1 yr postpartum. These factors may contribute to their risk of future CVD.

▶ The clinical features of preeclampsia rapidly resolve after delivery of the placenta. However, long-term morbidity has been associated with preeclampsia, the most notable association being an increased risk for CVD. The authors prospectively measured biomarkers known to be associated with preeclampsia, coronary artery disease, and insulin resistance more than 1 year after delivery. They found that women with recent preeclampsia had persistently increased sFlt-1 levels and $HOMA_{IR}$, a measure of insulin resistance. Although the study is limited by a small number of patients with a short follow-up, this study demonstrates plausible mechanisms for future CVD from preeclampsia. It will be exciting to see future studies that corroborate these findings more remote from delivery.

S. Thung, MD

Increased Cerebral Blood Flow in Preeclampsia With Magnetic Resonance Imaging
Zeeman GG, Hatab MR, Twickler DM (Univ of Texas, Dallas)
Am J Obstet Gynecol 191:1425-1429, 2004   7–4

Objective.—The purpose of this study was to compare third trimester and nonpregnant cerebral blood flow of women with preeclampsia to normotensive control subjects with the use of magnetic resonance imaging techniques.

Study Design.—Nine normotensive pregnant women and 12 untreated women with preeclampsia underwent velocity-encoded phase contrast magnetic resonance imaging of the bilateral middle and posterior cerebral arteries in the third trimester and at 6 to 8 weeks after delivery. The Student *t* test was used for comparison, with a probability value of <.05 considered significant.

Results.—Third-trimester large cerebral artery blood flow was significantly higher in preeclampsia. Mean vessel diameter was unchanged, except for the left posterior cerebral artery. There was no difference in mean vessel diameter or cerebral blood flow between the 2 groups while the women were not pregnant.

Conclusion.—Cerebral blood flow is increased significantly in preeclampsia. We hypothesize that increased cerebral blood flow ultimately could lead to eclampsia through hyperperfusion and the development of vasogenic edema.

▶ This study evaluated cerebral blood flow patterns in normotensive and preeclamptic women by MRI. The authors found that large cerebral artery blood flow was increased in preeclamptic women compared with normotensive women, with no differences noted in vessel diameters. The authors hypothesized that increased cerebral flow could lead to eclampsia through hyperperfusion and the development of vasogenic edema that could ultimately reduce cerebral perfusion and cause focal ischemia. These findings may lead to new treatment options to prevent eclampsia in women with preeclampsia.

P. P. van den Berg, MD, PhD

Urinary Placental Growth Factor and Risk of Preeclampsia

Levine RJ, Thadhani R, Qian C, et al (Natl Inst of Child Health and Human Development, Bethesda, Md; Harvard Med School, Boston; Allied Technology Group, Rockville, Md; et al)
JAMA 293:77-85, 2005   7–5

Context.—Preeclampsia may be caused by an imbalance of angiogenic factors. We previously demonstrated that high serum levels of soluble fms-like tyrosine kinase 1 (sFlt1), an antiangiogenic protein, and low levels of placental growth factor (PlGF), a proangiogenic protein, predict subsequent development of preeclampsia. In the absence of glomerular disease leading to proteinuria, sFlt1 is too large a molecule to be filtered into the urine, while PlGF is readily filtered.

Objective.—To test the hypothesis that urinary PlGF is reduced prior to onset of hypertension and proteinuria and that this reduction predicts preeclampsia.

Design, Setting, and Patients.—Nested case-control study within the Calcium for Preeclampsia Prevention trial of healthy nulliparous women enrolled at 5 US university medical centers during 1992-1995. Each woman with preeclampsia was matched to 1 normotensive control by enrollment site, gestational age at collection of the first serum specimen, and sample storage time at $-70°C$. One hundred twenty pairs of women were randomly chosen for analysis of serum and urine specimens obtained before labor.

Main Outcome Measure.—Cross-sectional urinary PlGF concentrations, before and after normalization for urinary creatinine.

Results.—Among normotensive controls, urinary PlGF increased during the first 2 trimesters, peaked at 29 to 32 weeks, and decreased thereafter. Among cases, before onset of preeclampsia the pattern of urinary PlGF was similar, but levels were significantly reduced beginning at 25 to 28 weeks. There were particularly large differences between controls and cases of preeclampsia with subsequent early onset of the disease or small-for-gestational-age infants. After onset of clinical disease, mean urinary PlGF in women with preeclampsia was 32 pg/mL, compared with 234 pg/mL in controls with fetuses of similar gestational age ($P<.001$). The adjusted odds ratio for the risk of preeclampsia to begin before 37 weeks of gestation for specimens obtained at 21 to 32 weeks, which were in the lowest quartile of control PlGF concentrations (<118 pg/mL), compared with all other quartiles, was 22.5 (95% confidence interval, 7.4-67.8).

Conclusion.—Decreased urinary PlGF at mid gestation is strongly associated with subsequent early development of preeclampsia.

▶ Preeclampsia is a major contributor to maternal and fetal morbidity/mortality, and the pathophysiology remains elusive. Although many explanations have been proposed, no unifying theory currently exists. Dysfunctional endothelial function appears to be a major factor in the initiation of disease. The authors have previously demonstrated that an imbalance of serum angiogenic factors, namely elevated sFlt-1 and decreased PlGF, were associated with preeclampsia.[1] In this study, urinary PlGF, a potent angiogenic agent, was also found at significantly lower concentrations in women destined to have clinical preeclampsia when compared with women who did not develop the disease. These differences were found before clinical disease, starting as early as 25 to 29 weeks' gestation. Interestingly, the authors also found progressively lower levels of PlGF when additional indicators of more severe preeclampsia such as fetal growth restriction or preterm birth were identified.

This is an important study because it identifies a potential biomarker for preeclampsia screening. Although there are no preventive therapies currently available, a biomarker such as urinary PlGF may be helpful in identifying high-risk patients for more intensive prenatal surveillance as well as for enrollment in future research trials.

S. Thung, MD

Reference

1. Levine RJ, Maynard SE, Qian C, et al: Circulating angiogenic factors and the risk of preeclampsia. *N Engl J Med* 350:672-683, 2004.

Urinary Angiogenic Factors Cluster Hypertensive Disorders and Identify Women With Severe Preeclampsia

Buhimschi CS, Norwitz ER, Funai E, et al (Yale Univ, New Haven, Conn)
Am J Obstet Gynecol 192:734-741, 2005   7–6

Objective.—Serum levels of soluble fms-like tyrosine kinase 1 (sFlt-1), vascular endothelial growth factor (VEGF), and placental growth factor (PlGF) are altered in women with clinical preeclampsia. We sought to identify whether similar alterations in urinary levels of these proteins cluster hypertensive disorders in pregnancy, and identify women with severe preeclampsia (sPE).

Study Design.—Free urinary levels of sFlt-1, VEGF, and PlGF were measured by immunoassay in 68 women enrolled prospectively in the following groups: nonpregnant reproductive age (NP-CTR n = 14), healthy pregnant control (P-CTR n = 16), pregnant hypertensive and proteinuric women who did not meet criteria for severe preeclampsia (pHTN n = 21), and women with sPE (n = 17).

Results.—There was no difference in gestational age at the time of enrollment among groups (median [range]: sPE: 31 [24-40], pHTN: 34 [16-40], P-CTR: 28 [7-39] wks). Urinary excretion of VEGF was significantly increased in sPE women compared with NP-CTR ($P = 023$), but did not differ among pregnant groups. Urinary PlGF levels were significantly increased in pregnant compared with nonpregnant women, but were decreased in all hypertensive women compared with healthy P-CTR ($P < .001$). Urinary sFlt-1 concentrations were significantly increased in women with sPE relative to all other groups ($P < .001$). pHTN women had higher sFlt-1 urinary output compared with P-CTR group ($P = .001$). A cutoff >2.1 in the ratio log [sFlt-1/PlGF] had 88.2% sensitivity and 100% specificity in differentiating women with sPE from normotensive controls. We also described that the log[sFlt-1/PlGF] ratio identified women with sPE better than proteinuria alone (*P* = .03). Our regression model revealed that uric acid correlated best with log[sFlt-1/PlGF] ratio (*r* = 0.628; *P* = .005).

Conclusion.—sPE is associated with increased urinary output of the anti-angiogenic factor sFlt-1 and a decreased output of PlGF at the time of clinical manifestation, providing a rapid noninvasive screening of hypertensive women based on a sFlt/PlGF ratio. This ratio may be used as representation for severity of the disease, and appears to be superior to random urinary protein measurements.

► Diagnosing preeclampsia and assessing its severity is primarily a clinical endeavor. As such, there are many clinical scenarios when the criteria commonly used are not adequate and the diagnosis remains in question. Unlike the previous study (Abstract 7–5), this prospective analysis evaluated angiogenic factors in the setting of clinically evident disease. The authors demonstrated lower PlGF levels in women with hypertensive disorders but could not differentiate between preeclampsia and gestational hypertension. However, they also showed that elevated urinary levels of sFlt-1 could be used to differentiate sPE from milder forms. The authors devised an sFlt-1/PlGF ratio (uFP) to take advantage of the changes associated with preeclampsia and found that the uFP was significantly higher in sPE than in women with mild disease or normal pregnancies. After confirmatory studies have been performed, the uFP ratio may be the much needed objective tool to help clinicians differentiate sPE from other hypertensive disorders.

S. Thung, MD

Increased Biological Oxidation and Reduced Anti-oxidant Enzyme Activity in Pre-eclamptic Placentae

Vanderlelie J, Venardos K, Clifton VL, et al (Griffith Univ, Southport, Australia; Hunter Med Research Inst, Newcastle, Australia; Royal Women's Hosp, Carlton, VIC, Australia)
Placenta 26:53-58, 2005   7–7

Background.—Several reports have examined the by-products of excessive cellular oxidation in preeclamptic placentae, including the measurement of lipid hydroperoxides, protein carbonyls, and nitrotyrosine residues. Most of these studies have shown increased levels of lipid and protein oxidation in preeclamptic placentae, and most researchers believe that there is excessive production of key antioxidant proteins in the human placenta during preeclampsia. The placental oxidative state and the activity of important antioxidant enzymes were evaluated in tissue homogenates of placental samples obtained from age-matched preeclamptic and normal pregnancies.

Methods.—Pregnant women were recruited at 2 Australian hospitals. Preeclamptic patients were selected for study. All preeclamptic pregnancies were delivered prematurely by cesarean section. Gestationally age-matched placental samples were collected from nonhypertensive pregnant women, which were delivered prematurely after various complications. The samples were assayed for tissue levels of the endogenous antioxidant proteins superoxide dismutase, glutathione peroxidase, thioredoxin reductase, and thioreductin and the level of lipid and protein oxidation.

Results.—Preeclamptic tissue homogenates showed significantly increased levels of lipid peroxidation and a trend toward increased protein carbonyl concentration when compared with control subjects. The levels and activities of superoxide dismutase, thioredoxin reductase, thioredoxin, and glutathione peroxidase were all significantly reduced when comparing preeclamptic placental tissue to gestational age-matched control placentae from non-preeclamptic pregnancies.

Conclusions.—Decreased enzymatic antioxidant capacity and increased oxidation were found in placental tissues from preeclamptic women. These factors may be components in the pathogenesis of preeclampsia.

▶ The etiology of preeclampsia is still largely unknown. An imbalance between the cellular generation of reactive oxygen species and the capacity of the exogenous antioxidants, such as vitamins E, C, and A and endogenous antioxidants such as glutathione, ubiquinone, and uric acid, results in oxidative stress. This study demonstrates an inability of the antioxidant systems to control increased oxidative stress in placentas of preeclamptic women. Oxidative stress in the human conceptus in the first trimester of pregnancy is nowadays believed to be related to deficient trophoblast invasion, ultimately resulting in generalized endothelial cell dysfunction and the clinical syndrome of preeclampsia.[1,2] Oxidative stress may also be related to increased placental apoptosis and shedding of placental fragments in the maternal circulation. As this study was performed on largely third-trimester placentae, it is unknown whether these findings also reflect such aberrations in the modulation of local oxidative stress in the first weeks of pregnancy. It is therefore impossible to determine whether the findings of an increased placental oxidative state and decreased antioxidant enzyme capacity are etiologically involved or are phenomena secondary to the disease. Although difficult to perform, studies on first-trimester trophoblasts must be performed to gain more insight of the etiology of preeclampsia.

E. A. P. Steegers, MD, PhD

References

1. Burton GJ, Jauniaux E: Placental oxidative stress: From miscarriage to preeclampsia. *J Soc Gynecol Investig* 11:342-352, 2004.
2. Raijmakers MTM, Peters WHM, Steegers EAP, et al: Amino thiols, detoxification and oxidative stress in preeclampsia and other disorders of pregnancy. *Curr Pharm Des* 11:711-734, 2005.

Antibodies From Preeclamptic Patients Stimulate Increased Intracellular Ca²⁺ Mobilization Through Angiotensin Receptor Activation
Thway TM, Shlykov SG, Day M-C, et al (Univ of Texas, Houston)
Circulation 110:1612-1619, 2004   7–8

Background.—Preeclampsia is a serious disorder of pregnancy character- ized by hypertension, proteinuria, edema, and coagulation and vascular ab- normalities. At the cellular level, abnormalities include increased calcium concentration in platelets, lymphocytes, and erythrocytes. Recent studies have shown that antibodies directed against angiotensin II type I (AT_1) re- ceptors are also highly associated with preeclampsia.

Method and Results.—We tested the hypothesis that AT_1 receptor- agonistic antibodies (AT_1-AAs) could activate AT_1 receptors, leading to an increased intracellular concentration of free calcium and to downstream ac- tivation of Ca^{2+} signaling pathways. Sera of 30 pregnant patients, 16 diag- nosed with severe preeclampsia and 14 normotensive, were examined for the presence of IgG capable of stimulating intracellular Ca^{2+} mobilization. IgG from all preeclamptic patients activated AT_1 receptors and increased in- tracellular free calcium. In contrast, none of the normotensive individuals had IgG capable of activating AT_1 receptors. The specific mobilization of in- tracellular Ca^{2+} by AT_1-AAs was blocked by losartan, an AT_1 receptor an- tagonist, and by a 7-amino-acid peptide that corresponds to a portion of the second extracellular loop of the AT_1 receptor. In addition, we have shown that AT_1-AA-stimulated mobilization of intracellular Ca^{2+} results in the ac- tivation of the transcription factor, nuclear factor of activated T cells.

Conclusions.—These results suggest that maternal antibodies capable of activating AT_1 receptors are likely to account for increased intracellular free Ca^{2+} concentrations and changes in gene expression associated with pre- eclampsia.

▶ This study explores an interesting mechanism for the development of pre- eclampsia in an in vitro setting. The authors explored the hypothesis that AT_1- AA in the serum of women with preeclampsia could have agonist properties on angiotensin receptors and result in increased intracellular calcium concentra- tions, similar to what is found in the platelets and erythrocytes of preeclamptic women. The authors found that IgG from preeclamptic women could increase intracellular calcium in Chinese hamster ovary cells in a dose dependent man- ner, and this action was blocked by an angiotensin receptor inhibitor. IgG from nonpreeclamptic women did not alter calcium concentrations. Although these experiments do show inducible changes that seem to mimic changes associ- ated with preeclampsia, by no means does it prove that AT_1-AA causes pre- eclampsia. This study highlights the fact that preeclampsia may not only be a condition of abnormal angiogenesis but in some women may be an immuno- logic disorder that results from the presence of activating immunoglobulin found in preeclamptic women.

S. Thung, MD

A Prospective Randomized Trial of Magnesium Sulfate in Severe Preeclampsia: Use of Diuresis as a Clinical Parameter to Determine the Duration of Postpartum Therapy

Fontenot MT, Lewis DF, Frederick JB, et al (Florida Perinatal Associates, Tampa; Louisiana State Univ, Shreveport; Univ of Kentucky, Lexington; et al)
Am J Obstet Gynecol 192:1788-1794, 2005   7–9

Objective.—The purpose of this study was to assess the use of the onset of diuresis in the determination of the duration of postpartum magnesium sulfate therapy among patients with severe preeclampsia.

Study Design.—A prospective randomized trial of postpartum therapy with magnesium sulfate was conducted. The control group received 24 hours of therapy, and the study group received therapy until the onset of diuresis (urine output >100 mL/hr for 2 consecutive hours). The Student t test, χ^2 test, and Fisher's exact test were used for analysis of data; a probability value of <.05 was considered statistically significant.

Results.—There were 50 patients in the control group and 48 patients in the study group. There was no difference in maternal demographic data, severe disease criteria, blood pressure, 24-hour postpartum urine output, or need for antihypertensive therapy. The study group had a significantly shorter duration of therapy, and no patient had eclampsia or required the re-initiation of therapy.

Conclusion.—The use of the onset of diuresis in the postpartum period as the determinant clinical parameter for the discontinuation of magnesium sulfate in patients with severe preeclampsia was associated with no untoward outcomes or need for the re-initiation of treatment.

▶ A common clinical question that has been inadequately studied is the optimal duration of postpartum magnesium therapy to prevent eclamptic seizures. Most clinicians arbitrarily continue magnesium infusions for at least 24 hours after delivery, thought to be the time when seizures are most common. Magnesium infusion, although thought to be safe, is associated with maternal complications commonly associated with excessive magnesium levels. Reducing the length of time on magnesium could result in fewer complications and lower costs. This study was a randomized trial that used the onset of diuresis as the end point for magnesium prophylaxis. Interestingly, the study did demonstrate a significant decrease in the time on magnesium and did not reveal an increased incidence of eclampsia. Although the study was too small to identify more subtle increases in eclampsia, it does provide an excellent starting point for a larger randomized trial.

S. Thung, MD

8 Infectious Disease

Multicenter Study of a Rapid Molecular-Based Assay for the Diagnosis of Group B *Streptococcus* Colonization in Pregnant Women
Davies HD, Miller MA, Faro S, et al (Univ of Calgary, Alberta, Canada; McGill Univ, Montreal; Univ of Texas, Austin; et al)
Clin Infect Dis 39:1129-1135, 2004   8–1

Background.—Current prevention of infection due to group B *Streptococcus* (GBS) involves giving intrapartum antibiotics to women on the basis of either antenatal culture colonization status or presence of risk factors.

Methods.—We prospectively compared the performance characteristics of a rapid molecular diagnostic test (IDI-Strep B; Infectio Diagnostic) with culture for intrapartum GBS detection after 36 weeks' gestation in 5 North American centers during the period September 2001–May 2002. Antenatal GBS screening was done according to the usual practice of participating hospitals. Two combined vaginal/anal specimens were obtained from participants during labor by use of standard techniques and processed by the same laboratories that processed the antenatal specimens. Each swab sample was processed simultaneously by culture and with IDI-Strep B. The collected specimens were randomized for order of testing of the swab samples by culture or the rapid test.

Results.—Of enrolled women, 803 (91.1%) were eligible for analysis. The overall intrapartum GBS colonization rate by culture was 18.6% (range, 9.1%-28.7%). Compared with intrapartum culture, the molecular test had a sensitivity of 94.0% (range, 90.1%-97.8%), specificity of 95.9% (range, 94.3%-97.4%), positive predictive value of 83.8% (range, 78.2%-89.4%), and negative predictive value of 98.6% (range, 97.7%-99.5%). The molecular test was superior to antenatal cultures (sensitivity, 94% vs. 54%; $P < .0001$) and prediction of intrapartum status on the basis of risk factors (sensitivity, 94% vs. 42%; $P < .0001$).

Conclusion.—Use of this test for determination of GBS colonization during labor is highly sensitive and specific and may lead to a further reduction in rates of neonatal GBS disease.

▶ GBS is the leading cause of infectious morbidity and mortality among newborns in North America. The prevalence of GBS colonization in pregnant women varies from 15% to 40% and prevention of infection caused by GBS involves intrapartum antibiotics. Such interventions have their own risks and involve providing antibiotics to many women who will not go on to transmit the infection to their fetuses. The authors evaluated a rapid molecular diagnostic test for GBS and compared it with conventional culture. They found that this rapid test was highly sensitive and specific and could lead to further reductions in the rates of neonatal GBS disease, a highly desired outcome for a condition that has been increasing in neonates in the past decade.

J. M. G. van Vugt, MD, PhD

Diagnosis of Intra-amniotic Infection by Proteomic Profiling and Identification of Novel Biomarkers
Gravett MG, Novy MJ, Rosenfeld RG, et al (Oregon Natl Primate Research Ctr, Beaverton; Oregon Health and Science Univ, Portland; ProteoGenix Inc, Portland, Ore; et al)
JAMA 292:462-469, 2004   8–2

Context.—Intra-amniotic infection (IAI) is commonly associated with preterm birth and adverse neonatal sequelae. Early diagnosis of IAI, however, has been hindered by insensitive or nonspecific tests.

Objective.—To identify unique protein signatures in rhesus monkeys with experimental IAI, a proteomics-based analysis of amniotic fluid was used to develop diagnostic biomarkers for subclinical IAI in amniotic fluid and blood of women with preterm labor.

Design, Setting, and Participants.—Surface-enhanced laser desorption-ionization/time-of-flight mass spectrometry, gel electrophoresis, and tandem mass spectrometry were used to characterize amniotic fluid peptides in 19 chronically instrumented pregnant rhesus monkeys before and after experimental IAI. Candidate biomarkers were determined by liquid chromatography-tandem mass spectrometry. Polyclonal antibodies were generated from synthetic peptides for validation of biomarkers of IAI. Amniotic fluid peptide profiles identified in experimental IAI were subsequently tested in a cohort of 33 women admitted to Seattle, Wash, hospitals between June 25, 1991, and June 30, 1997, with preterm delivery at 35 weeks or earlier associated with subclinical IAI (n = 11), preterm delivery at 35 weeks or earlier without IAI (n = 11), and preterm contractions with subsequent term delivery at later than 35 weeks (n = 11).

Main Outcome Measures.—Identification of peptide biomarkers for occult IAI.

Results.—Protein expression profiles in amniotic fluid showed unique signatures of overexpression of polypeptides in the 3- to 5-kDa and 10- to 12-kDa molecular weight ranges in all animals after infection and in no animal prior to infection. In women, the 10- to 12-kDa signature was identified in all 11 patients with subclinical IAI, in 2 of 11 with preterm delivery without IAI, and in 0 of 11 with preterm labor and term delivery without infection ($P<.001$). Peptide fragment analysis of the diagnostic peak in amniotic fluid identified calgranulin B and a unique fragment of insulinlike growth factor binding protein 1, which were also expressed in maternal serum. Mapping of other amniotic fluid proteins differentially expressed in IAI identified several immunoregulators not previously described in amniotic fluid.

Conclusions.—This proteomics-based characterization of the differential expression of amniotic fluid proteins in IAI identified a distinct proteomic profile in an experimental primate chorioamnionitis model that detected subclinical IAI in a human cohort with preterm labor. These diagnostic protein expression signatures, complemented by immunodetection of specific biomarkers in amniotic fluid and in maternal serum, might have application in the early detection of IAI.

▶ Proteomic profiling of amniotic fluid in women with IAI produced unique patterns of protein expression. A potentially exciting preliminary finding showed that some of the identified proteins may also be differentially present in serum samples of infected versus noninfected mothers. These findings provided important clues for the pathophysiology of preterm labor associated with IAI and also may serve to develop a serum test to diagnose subclinical IAI. Such a test would presumably allow for the premorbid detection of women at risk for preterm labor from IAI and thus serve to improve maternal and neonatal outcomes.

S. E. Bulun, MD

Genital Herpes Complicating Pregnancy
Brown ZA, Gardella C, Wald A, et al (Univ of Washington, Seattle)
Obstet Gynecol 106:845-856, 2005   8–3

Abstract.—Approximately 22% of pregnant women are infected with herpes simplex virus (HSV)-2, and 2% of women will acquire HSV during pregnancy. Remarkably, up to 90% of these women are undiagnosed because they are asymptomatic or have subtle symptoms attributed to other vulvovaginal disorders. Diagnosis of genital herpes relies on laboratory confirmation with culture or polymerase chain reaction assay of genital lesions and type-specific glycoprotein G–based serologic testing. Neonatal herpes is the most severe complication of genital HSV infection and is caused by contact with infected genital secretions at the time of labor. Maternal acquisition of HSV in the third trimester of pregnancy carries the highest risk of neonatal transmission. Despite advances in the diagnosis and treatment of neonatal herpes, little change in the incidence or serious sequelae from this infection has occurred. As such, prevention of the initial neonatal infection is critically important. Obstetricians are in a unique position to prevent vertical HSV transmission by identifying women with genital lesions at the time of labor for cesarean delivery, prescribing antiviral suppressive therapy as appropriate, and avoiding unnecessary invasive intrapartum procedures in women with genital herpes. Enhanced prevention strategies include identification of women at risk for HSV acquisition during pregnancy by testing women and possibly their partners for HSV antibodies and providing counseling to prevent transmission to women in late pregnancy.

▶ The prevalence of genital and neonatal herpes continues to rise in both the industrialized and developing world. More than 1.5 million cases of genital herpes occur annually, and about one quarter of all pregnant women are seropositive for HSV. In addition, about 2% of women acquire genital herpes during pregnancy. Because of the high prevalence of HSV infection in women of reproductive age, obstetricians must be able to diagnose and manage HSV in pregnancy. Interestingly, up to 90% of women positive for HSV-2 are undiagnosed either because they are asymptomatic or because they have subtle symptoms attributable to other vulvovaginal disorders. Obstetricians are in a unique position to prevent vertical HSV transmission by identifying women with genital lesions at the time of labor for cesaerean delivery, as well as prescribing antiviral suppressive therapy when appropriate. It is hoped that enhanced prevention strategies will reduce the perinatal morbidity and mortality associated with fetal and neonatal HSV infections.

J. M. G. van Vugt, MD, PhD

Poor Correlation Between Genital Lesions and Detection of Herpes Simplex Virus in Women in Labor
Gardella C, Brown ZA, Wald A, et al (Univ of Washington, Seattle)
Obstet Gynecol 106:268-274, 2005   8–4

Objective.—To estimate the accuracy of clinical diagnosis of genital herpes for herpes simplex virus (HSV) detection among women in labor.

Methods.—Viral detection by culture and HSV DNA polymerase chain reaction (PCR) among women who underwent cesarean delivery for genital herpes was compared with women without HSV symptoms in labor who had genital swabs collected for HSV culture and to a subset of these women who had genital specimens available for PCR analysis, regardless of culture results.

Results.—From 1989 to 1999, 126 of 19,568 (0.6%) women underwent cesarean delivery for HSV. Twenty-six percent of 110 of these women had HSV detected by culture from at least 1 genital specimen and 46% of 70 of these women had HSV detected by PCR. During the same period, 61 of 12,623 (0.5%) asymptomatic women had HSV detected by culture. Between 1995 and 1996, 57 of 2,109 (2.7%) asymptomatic women had HSV detected by PCR. Thus, the presence of genital lesions had a sensitivity for HSV detection of 37% by culture and 41% by PCR. The amount of HSV present in asymptomatic women with HSV detected in genital secretions by PCR was often as high as those with genital lesions, although the median amount of HSV DNA detected was greater in women with lesions.

Conclusion.—Clinical diagnosis of genital herpes at the time of labor correlates relatively poorly with HSV detection from genital sites or lesions by culture or PCR and fails to identify asymptomatic women who have HSV in their genital secretions at the time of labor.

▶ Current guidelines for neonatal HSV prevention recommend cesarean delivery for women with genital lesions at the time of labor, because the lesions are presumed to indicate the presence of infectious HSV. The findings of this longitudinal cohort observed over 10 years describe the outcomes in 126 women who underwent cesarean delivery for suspicious genital lesions. The presence of genital lesions had a sensitivity for HSV detection of only 37% by culture and 41% by PCR. More concerning was that the amount of virus found in the lesions was comparable to the HSV detected by quantitative PCR among others in the cohort who only had asymptomatic shedding of HSV. However, the median amount of HSV DNA detected was greater in women with lesions overall. The authors conclude that the clinical diagnosis of genital herpes at the time of labor correlates relatively poorly with HSV detection from genital lesions in culture or PCR, and fails to identify asymptomatic women who have HSV in their genital secretions at the time of labor from asymptomatic lesions.

G. D. Wendel, Jr, MD

Periodontal Disease and Upper Genital Tract Inflammation in Early Spontaneous Preterm Birth
Goepfert AR, Jeffcoat MK, Andrews WW, et al (Univ of Alabama at Birmingham; Univ of Pennsylvania, Philadelphia)
Obstet Gynecol 104:777-783, 2004   8–5

Objective.—To estimate the relationship between maternal periodontal disease and both early spontaneous preterm birth and selected markers of upper genital tract inflammation.

Methods.—In this case-control study, periodontal assessment was performed in 59 women who experienced an early spontaneous preterm birth at less than 32 weeks of gestation, in a control population of 36 women who experienced an early indicated preterm birth at less than 32 weeks of gestation, and in 44 women with an uncomplicated birth at term ($\geq$37 weeks). Periodontal disease was defined by the degree of attachment loss. Cultures of the placenta and umbilical cord blood, cord interleukin-6 levels, and histopathologic examination of the placenta were performed for all women.

Results.—Severe periodontal disease was more common in the spontaneous preterm birth group (49%) than in the indicated preterm (25%, $P = .02$) and term control groups (30%, $P = .045$). Multivariable analyses, controlling for possible confounders, supported the association between severe periodontal disease and spontaneous preterm birth (odds ratio 3.4, 95% confidence interval 1.5-7.7). Neither histologic chorioamnionitis, a positive placental culture, nor an elevated cord plasma interleukin-6 level was significantly associated with periodontal disease (80% power to detect a 50% difference in rate of histological chorioamnionitis, $\alpha = 0.05$).

Conclusion.—Women with early spontaneous preterm birth were more likely to have severe periodontal disease than women with indicated preterm birth or term birth. Periodontal disease was not associated with selected markers of upper genital tract inflammation.

▶ Preterm birth complicates about 1 in 8 pregnancies and is a leading cause of infant morbidity and mortality. Periodontal disease is a chronic anaerobic inflammatory condition that affects up to 50% of pregnant women in our country. An association has been observed between maternal periodontal disease and multiple adverse pregnancy outcomes, including preterm birth. The mechanism by which periodontal disease and preterm birth is associated is not clear. It has been hypothesized that severe periodontal disease results in dissemination of organisms hematogenously that may target the placenta membranes and fetus, resulting in increased cytokine expression and preterm labor.

These authors investigated whether women who had a preterm birth (<32 weeks' gestation) were more likely to have periodontal disease than women with an indicated preterm birth at the same gestational age or women with a term birth. They also examined selected markers of upper genital tract inflammation for an association with periodontal disease. The authors found that severe periodontal disease was nearly twice as common among the women with a spontaneous early preterm birth compared with those with an indicated preterm birth or term controls. However, they did not find that histologic chorioamnionitis, a positive placental culture, or an elevated cord plasma interleukin-6 level was significantly associated with periodontal disease. The investigators could not demonstrate any association between these markers of upper genital tract inflammation at the time of birth and moderate to severe periodontal disease.

Their data suggest that the potential mechanisms of periodontal disease–associated preterm birth are not hematogenous spread of the periodontal organisms to the placenta with colonization and subsequent inflammation precipitating preterm labor or premature rupture of the membranes. Their data further suggest that if preterm birth associated with periodontal disease is inflammation mediated, the levels of inflammation are lower than those seen with infection-mediated preterm birth previously studied. Further investigation into the potential etiology of the association between periodontal disease and preterm birth is warranted.

G. D. Wendel Jr, MD

Markers of Periodontal Infection and Preterm Birth
Jarjoura K, Devine PC, Perez-Delboy A, et al (Columbia Univ, New York)
Am J Obstet Gynecol 192:513-519, 2005   8–6

Objective.—This study was undertaken to explore the relationship between clinical, microbiologic, and serologic markers of periodontitis and preterm birth (PTB).

TABLE 2.—Pregnancy-Related Variables in Cases and Controls

	Controls	Cases	P Values
Gestational age (wk); mean (SD)	39.3 (1.1)	33.2 (3.2)	
Birth weight (g); mean, (SD)	3,366.6 (554.4)	2,208.5 (790.1)	< .0001
Parity (median) (range)	1 (0 - 9)	0.5 (0 - 7)	.184
BMI, mean, (SD)	30.0 (6.3)	27.7 (6.1)	.019
Previous preterm delivery (n) (%)	1 (0.8)	7 (8.4)	.001
Preterm premature rupture of membranes (n) (%)	23 (19.2)	46 (55.4)	< .0001
UTI (n) (%)	24 (20.0)	14 (16.9)	.574
Clinical chorio-amnionitis (n) (%)	3 (2.5)	16 (19.3)	< .0001
Fetal growth restriction (n) (%)	3 (2.5)	4 (4.8)	.373

Abbreviations: BMI, Body mass index; *UTI*, urinary tract infection.
(Courtesy of Jarjoura K, Devine PC, Perez-Delboy A, et al: Markers of periodontal infection and preterm birth. Am J Obstet Gynecol 192:513-519, 2005. Copyright 2005 by Elsevier. Reprinted by permission.)

Study Design.—We compared women with a singleton gestation giving birth before the 37th week (cases, n = 83) with term delivery controls (n = 120) (Table 2). Periodontal examination and collection of dental plaque and blood samples were performed within 48 hours after delivery. Microbial levels and maternal immunoglobulin G titers to oral bacteria were analyzed. Multivariate regression models were fitted controlling for common covariates.

Results.—Cases showed greater mean attachment loss (1.7 vs 1.5 mm, $P = .003$) and higher prevalence of periodontitis (30.1% vs 17.5%, $P = .027$). No differences in microbial or serum antibody levels were detected between the groups. Logistic regression revealed that PTB was associated with attachment loss (adjusted odds ratio: 2.75, 95% CI: 1.01-7.54). Linear regression indicated a significant ($P = .04$) association between attachment loss and low birth weight (LBW).

Conclusion.—The data support the notion that periodontitis is independently associated with PTB and LBW.

▶ Infection plays an important role in the pathogenesis of PTB. Evidence of intrauterine infection has been reported in approximately 25% of women with singleton gestation and PTB. The pathophysiology of intrauterine infection is not well known, and the authors of this article sought to determine whether periodontal disease was a positive factor for PTB. The authors found that periodontitis was independently associated with PTB and LBW. Accordingly, pregnant women who have a history or evidence of periodontal disease should be referred for appropriate dental evaluation and care.

J. M. G. van Vugt, MD, PhD

Diagnosis of and Screening for Cytomegalovirus Infection in Pregnant Women

Munro SC, Hall B, Whybin LR, et al (SEALS Prince of Wales Hosp, Randwick, New South Wales, Australia; Univ of New South Wales, Kensington, Australia; Royal Hosp for Women, Randwick, New South Wales, Australia; et al)

J Clin Microbiol 43:4713-4718, 2005   8–7

Abstract.—No single diagnostic test for cytomegalovirus (CMV) infection is currently available for pregnant women at all stages of gestation. Improved accuracy in estimating the timing of primary infections can be used to identify women at higher risk of giving birth to congenitally infected infants. A diagnostic algorithm utilizing immunoglobulin G (IgG), IgM, and IgG

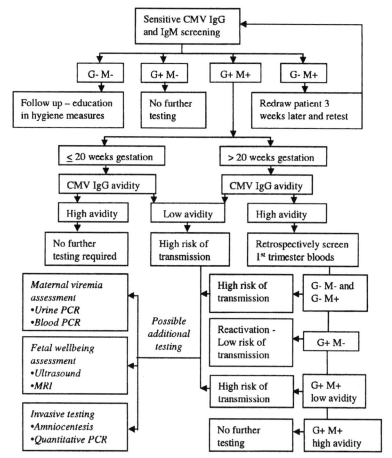

FIGURE 1.—Proposed diagnostic algorithm for cytomegalovirus (CMV) serology screening in pregnant women. *Abbreviation: PCR*, Polymerase chain reaction. (Courtesy of Munro SC, Hall B, Whybin LR, et al: Diagnosis of and screening for cytomegalovirus infection in pregnant women. *J Clin Microbiol* 43:4713-4718. Copyright 2005, American Society for Microbiology.)

avidity was used to prospectively screen serum from 600 pregnant women enrolled from two groups: ≤20 weeks gestation (*n* = 396) or >20 weeks gestation (*n* = 204) (Fig 1). PCR testing of urine and/or blood was performed on all seropositive women (n = 341). The majority (56.8%) of women were CMV IgG seropositive, with 5.5% being also CMV IgM positive. In the IgM-positive women, 1.2% had a low-avidity IgG, indicating a primary CMV infection and a high risk of intrauterine transmission. Two infants with asymptomatic CMV infection were born of mothers who had seroconverted in the second trimester of pregnancy. Baseline, age-stratified CMV serostatus was established from 1,018 blood donors. Baseline seropositivity from a blood donor population increased with age from 34.9% seroprevalence at less than 20 years of age to 72% seroprevalence at 50 years of age. Women at high risk of intrauterine transmission of CMV were identified at all stages of gestation. Women infected with CMV during late gestation may be more likely to transmit the virus, so failure to detect seroconversions in late gestation may result in failure to detect infected neonates.

▶ Human CMV is the most common cause of congenital malformation resulting from viral intrauterine infection in the industrialized world. Unfortunately, no single diagnostic test for CMV is currently available for pregnant women at all stages of gestation. The authors evaluated a diagnostic algorithm utilizing IgG, IgM, and IgG avidity to prospectively screen serum from 600 pregnant women enrolled in 2 groups: those at 20 weeks' gestation or less and those at greater than 20 weeks' gestation. The authors found that this diagnostic algorithm was effective in identifying women at high risk of intrauterine transmission. Although effective prevention and intervention approaches have not yet been determined, identifying those women who are at increased risk for CMV transmission or CMV infection could provide important information to obstetricians seeking to identify women at risk for having fetuses with abnormalities resulting from CMV infections.

J. M. G. van Vugt, MD, PhD

Perinatal or Early-Postnatal Cytomegalovirus Infection in Preterm Infants Under 34 Weeks Gestation Born to CMV-Seropositive Mothers Within a High-Seroprevalence Population

Mussi-Pinhata MM, Yamamoto AY, Aparecida do Carmo Rego M, et al (Univ of São Paulo, Brazil)
J Pediatr 145:685-688, 2004   8–8

Abstract.—In a prospective study, we evaluated the frequency, correlates, and clinical significance of perinatal or early-postnatal cytomegalovirus (CMV) infection in <34-week-gestation infants (n = 95) born to CMV-seropositive mothers. None had congenital CMV infection. Overall, 21 (22.1%; 95% CI = 14.2-31.8) infants were found to be infected; 10 excreted CMV at <60 days, and 11 had later excretion. Blood transfusion, birth weight, and vaginal delivery were not associated factors. Receiving natural

TABLE 1.—Anthropometric, Obstetric, and Neonatal Data According to
CMV Infection of 95 Infants

	CMV-Infected (n = 21; 22.1%)	CMV-Uninfected (n = 74; 77.9%)	*P* Value
Median birth weight (g), n (range)	1195 (760-1715)	1147 (710-2165)	.44
Birth weight <1200 g, n (%)	5 (23.8)	24 (32.4)	.31
Median gestational age (wk), n (range)	31 (27-34)	31 (26-34)	.71
Gestational age ≤30 wk, n (%)	9 (42.9)	33 (44.6)	.54
Vaginal delivery, n (%)	9 (42.9)	27 (36.5)	.38
Tracheal intubation at birth, n (%)	8 (38.1)	35 (47.3)	.29
Banked breast milk, n (%)	21 (100.0)	74 (100.0)	—
Natural breast milk, n (%)	13 (61.9)	36 (48.6)	.20
Median number of days receiving natural breast milk, n (range)	80 (16-180)	20 (1-300)	.01
Natural breast milk at <30 d of age, n (%)	9 (42.9)	12 (33.3)	.02
Blood transfusion, n (%)	14 (66.6)	49 (66.2)	.49
Median blood transfusions, n (range)	1 (0-14)	2 (0-70)	.43
Median volume of transfused blood (mL), n (range)	15 (0-175)	20 (0-970)	.26
Blood transfusion at age <30 d, n (%)	11 (52.4)	48 (64.9)	.21
Median volume (mL) of blood transfused at age <30 d, n (range)	10 (0-160)	17.5 (0-180)	.25
Median neutralizing anti-CMV antibody titer at birth, n (range)*	128 (8-1024)	128 (8-1024)	.51

*Neutralization titer was considered to be the highest serum dilution showing complete inhibition of the cytopathic effect.
Abbreviation: CMV, Cytomegalovirus.
(Courtesy of Mussi-Pinhata MM, Yamamoto AY, Aparecida do Carmo Rego M, et al: Perinatal or early-postnatal cytomegalovirus infection in preterm infants under 34 weeks gestation born to CMV-seropositive mothers within a high-seroprevalence population. *J Pediatr* 145:685-688. Copyright 2004 by Elsevier.)

breast milk within the first 30 days (OR = 4.5, *P* = .02) or for >30 days (OR = 7.9, *P* < .01) was associated with infection (Table 1). Only one (4.8%) of the infected infants was symptomatic. For <34-week-gestation infants, frequency of perinatal and early-postnatal CMV infection is high. Early or prolonged exposure to breast milk is an associated factor. However, most infections are asymptomatic, indicating that CMV infection in preterm infants within such a population is a serious problem infrequently.

Intrapartum Fetal Heart Rate Monitoring in Cases of Cytomegalovirus Infection

Kaneko M, Sameshima H, Ikeda T, et al (Miyazaki Med College, Japan; Aisenkai Nichinan Hosp, Miyazaki, Japan)
Am J Obstet Gynecol 191:1257-1262, 2004   8–9

Objective.—Several studies have shown that abnormal intrapartum fetal heart rate patterns are the results from pre-existing fetal brain damage. We evaluated intrapartum fetal heart rate pattern of cytomegalovirus-infected fetuses and correlated the patterns with neurologic outcomes.

Study Design.—Between 1991 and 2001, there were 20 cytomegalovirus-infected fetuses. We selected 40 fetuses as control subjects that were matched for gestational age and birth weight. Fetal heart rate was interpreted accord-

TABLE 2.—Incidence of FHR Deceleration in Patients With Cytomegalovirus and Control Subjects

Deceleration	Cytomegalovirus (n = 20)	Control Subjects (n = 40)	*P* Value
Prolonged	7	1	<.05
Recurrent late	1	2	NS
Occasional late	2	2	NS
Moderate variable	1	4	NS
Mild variable	1	10	NS
None	8	21	NS

Abbreviations: FHR, Fetal heart rate; *NS*, not significant.
(Courtesy of Kaneko M, Sameshima H, Ikeda T, et al: Intrapartum fetal heart rate monitoring in cases of cytomegalovirus infection. *Am J Obstet Gynecol* 191:1257-1262, 2004. Copyright 2004 by Elsevier. Reprinted by permission.)

ing to the guidelines of the National Institute for Child and Human Development. The incidence of abnormal fetal heart rate pattern and umbilical blood gases were compared between both groups. We also investigated the factors that contributed to abnormal fetal heart rate pattern in the cytomegalovirus group.

Results.—Nonreassuring fetal heart rate patterns (prolonged deceleration and recurrent late deceleration) were observed in 8 of 20 fetuses (prolonged deceleration, 7 fetuses; recurrent late deceleration, 1 fetus) in the cytomegalovirus group and in 3 of 41 fetuses (prolonged deceleration, 1 fetus; recurrent late deceleration, 2 fetuses) in the control group ($P < .05$, Fisher test) (Table 2). Baseline fetal heart rate variability was minimal in 4 of the 7 prolonged deceleration cases in the cytomegalovirus group. Umbilical pH <7.1 was found for 1 fetus in the cytomegalovirus group. The average umbilical arterial pH values were similar in both the groups. In the cytomegalovirus group, there were no differences in the incidence of contributing factors between 8 fetuses with abnormal fetal heart rate pattern (prolonged deceleration and recurrent late deceleration) and 8 fetuses with no change. There were 3 fetuses with cerebral palsy: 2 fetuses in the no change group and 1 fetus in the prolonged deceleration group. Antigenemia was positive exclusively in 4 cases with abnormal fetal heart rate pattern ($P < .05$).

Conclusion.—Cytomegalovirus-infected fetuses are more likely to show abnormal intrapartum fetal heart rate patterns than low-risk control fetuses, which suggests that the perinatal detection of cytomegalovirus is necessary to distinguish hypoxic-ischemic encephalopathy.

▶ In the industrialized world, human cytomegalovirus (CMV) is the most common cause of congenital malformation resulting from a viral intrauterine infection. Primary sources of the virus are maternal genital tract secretions, breast milk, and blood transfusions. The authors of the first article (Abstract 8–8), from the University of São Paulo in Brazil, found that among preterm infants born before 34 weeks' gestation, CMV infections were common (22% of the cohort), although most (95%) were asymptomatic. In that study, the authors found that CMV was most likely to be transmitted by breast milk. The authors believed that CMV was not a serious problem and that analysis of antibodies was likely the best approach to accurate diagnosis. In the second article (Abstract 8–9), the authors from Miyazaki Medical College in Japan found that CMV-infected fetuses were more likely to demonstrate abnormal fetal heart rate patterns than low-risk control fetuses. In these cases, an accurate diagnosis of CMV would be warranted in order to distinguish a heart rate pattern associated with hypoxia from one associated with CMV infection. These articles highlight the challenges of accurately diagnosing CMV infection and predicting uncommon adverse outcomes among relatively common CMV infections in newborns.

J. M. G. van Vugt, MD, PhD

Passive Immunization During Pregnancy for Congenital Cytomegalovirus Infection
Nigro G, for the Congenital Cytomegalovirus Collaborating Group (La Sapienza Univ, Rome; et al)
N Engl J Med 353:1350-1362, 2005   8–10

Background.—Currently, there is no effective intervention for a primary cytomegalovirus (CMV) infection during pregnancy.

Methods.—We studied pregnant women with a primary CMV infection. The therapy group comprised women whose amniotic fluid contained either CMV or CMV DNA and who were offered intravenous CMV hyperimmune globulin at a dose of 200 U per kilogram of maternal weight. A prevention group, consisting of women with a recent primary infection before 21 weeks' gestation or who declined amniocentesis, was offered monthly hyperimmune globulin (100 U per kilogram intravenously).

Results.—In the therapy group, 31 women received hyperimmune globulin, only 1 (3 percent) of whom gave birth to an infant with CMV disease (symptomatic at birth and handicapped at two or more years of age), as compared with 7 of 14 women who did not receive hyperimmune globulin (50 percent). Thus, hyperimmune globulin therapy was associated with a significantly lower risk of congenital CMV disease (adjusted odds ratio, 0.02; 95 percent confidence interval, $-\infty$ to 0.15; P<0.001). In the prevention group, 37 women received hyperimmune globulin, 6 (16 percent) of whom had infants with congenital CMV infection, as compared with 19 of 47 women (40 percent) who did not receive hyperimmune globulin. Thus, hyperimmune globulin therapy was associated with a significantly lower risk of congenital CMV infection (adjusted odds ratio, 0.32; 95 percent confidence interval, 0.10 to 0.94; P=0.04). Hyperimmune globulin therapy significantly (P<0.001) increased CMV-specific IgG concentrations and avidity and decreased natural killer cells and HLA-DR+ cells and had no adverse effects.

Conclusions.—Treatment of pregnant women with CMV-specific hyperimmune globulin is safe, and the findings of this nonrandomized study suggest that it may be effective in the treatment and prevention of congenital CMV infection. A controlled trial of this agent may now be appropriate.

▶ CMV is a common serious infection that occurs in approximately 1% of all newborns. Infection can be symptomatic at birth in about 10% of these infants, and an additional 8% to 13% develop neurologic deficits. Primary infection during pregnancy conveys the highest risk of infection (approximately 40%). Although prenatal diagnosis is possible, there is no current therapy to prevent or cure fetal infection. These investigators report on a cohort of women with diagnosed primary infection and fetal infection during pregnancy who were treated with an IV CMV hyperimmune globulin. The control or prevention group consisted of women with a similar documented primary infection or who declined amniocentesis, and were given monthly standard immunoglobulin injections. Hyperimmune globulin therapy was associated with a significantly lower risk of congenital CMV infection and disease. This preliminary nonrandomized study indicates that further investigation in a controlled trial may be appropriate to better study the role of passive immunization to prevent congenital CMV infection. If further studies are shown effective, significant consideration may be given to prenatal screening for maternal CMV infection in early pregnancy.

G. D. Wendel, Jr, MD

Neonatal Cerebral White Matter Injury in Preterm Infants Is Associated With Culture Positive Infections and Only Rarely With Metabolic Acidosis
Graham EM, Holcroft CJ, Rai KK, et al (Johns Hopkins Univ, Baltimore, Md; Ross Med School, Dominica, West Indies)
Am J Obstet Gynecol 191:1305-1310, 2004   8–11

Objective.—Neonatal cerebral white matter injury represents a major precursor for neurological impairment and cerebral palsy. Our objective was to identify risk factors associated with its development.

Study Design.—This retrospective case-control study of all births between 23 and 34 weeks gestation at a single university hospital between May 1994 and September 2001 identified 150 cases with white matter injury characterized by periventricular leukomalacia or ventricular dilatation from white matter atrophy that were chromosomally normal and did not have other congenital anomalies. Cases were matched to controls without brain injury by the next delivery within 7 days of their gestational age.

Results.—There were small differences between controls and cases in gestational age (27.5 ± 2.7, 27.4 ± 2.6 weeks, $P = .01$) and birth weight (1053 ± 402, 966 ± 285 g, $P = 002$) that were statistically but not clinically significant. There was no difference in the percentage of controls and cases delivered by cesarean (45%, 49%, $P = .64$). There were no differences between controls and cases in umbilical arterial pH (7.27 ± 0.11, 7.25 ± 0.15, $P = .19$), base excess (-2.1 ± 2.7, -3.0 ± 4.1 mmol/L, $P = .28$), pH less than 7.0 (2/122 [2%], 3/107 [3%], $P = 1.0$), or base excess less than -12 mmol/L (4/121 [3%], 6/106 [6%], $P = 75$). The cases had a significant increase in positive blood (19%, 29%, $P = .036$), cerebrospinal fluid (6%, 17%, $P = .002$), and tracheal (9%, 22%, $P = .003$) cultures during the neonatal period. Conditional logistic regression showed a significant association among multiple gestations ($P = .02$), intraventricular hemorrhage ($P < .001$), and positive tracheal cultures ($P = .02$) with cerebral white matter injury.

Conclusion.—Culture-positive infection was associated with an increased risk of cerebral white matter injury in preterm neonates. Intrapartum hypoxia-ischemia as manifested by metabolic acidosis was rarely associated with white matter injury and was not different from the incidence in premature neonates without injury.

▶ Hypoxia during pregnancy is still believed to be the primary cause of neonatal white matter injury characterized by periventricular leukomalacia (PVL), leading to neurologic morbidity. In this study, metabolic acidosis (base excess < −12 mmol/L) was weakly associated with PVL, but culture-positive infection in neonatal life was strongly associated with PVL. Such studies provide important information concerning the etiology of PVL and thus allow for the development of more effective diagnostic and therapeutic protocols that will hopefully reduce adverse clinical outcomes.

P. P. van den Berg, MD, PhD

Risk Factors for *Toxoplasma gondii* Infection in Mothers of Infants With Congenital Toxoplasmosis: Implications for Prenatal Management and Screening
Boyer KM, for the Toxoplasmosis Study Group (Rush Univ, Chicago; et al)
Am J Obstet Gynecol 192:564-571, 2005   8–12

Objective.—The purpose of this study was to determine whether demographic characteristics, history of exposure to recognized transmission vehicles, or illness that was compatible with acute toxoplasmosis during gestation identified most mothers of infants with congenital toxoplasmosis.

Study Design.—Mothers of 131 infants and children who were referred to a national study of treatment for congenital toxoplasmosis were characterized demographically and questioned concerning exposure to recognized risk factors or illness.

Results.—No broad demographic features identified populations that were at risk. Only 48% of mothers recognized epidemiologic risk factors (direct or indirect exposure to raw/undercooked meat or to cat excrement) or gestational illnesses that were compatible with acute acquired toxoplasmosis during pregnancy (Table 6).

Conclusion.—Maternal risk factors or compatible illnesses were recognized in retrospect by fewer than one half of North American mothers of infants with toxoplasmosis. Educational programs might have prevented acquisition of Toxoplasma gondii by those mothers who had clear exposure risks. However, only systematic serologic screening of all pregnant women at prenatal visits or of all newborn infants at birth would prevent or detect a higher proportion of these congenital infections.

TABLE 6.—Summary Epidemiologic Factors of Maternal
Exposure and Illness History

Factor	Percentage
Any exposure to cats	65
Any exposure to undercooked or uncooked meat	50
Any exposure to cats or undercooked or uncooked meat	75
Specific exposure to cat litter or uncooked meat	39
Unexplained febrile illness or lymphadenopathy during pregnancy	48
Exposure to cat litter, uncooked meat, or toxoplasmosis-like illness during pregnancy	48

(Courtesy of Boyer KM, for the Toxoplasmosis Study Group: Risk factors for *Toxoplasma gondii* infection in mothers of infants with congenital toxoplasmosis: Implications for prenatal management and screening. *Am J Obstet Gynecol* 192:564-571, 2005. Copyright 2005 by Elsevier. Reprinted by permission.)

▶ Neonatal toxoplasmosis affects an estimated 500 to 5000 newborn infants in the United States each year, and also causes problems in the developing world. Most infected infants have no apparent physical abnormalities at birth, but without treatment, most will develop significant morbidity related to chorioretinitis, hydrocephalus, or neurologic damage. To this end, the authors sought to determine whether demographic characteristics, history of exposure, or illness that was compatible with acute toxoplasmosis during gestation were able to identify most mothers of infants with congenital toxoplasmosis. The authors found that only one half of North American mothers of infants with toxoplasmosis exhibited any of the risk factors or compatible illnesses. The authors conclude that only systematic serologic screening of all pregnant women would prevent or detect a higher proportion of affected pregnancies.

J. M. G. van Vugt, MD, PhD

9 HIV

HIV and Pregnancy

Great strides in the treatment of HIV-infected pregnant women have led to a remarkable reduction in perinatal transmission, and for the first time, talk of actually eliminating pediatric HIV/AIDS in the United States. If pediatric HIV/AIDS is to truly be eliminated, the safety net of prevention must be extended to women without prenatal care. Rapid HIV testing in the intrapartum period represents a remarkable opportunity to include these newly diagnosed women and exposed neonates in prevention efforts. Hence, the new recommendations for rapid testing promulgated by ACOG.[1] While treatment throughout pregnancy, labor, and the neonatal period is most efficacious, antiretroviral therapy as late as labor or the newborn period can still significantly reduce perinatal transmission. As more women are treated with a greater number of potentially toxic medications, there is a need to ensure that treatment during pregnancy does bring more good than harm for both women and children. Several reports published this year attest to the fact that the benefits of highly active antiretroviral therapy (HAART) during pregnancy outweigh the potential risks, though special caution with certain antiretroviral medications is warranted.

Patricia M. Garcia, MD, MPH

Reference

1. American College of Obstetricians and Gynecologists Committee Opinion No. 304: Prenatal and perinatal human immunodeficiency virus testing: Expanded recommendations. *Obstet Gynecol* 104:1119-1124, 2004.

Decline in Perinatal HIV Transmission in New York State (1997-2000)
Wade NA, Zielinski MA, Butsashvili M, et al (AIDS Inst, Albany, NY; Bureau of HIV/AIDS Epidemiology, Albany, NY; New York State Dept of Health, Albany; et al)
J Acquir Immune Defic Syndr 36:1075-1082, 2004
9–1

Background.—Perinatal HIV transmission has declined significantly in New York State (NYS) since implementation of a 3-part regimen of zidovudine prophylaxis in the antenatal, intrapartum, and newborn periods. This study describes the factors associated with perinatal transmission in NYS from 1997 to 2000, the first 4 years of NYS's comprehensive program in which all HIV-exposed newborns were identified through universal HIV testing of newborns.

Methods.—This population-based observational study included all HIV-exposed newborns whose infection status was known and their mothers identified in NYS through the universal Newborn HIV Screening Program (NSP) from February 1997 to December 2000. Antepartum, intrapartum, newborn, and pediatric medical records of HIV-positive mothers/infants were reviewed for history of prenatal care, antiretroviral therapy (ART), and infant infection status. Risks associated with perinatal HIV transmission were examined.

Results.—Perinatal HIV transmission declined significantly from 11.0% in 1997 to 3.7% in 2000 ($P < 0.05$). Prenatal ART was associated with a decline in perinatal HIV transmission both for monotherapy (5.8%, relative risk [RR] = 0.3, 95% confidence interval: 0.2%–0.5%) and combination therapy (2.4%, RR = 0.1, 95% confidence interval: 0.1%–0.2%) compared with no prenatal antiretroviral prophylaxis ($P < 0.05$).

Conclusions.—Public health policies to improve access to care for pregnant women and advances in clinical care, including receipt of appropriate preventive therapies, have contributed to declines in perinatal HIV transmission in NYS.

▶ The efficacy of antiretroviral therapy (ART) in reducing perinatal transmission is demonstrated from observational statewide data from NYS. Starting in 1996, NYS implemented a comprehensive HIV perinatal prevention program that requires universal testing of newborns and expedited testing of mothers and newborns in the labor/delivery setting with follow-up of all exposed newborns. Wade et al report on perinatal transmission rates in NYS from February 1997 through December 2000, the first 4 years of this important model program. They document a significant reduction in perinatal transmission during each year (11.0% in 1997, 8.6% in 1998, 7.1% in 1999, 3.7% in 2000). A 3-part ART regimen (medications administered in the antepartum, intrapartum, and neonatal periods) was associated with the lowest transmission rate (3.3%; RR, 0.2; 95% confidence interval, 0.1-0.2) compared with more limited regimens. However, as has been consistently seen in many studies, even abbreviated ART regimens administered in the intrapartum/neonatal periods were associated with a reduction in transmission compared with no therapy. Other factors significantly associated with transmission were maternal age (2.1 RR of transmission for women older than 40 years), route of delivery (elective cesarean section was barely significantly associated with a reduction in transmission; RR, 0.6 [0.4-1.0]); maternal race (white women had an unexplained greater risk of transmission; RR, 2.6 [1.6-4.3] despite having higher rates of prenatal care and 3-part ART use), maternal residence (New York City residents had a higher rate of transmission compared with the rest of the state), and birth weight (infants weighing less than 1500 g were 2.5 times as likely to be associated with transmission).

P. M. Garcia, MD, MPH

Increased Risk of Incident HIV During Pregnancy in Rakai, Uganda: A Prospective Study

Gray RH, Li X, Kigazi G, et al (Johns Hopkins Univ, Baltimore, Md; Uganda Virus Research Inst, Entebbe; Makerere Univ, Kampala, Uganda; et al)

Lancet 366:1182-1188, 2005   9–2

Background.—HIV acquisition is significantly higher during pregnancy than in the postpartum period. We did a prospective study to estimate HIV incidence rates during pregnancy and lactation.

Methods.—We assessed 2188 HIV-negative sexually active women with 2625 exposure intervals during pregnancy and 2887 intervals during breast-feeding, and 8473 non-pregnant and non-lactating women with 24,258 exposure intervals. Outcomes were HIV incidence rates per 100 person years and incidence rate ratios estimated by Poisson multivariate regression, with the non-pregnant or non-lactating women as the reference group. We also assessed the husbands of the married women to study male risk behaviours.

Findings.—HIV incidence rates were 2.3 per 100 person years during pregnancy, 1.3 per 100 person years during breastfeeding, and 1.1 per 100 person years in the non-pregnant and non-lactating women. The adjusted incidence rate ratios were 2.16 (95% CI 1.39-3.37) during pregnancy and 1.16 (0.82-1.63) during breastfeeding. Pregnant women and their male partners reported significantly fewer external sexual partners than did the other groups. In married pregnant women who had a sexual relationship with their male spouses, the HIV incidence rate ratio was 1.36 (0.63-2.93). In married pregnant women in HIV-discordant relationships (ie, with HIV-positive men) the incidence rate ratio was 1.76 (0.62-4.03).

Interpretation.—The risk of HIV acquisition rises during pregnancy. This change is unlikely to be due to sexual risk behaviours, but might be attributable to hormonal changes affecting the genital tract mucosa or immune responses. HIV prevention efforts are needed during pregnancy to protect mothers and their infants.

▶ This study addresses the observation that HIV acquisition is higher in pregnancy than in the postpartum period. The investigators followed up a prospective cohort of sexually active women during pregnancy and breast-feeding, and they compared them with a cohort of nonpregnant, nonlactating women. They surprisingly found that the HIV incidence rates were nearly twice as high during pregnancy compared with during breast-feeding or the nonpregnant state. This increased risk of HIV acquisition during pregnancy seemed at odds with the demographic information of this cohort, because the authors were able to control for sexual behavior to a greater extent than in previous reports. They found little effect of behavioral factors on the increased risk of HIV acquisition during pregnancy, suggesting that biologic changes during pregnancy may have a more important role. The increased risk may be attributable to hormonal changes affecting the genital tract mucosa or maternal immune responses.

Public health implications of this study are important. Most importantly, primary HIV infection during pregnancy is associated with an increased risk of mother-to-child transmission of HIV. Pregnant women in high-risk geographic areas or high-risk situations (discordant HIV couples) need to be aware of the increased potential for HIV infection during pregnancy and should be given information on protective strategies. The findings also raise a question about HIV testing strategies during pregnancy. Most states recommend HIV testing during pregnancy; however, it is unclear whether repeat testing in late pregnancy is cost-effective. Clearly, antenatal care is improved by HIV testing, but it is also important to provide education about a potentially increased risk of transmission during pregnancy. Further research is needed to evaluate the cost-effectiveness of repeat testing late in pregnancy or even at delivery.

G. D. Wendel, Jr, MD

Early Invasive Diagnostic Techniques in Pregnant Women Who Are Infected With the HIV: A Multicenter Case Series
Somigliana E, for the Italian Collaborative Study on HIV Infection in Pregnancy ("L Mangiagalli" Hosp, Milan, Italy; et al)
Am J Obstet Gynecol 193:437-442, 2005   9–3

Objective.—Studies that mostly were conducted before the widespread use of combination antiretroviral treatments have reported that antenatal invasive procedures markedly increase the risk of human immunodeficiency virus vertical transmission. We aimed to evaluate the vertical transmission rate and other maternal and neonatal complications among women who were infected with human immunodeficiency virus who underwent antenatal invasive procedures during the second trimester of pregnancy and who were delivered after the advent of antiretroviral regimens.

Study Design.—We conducted a multicenter case series of women who were infected with human immunodeficiency virus who underwent amniocentesis or chorionic villus sampling or cordocentesis during the second trimester of pregnancy and who were delivered after January 1, 1997.

Results.—Sixty-three of 775 recruited women (8.1%) had performed early invasive diagnostic techniques . This rate has improved progressively from 4% in 1997 to 14%. Two of 60 viable infants (3.3%; 95% CI, 0.6%-10.1%) were infected with the human immunodeficiency virus. This rate did not differ significantly from the transmission rate that was observed in women who did not undergo antenatal invasive techniques (1.7%; $P = .30$).

Conclusion.—The current risk of human immunodeficiency virus vertical transmission that is associated with early invasive diagnostic techniques is lower than previously reported.

▶ In recent years, the use of highly active antiretroviral therapy has significantly reduced the rates of HIV mortality and disease progression. However, earlier studies that were mostly conducted before the widespread use of these antiretroviral therapies showed that invasive diagnostic procedures were associated with considerable increases in the risk of vertical transmission of HIV from mother to fetus. Accordingly, many called for the use of these invasive procedures only in situations of the highest risk for fetal abnormality. The authors of this study sought to determine whether more current use of invasive prenatal testing would similarly increase the risk of vertical transmission, given the more widespread use of highly effective antiretroviral therapies. The authors found that the current risk of HIV vertical transmission associated with early invasive diagnostic techniques (chorionic villus sampling, amniocentesis) was considerably lower than had been previously reported. Indeed, the authors observed only 2 cases of HIV infection of 60 viable newborn infants who had been exposed to early prenatal diagnosis. Although the possibility of vertical transmission must be a part of the counseling of women who are HIV positive and are at increased risk of detectable fetal abnormalities, this study gives important new information to those clinicians who care for HIV-positive pregnant women and may allay the fears of women and clinicians who are dealing with 2 important health-related issues that can affect mother and fetus.

L. P. Shulman, MD

Rapid HIV-1 Testing During Labor: A Multicenter Study
Bulterys M, for the Mother-Infant Rapid Intervention at Delivery (MIRIAD) Study Group (Ctrs for Disease Control and Prevention, Atlanta, Ga; et al)
JAMA 292:219-223, 2004   9–4

Context.—Timely testing of women in labor with undocumented human immunodeficiency virus (HIV) status could enable immediate provision of antiretroviral prophylaxis.

Objectives.—To determine the feasibility and acceptance of rapid HIV testing among women in labor and to assess rapid HIV assay performance.

Design, Setting, and Patients.—The Mother-Infant Rapid Intervention At Delivery (MIRIAD) study implemented 24-hour counseling and voluntary rapid HIV testing for women in labor at 16 US hospitals from November 16, 2001, through November 15, 2003. A rapid HIV-1 antibody test for whole blood was used.

Main Outcome Measures.—Acceptance of HIV testing; sensitivity, specificity, and predictive value of the rapid test; time from blood collection to patient notification of results.

Results.—There were 91,707 visits to the labor and delivery units in the study, 7381 of which were by eligible women without documentation of HIV testing. Of these, 5744 (78%) women were approached for rapid HIV testing and 4849 (84%) consented. HIV-1 test results were positive for 34 women (prevalence = 7/1000). Sensitivity and specificity of the rapid test were 100% and 99.9%, respectively; positive predictive value was 90% compared with 76% for enzyme immunoassay (EIA). Factors independently associated with higher test acceptance included younger age, being black or Hispanic, gestational age less than 32 weeks, and having had no prenatal care. Lower acceptance was associated with being admitted between 4 pm and midnight, particularly on Friday nights, but this may be explained in part by fewer available personnel. Median time from blood collection to patient notification of result was 66 minutes (interquartile range, 45-120 minutes), compared with 28 hours for EIA (*P* < .001).

Conclusions.—Rapid HIV testing is feasible and delivers accurate and timely test results for women in labor. It provides HIV-positive women prompt access to intrapartum and neonatal antiretroviral prophylaxis, proven to reduce perinatal HIV transmission, and may be particularly applicable to higher-risk populations.

▶ If pediatric HIV infection is to be eliminated in the United States, pregnant women without prenatal care (who are at increased risk of HIV infection) must be included in prevention efforts. Antiretroviral therapy given to women in labor who are newly diagnosed can still significantly reduce transmission. The MIRIAD study demonstrated that rapid HIV testing (with the OraQuick Rapid Test, Orasure Technologies) was feasible; 84% of women who presented with an undocumented HIV test that were offered participation in the study consented to rapid testing. The test was highly sensitive (100%) and specific (99.9%) with a good positive predictive value (90%). Because many women without prenatal care present in advanced labor, a quick turnaround time is essential. The median time from blood collection to patient notification of result was 66 minutes compared with 28 hours for the standard EIA test (*P* < .001). Rapid HIV testing in the labor and delivery setting should be implemented in all birthing hospitals.

P. M. Garcia, MD, MPH

Assessing the Risk of Birth Defects Associated With Antiretroviral Exposure During Pregnancy
Watts DH, Covington DL, Beckerman K, et al (Natl Inst of Child Health and Human Development, Bethesda, Md; Inveresk, Wilmington, NC; Newark Beth Israel Medical Ctr, NJ; et al)
Am J Obstet Gynecol 191:985-992, 2004   9–5

Objective.—The purpose of this study was to examine teratogenic risk of antiretroviral (ARV) drugs.

Study Design.—The Antiretroviral Pregnancy Registry (APR) monitors prenatal exposures to ARV drugs and pregnancy outcome through a prospective exposure-registration cohort. Statistical inference uses exact methods for binomial proportions.

Results.—Through July 2003, APR has monitored 3583 live births exposed to ARV. Among 1391 first trimester exposures, there were 38 birth defects, prevalence of 2.7% (95% CI 1.9–3.7), not significantly higher than the CDC's population surveillance rate, 3.1 per 100 live births (95% CI 3.1–3.2). For lamivudine, nelfinavir, nevirapine, stavudine, and zidovudine, sufficient numbers of live births (>200) following first-trimester exposures have been monitored to allow detection of a 2-fold increase in risk of birth defects overall; no increases have been detected.

Conclusion.—APR data demonstrate no increase in prevalence of birth defects overall or among women exposed to lamivudine, nelfinavir, nevirapine, stavudine, and zidovudine.

▶ To counsel pregnant HIV-infected women accurately and fairly with regard to the risks and benefits of antiretroviral drug use in pregnancy, both maternal and neonatal toxicity data are needed. The APR is an important source of information for the risk of birth defects associated with antiretroviral use in pregnancy. The registry now has birth outcomes data from 3583 live births exposed to antiretroviral drugs, including 1391 first-trimester exposures. In their latest publication, they update birth defect reports related to the use of lamivudine, nelfinavir, nevirapine, stavudine, and zidovudine. Overall, there were 38 birth defects in liveborn infants reported among the 1391 first trimester-exposed pregnancies (2.7% prevalence rate; 95% confidence interval, 1.9-3.7). This compares favorably with the CDC population surveillance rate of 3.1 per 100 live births (95% confidence interval, 3.1-3.2). For each drug individually, there were more than 200 first-trimester exposures (a sample size sufficient to detect a 2-fold increase in the overall risk of birth defects) and no such increase was detected. Complete details on all ARV drugs and specific defects in the registry can be found online at www.APRegistry.com.

P. M. Garcia, MD, MPH

Maternal Toxicity and Pregnancy Complications in Human Immunodeficiency Virus–Infected Women Receiving Antiretroviral Therapy: PACTG 316
Watts DH, for the PACTG 316 Study Team (Natl Inst of Child Health and Human Development, Bethesda, Md; et al)
Am J Obstet Gynecol 190:506-516, 2004   9–6

Objective.—The purpose of this study was to evaluate rates of maternal toxicity, pregnancy complications, and peripartum morbidity by type and duration of antiretroviral therapy (ART) during pregnancy.

Study Design.—The Pediatric AIDS Clinical Trials Group (PACTG) Protocol 316 (PACTG 316) study evaluated the addition of intrapartum/neonatal nevirapine to background ART to reduce perinatal transmission of human immunodeficiency virus-1 (HIV-1). For this secondary analysis, women were categorized into one of six groups on the basis of ART during pregnancy (monotherapy [monoRx], combination without protease inhibitor [PI], combination with PI), and start time (early: before or during first trimester; late: second or third trimester).

Results.—One thousand four hundred seven women were included: 288 monoRx late, 34 monoRx early, 327 combo, no PI late, 175 combo, no PI early, 320 combo, PI late, and 263 combo, PI early. Symptoms and laboratory abnormalities of moderate grade or more occurred in less than 5% of women. Only gestational diabetes (highest in combo PI early) varied significantly by therapy group.

Conclusion.—In HIV-infected women receiving prenatal care and ART, adverse events were uncommon.

▶ The general tolerability of complex ART regimens is documented in the report from PACTG 316, an NIH-sponsored trial that evaluated the addition of intrapartum/neonatal nevirapine to background antiretroviral therapy to reduce perinatal transmission. Their analysis looked at toxicity and pregnancy complications among 1407 women enrolled in the study who were on various ART regimens (23% monotherapy, 36% combination therapy without PIs, and 41% combination therapy with PIs). In general, toxicities (clinical symptoms and laboratory abnormalities) were low among these women and did not differ among the treatment groups, suggesting that even complex therapies were well tolerated. Less than 5% of women experienced significant symptoms or abnormalities (at least moderate-grade toxicities). The most common symptoms were nausea and vomiting (3.1%), headache (2.6%), and abdominal pain (3.1%). Hemoglobin levels less than 8 g/dL were noted in 8.9% of women in the early monotherapy group. The overall rate of gestational diabetes was 2.1%, well within the range of 2% to 3% reported for the general population. However, as reported in other studies, there was a significantly higher rate of glucose intolerance reported in women on long-term PI therapy (4.6%). The rate of antenatal hospitalizations (17.3/100 deliveries) was no different than that reported for the general population (18/100 deliveries), again attesting to the general tolerability of ART regimens, including highly active antiviral therapy.

P. M. Garcia, MD, MPH

Maternal Toxicity With Continuous Nevirapine in Pregnancy: Results From PACTG 1022

Hitti J, for the PACTG 1022 Study Team (Univ of Washington, Seattle; et al)
J Acquir Immune Defic Syndr 36:772-776, 2004   9–7

Objective.—To compare the safety of nelfinavir and nevirapine-based antiretroviral treatment in HIV-1-infected pregnant women.

Methods.—In Pediatric AIDS Clinical Trials Group Protocol 1022, 38 antiretroviral-naive pregnant women at 10-30 weeks' gestation were randomized to nelfinavir or nevirapine with zidovudine plus lamivudine. The study was suspended because of greater than expected toxicity and changes in nevirapine prescribing information. The incidence of treatment-limiting hepatic or cutaneous toxicity was compared between groups for all subjects and for the subset with CD4 cell counts greater than 250 cells/µL at study entry.

Results.—Toxicity was seen in 1 (5%) of 21 subjects randomized to nelfinavir and 5 (29%) of 17 subjects randomized to nevirapine ($P = 0.07$). Within the nevirapine group, 1 subject developed fulminant hepatic failure and died, and another developed Stevens-Johnson syndrome. The one adverse event associated with nelfinavir occurred in a subject with a CD4 cell count less than 250 cells/μL. All 5 events among subjects with a CD4 cell count greater than 250 cells/μL were associated with nevirapine ($P = 0.04$).

Conclusions.—Continuous nevirapine may be associated with increased toxicity among HIV-1-infected pregnant women with CD4 cell counts greater than 250 cells/μL, as has been observed in non-pregnant women.

▶ Over the last few years, the unique susceptibility of women to the hepatotoxicity of nevirapine has been demonstrated. The report of Hitti and colleagues extends this observation to pregnant women. PACTG 1022 was a study of pregnant women randomized to either nevirapine or nelfinavir in addition to zidovudine plus lamivudine. During the course of the study, a Food and Drug Administration alert was issued with regard to the increased toxicity of nevirapine in women (those with CD4 counts >250 cells/μL), and accrual was halted. A greater than expected rate of treatment-limiting toxicity associated with nevirapine use as compared with nelfinavir was seen (5 of 17 [29%] vs 1 of 21 [5%], $P = .07$). Among the subset of women with CD4 counts greater than 250 cells/μL, the rate of toxicity leading to discontinuation of treatment was 36% for the nevirapine group (5 of 14) and zero for the nelfinavir group (0 of 14). Treatment-limiting toxicities included one subject with Stevens-Johnson syndrome and tragically, one subject who developed fulminant hepatic failure and died. Five additional cases of maternal death have been reported among pregnant women treated with nevirapine. All were associated with fulminant hepatic failure that presented 4 to 5 weeks after initiating nevirapine in previously healthy individuals (normal liver function tests and no history of hepatitis B or C). Pregnant patients with CD4 counts greater than 250 cells/μL should not be prescribed nevirapine for continuous use. However, these data should not be extrapolated to the use of a single maternal dose of nevirapine for the prevention of perinatal HIV transmission, as 3 large trials of over 1600 pregnant women given a single dose of neviripine in labor have not demonstrated any increase in toxicity.

P. M. Garcia, MD, MPH

10 Medical Complications

Safety of Influenza Vaccination During Pregnancy
Munoz FM, Greisinger AJ, Wehmanen OA, et al (Kelsey Research Found, Houston)
Am J Obstet Gynecol 192:1098-1106, 2005   10–1

Objective.—The purpose of this study was to evaluate the safety of influenza vaccine that is administered in the second or third trimester of gestation.

Study Design.—A retrospective electronic database search of 5 influenza seasons (July 1, 1998, to June 30, 2003) was performed at a large multispecialty clinic in Houston, Texas. Immunization rates were calculated, and outcomes of pregnancy were compared between a cohort of healthy women who received influenza vaccine and a control group of healthy unvaccinated women who were matched by age, month of delivery, and type of medical insurance.

Results.—Among 7183 eligible mother-infant pairs, only 252 pregnant women (3.5%) received the influenza vaccine. Women with medical insurance were more likely to be vaccinated, although the rates for women with chronic underlying conditions were similar to those of healthy women, regardless of insurance status. The mean gestational age at the time of influenza vaccination was 26.1 weeks (range, 14-39 weeks). No serious adverse events occurred within 42 days of vaccination, and there was no difference between the groups in the outcomes of pregnancy (including cesarean delivery and premature delivery) and infant medical conditions from birth to 6 months of age.

Conclusion.—Influenza vaccine that was administered in the second or third trimester of gestation was safe in this study population.

► The increasing concern in public health circles concerning the possibility of pandemic flu outbreaks in the United States and around the world has led to an increasing interest in influenza vaccination to prevent these viral outbreaks. This study by Munoz et al assessed the safety of influenza vaccine during pregnancy. Their study evaluated 252 pregnant women who received influenza vaccine during their pregnancy. The authors found no serious adverse events had occurred within 42 days of vaccination, and there were no differences between the women who had received the vaccine and a comparative group of women who received no such vaccination. In addition, infant medical conditions were not different between the 2 groups from birth to 6 months of age. The safety of influenza vaccination during pregnancy is an obviously important issue to the large number of pregnant women who may be exposed to influenza during their pregnancy and who are seeking to reduce or eliminate the potential for influenza-related complications during their pregnancies.

L. P. Shulman, MD

Factors That Predict Prematurity and Preeclampsia in Pregnancies That Are Complicated by Systemic Lupus Erythematosus
Chakravarty EF, Colón I, Langen ES, et al (Stanford Univ, Palo Alto, Calif)
Am J Obstet Gynecol 192:1897-1904, 2005   10–2

Objective.—The purpose of this study was to describe the outcomes of a 10-year cohort of pregnancies in patients with systemic lupus erythematosus and to evaluate clinical and laboratory markers for adverse outcomes.

Study Design.—We reviewed all pregnancies in patients with systemic lupus erythematosus who were seen at Stanford University from 1991 to 2001. Univariate analyses were performed to identify potential risk factors for adverse outcomes.

Results.—Sixty-three pregnancies in 48 women were identified. Approximately 35% of the pregnancies occurred in women with previous renal disease and 10% in women with previous central nervous system disease. Flares occurred in 68% of the pregnancies, the majority of which were mild to moderate. Preeclampsia complicated 12 pregnancies. Factors that were associated with premature delivery included prednisone use at conception (relative risk, 1.8), the use of antihypertensive medications (relative risk, 1.8), and a severe flare during pregnancy (relative risk, 2.0). Thrombocytopenia was associated with an increased risk of preeclampsia (relative risk, 3.2).

Conclusion.—Flares, most of which were mild to moderate, occurred in most of the pregnancies in our cohort of patients with systemic lupus erythematosus. Thrombocytopenia, hypertension, and prednisone use may be predictive factors for particular adverse outcomes.

▶ The management of systemic lupus erythematosus (SLE) during pregnancy remains a challenge for obstetricians and maternal-fetal specialists. Most pregnancies that are complicated by SLE have good outcomes with few adverse outcomes for mother and infant, although poor outcomes still occur and may exceed rates that are expected in unaffected women. To this end, Chakravarty et al from Stanford University sought to delineate factors that predicted adverse maternal and perinatal outcomes in pregnant women with SLE. It was found that thrombocytopenia, hypertension, and prednisone use were associated with an increased risk for adverse outcomes. Nonetheless, women with SLE should not be discouraged from child bearing, but should be provided with accurate and comprehensive counseling concerning the risk to their health as well the potential impact of SLE on their pregnancy. According to the authors, optimal outcomes are most likely to arise from treatment by a team of experienced obstetricians and rheumatologists.

L. P. Shulman, MD

Low Ratio of S-adenosylmethionine to S-adenosylhomocysteine Is Associated With Vitamin Deficiency in Brazilian Pregnant Women and Newborns

Guerra-Shinohara, EM, Morita OE, Peres S, et al (Universidade de São Paulo, Brazil; Institutos de Pesquisas da Secretaria de Saúde do Estado de São Paulo, Brazil; Instituto Adolfo Lutz, São José do Rio Preto, Brazil; et al)
Am J Clin Nutr 80:1312-1321, 2004   10–3

Background.—Pregnant women with low cobalamin concentrations are unable to provide the necessary amount of cobalamin to their fetuses. The effect of low maternal cobalamin concentrations on transmethylation metabolism in pregnant women and their newborns is unknown.

Objective.—We investigated the relation between maternal and neonatal cobalamin concentrations and changes in total homocysteine (tHcy), S-adenosylmethionine (SAM), and S-adenosylhomocysteine (SAH).

Design.—Hematologic data and concentrations of cobalamin, red blood cell folate, serum folate, tHcy, methylmalonic acid, SAM, SAH, and other metabolites were measured in 119 serum specimens from pregnant Brazilian women (gestational age: 37-42 wk) and their newborns' placental veins at the time of delivery.

Results.—The tHcy concentrations were higher in placental vein serum from newborns whose mothers had low cobalamin. Serum SAH concentrations were elevated and serum SAM and methionine concentrations were decreased in pregnant women with lower cobalamin concentrations. SAM:SAH was significantly decreased in both cobalamin-deficient pregnant women and their newborns.

Conclusions.—Lower maternal cobalamin concentrations are associated with higher tHcy and lower SAM:SAH in newborns. Because SAM:SAH is closely linked with the activity of numerous enzymatic methylation reactions, these results suggest that methylation could be impaired in cobalamin-deficient pregnant women and their newborns.

▶ When cobalamin levels are low in pregnant women, their fetuses also have lower amounts. These authors assessed for low cobalamin levels and changes in homocysteine, SAM and SAH levels. This Brazilian study demonstrated that low cobalamin levels lead to higher homocysteine and lower SAM/SAH levels in the newborn. Further research is necessary to clearly correlate the potential for increased risk of congenital malformations, such as neural tube defects and intrauterine growth restriction, in women with low levels of cobalamin.

S. H. Ural, MD

Fertility and Pregnancy-Related Events in Women With Celiac Disease: A Population-Based Cohort Study
Tata LJ, Card TR, Logan RFA, et al (Univ of Nottingham, England; Nottingham City Hosp, England)
Gastroenterology 128:849-855, 2005   10–4

Background & Aims.—Previous studies have raised concern about reduced fertility and increased adverse pregnancy-related events in women with celiac disease, but none has estimated overall fertility compared with the general female population.

Methods.—We compared computerized primary care data for 1521 women with celiac disease with data for 7732 age- and practice-matched women without celiac disease. We estimated population-based rates of fertility and adverse pregnancy outcomes.

Results.—Crude fertility rates were 48.2 and 47.7 live births per 1000 person-years for women with and without celiac disease, respectively (rate ratio, 1.01; 95% confidence interval, 0.90-1.14). Age-specific fertility rates showed that women with celiac disease had lower fertility when younger but higher fertility when older compared with women without celiac disease. This increase in relative fertility with increasing age held whether women had treated or untreated celiac disease. Risks of cesarean section (odds ratio, 1.33; 95% confidence interval, 1.03-1.70) and miscarriage (rate ratio, 1.31; 95% confidence interval, 1.06-1.61) were moderately higher in women with celiac disease, but risks of assisted birth, breech birth, preeclampsia, postpartum hemorrhage, ectopic pregnancy, stillbirth, and termination were similar.

Conclusions.—Overall, women with celiac disease have fertility similar to that of the general female population, but they have their babies at an older age. Although our findings may reflect a disease effect, the age shift in fertility rates and the increase in cesarean section risk is consistent with socioeconomic or educational advantages of women with celiac disease.

▶ Celiac disease affects as much as 1% of the female population in Western Europe and North America. A large proportion of affected patients are undiagnosed. Only limited information is available on associations of this disease with fertility, adverse pregnancy outcomes such as miscarriage, intrauterine growth restriction, and congenital malformations such as neural tube defects. It has been suggested that these risks can be eliminated by treatment with a gluten-free diet. This has never been adequately studied. In this large, general population–based cohort study, the aforementioned issues have been addressed. It revealed that women with celiac disease have lower fertility when younger but catch up at later ages, resulting in the same overall fertility as women in the general population. This was true for women with treated as well as untreated celiac disease. The later increase in fertility and the increased proportion of cesarean sections in the older groups may reflect socioeconomic advantages of women with this disease. The risks of adverse pregnancy outcomes for women with celiac disease did not appear to be as high as previously reported. Only the rates of miscarriage and cesarean section were slightly increased. This may be partially explained by the findings that these women were more likely to have never smoked and to have a lower body mass compared with women without the disease. These factors are known to affect fertility and pregnancy outcome, and support the beneficial effects of a healthy lifestyle in general, but also in women with celiac disease.

Celiac disease is characterized by disturbances in nutrient absorption through which deficiencies can occur; of special concern are the levels of folate and zinc. The risk of having a child with a neural tube defect, however, was not significantly different as compared with that in the general population.

E. A. P. Steegers, MD, PhD

Pregnancy in Heart Transplant Recipients
Miniero R, Tardivo I, Centofanti P, et al (Univ of Turin, Italy; IRCCS San Matteo, Pavia, Italy; Ospedali Riuniti, Bergamo, Italy; et al)
J Heart Lung Transplant 23:898-901, 2004　　　　　　　　　　　　　　10–5

Abstract.—The aim of this report is to present data from Italian cardiac transplant centers assessing pregnancy after cardiac transplantation. Our retrospective survey included 10 pregnancies occurring in 7 patients during January 1991 to February 2002. Eight pregnancies were completed successfully and 2 abortions were reported (frequency rate 20%). No complications were observed during pregnancy or after delivery. Of 8 infants studied, 6 (75%) were born at term and 2 (25%) pre-term. One baby presented congenital talipes valgus. Pediatric development was uneventful. The data from the literature and our series show that a multidisciplinary approach is mandatory. The course of pregnancy is usually normal and the maternal and fetal outcomes are usually favorable. Although no fetal malformations have been reported, prolonged follow-up of these infants is required.

▶ Advances in surgical techniques and immunosuppressive therapy have allowed more women with cardiac transplantation to survive and lead a relatively normal life. Some may desire to become pregnant. Adequate preconception counseling is of the utmost importance in these high-risk women, during which balancing the risks of pregnancy for the mother and the fetus is crucial. Furthermore, the long-term results of cardiac transplantation as well as the etiology of the cardiac disease should be discussed before any pregnancy. The inheritance of certain conditions, such as cardiomyopathy, have been well established. The risks of pregnancy for the mother after heart transplantation include cardiovascular, infectious, and immune complications. Pregnancy, as well as the early puerperium, induces hemodynamic changes such as an increased cardiac workload. Immunosuppressive therapy increases the risks of bacterial, viral, mycotic, and opportunistic infections. Chances of rejection do not seem to be lower during pregnancy than in the nonpregnant state. Fetal risks include viral infectious, such as cytomegalovirus and rubella infections, resulting from the immunosuppressive therapy of the mother. Next to ethical issues involved, such as the uncertain life expectancy of these women, pregnancy outcome should be continuously monitored worldwide. Up to the year 2002, 86 cases of pregnancy after cardiac transplantation have been reported. Therapeutic abortion was performed in 12% of cases, and 8% spontaneously miscarried. Of the resulting pregnancies, 42% of babies were born prematurely and 58% at term. The most frequent maternal complications were hypertension, infection, and preeclampsia. In 8 pregnancies rejection was observed, and 2 of those women died. No structural congenital malformations were identified, but intrauterine growth restriction was more prevalent with immunosuppressive therapy. The results of an Italian retrospective survey show similar results. Management of pregnancies in heart transplant recipients does not seem to be very different from that in a healthy woman, but stringent multidisciplinary control of both the maternal and fetal condition is mandatory. In general, there is no contraindication to vaginal delivery. Breastfeeding is usually discouraged because of the neonatal exposure to immunosuppressive drugs.

E. A. P. Steegers, MD, PhD

Pregnancy Outcome in Women With Prosthetic Heart Valves
Nassar AH, Hobeika EM, Abd Essamad HM, et al (American Univ, Beirut, Lebanon)
Am J Obstet Gynecol 191:1009-1013, 2004   10–6

Objective.—This study was undertaken to evaluate the risks and pregnancy outcome in women with prosthetic heart valves on different anticoagulent regimens.

Study Design.—A retrospective chart review of 82 pregnancies in 33 women with mechanical valve prostheses at a tertiary referral center from 1987 to 2002. The main outcome measures were major maternal complications and perinatal outcome.

Results.—The valve replaced was mitral (60.6%), aortic (18.2%), and both (21.2%). Fifty-four pregnancies (65.9%) resulted in live births, 9 (11.0%) had stillbirths (all on warfarin), and 12 (14.6%) had spontaneous and 7 (8.5%) therapeutic abortions (all on warfarin). The rate of spontaneous abortion was highest in women on warfarin throughout pregnancy ($P < .01$). The live birth rate was higher in women on heparin compared with those on warfarin ($P < .01$), and in those on heparin/warfarin compared with warfarin alone ($P < .01$). There were no maternal deaths; however, 3 patients had mitral valve thrombosis (2 on heparin and 1 on warfarin) necessitating surgery in 1 patient and medical thrombolysis in 2 patients. Hemorrhagic complications occurred in 5 patients, 4 of whom required transfusion.

Conclusion.—No single anticoagulant regimen confers complete protection from thromboembolic phenomena in pregnancy. Despite a high maternal morbidity rate, the perinatal outcome is acceptable when pregnancy progresses beyond the first trimester.

▶ Women with mechanical prosthetic valves were often advised not to get pregnant because of their increased risk of pregnancy-associated thromboembolic complications, an increased risk of functional deterioration of the valve, and the concern about the teratogenicity of anticoagulant medication. In particular, warfarin is associated with embryopathy, spontaneous abortions, stillbirths, and less commonly, CNS defects and fetal bleeding with exposure beyond the first trimester. By using heparin only, fetal risks are eliminated at the expense of possibly significantly higher maternal morbidity and mortality rates secondary to valve thrombosis. In this study, single warfarin therapy resulted in a higher spontaneous abortion rate. Nonfatal valve thromboses occurred in 3 women, 2 of whom were receiving low molecular weight heparin (LMWH) throughout pregnancy. The risk of valve complications relies on many factors including type, number, and position of the valves, arrhythmias, previous thrombosis, and adequacy of anticoagulation. If unfractionated heparin (U-heparin) or LMWH is to be used in pregnant women with mechanical prosthetic heart valves, it should be administered in adequate dosages and monitored at least twice weekly. Despite warfarin being superior to heparin in protecting prosthetic valves, 78% of the patients elected to be on heparin because of its safety to their fetuses. On the other hand, 86% of the patients chose to continue on warfarin after the first trimester, despite the knowledge of the risks in the second and third trimester. Patients seem to balance the fetal and maternal risks, although a financial factor could not be ruled out.

Clinicians caring for these patients are faced with a dilemma because of the American College of Obstetricians and Gynecologists advisory against the use of LMWH, and the growing evidence of the lack of efficacy of U-heparin. These patients should be thoroughly counseled, preferably before pregnancy, regarding the balance of maternal and fetal risks with the available anticoagulants, allowing them to make an informed decision about whether to become pregnant, and in order to make an optimal plan of management for the periconceptional period, pregnancy, delivery, and the puerperium. To make evidence-based recommendations for these patients, well-designed studies should be performed.

E. A. P. Steegers, MD, PhD

11 Antepartum Surveillance

Use of Fetal Pulse Oximetry Among High-Risk Women in Labor: A Randomized Clinical Trial
Klauser CK, Christensen EE, Chauhan SP, et al (Univ of Mississippi, Jackson; Spartanburg Regional Med Ctr, SC; Naval Med Ctr Portsmouth, Va)
Am J Obstet Gynecol 192:1810-1819, 2005   11–1

Objective.—The purpose of this study was to determine the clinical role of fetal pulse oximetry to reduce cesarean delivery for a nonreassuring fetal heart rate tracing.

Study Design.—Singletons ≥28 weeks were randomized to fetal pulse oximetry plus electronic fetal heart rate monitoring (monitoring+fetal pulse oximetry) or monitoring alone.

Results.—Overall, 360 women in labor were recruited: 150 cases with monitoring+fetal pulse oximetry and 177 cases with monitoring alone were analyzed. Most demographic, obstetric, and neonatal characteristics were similar. Specifically, the gestational age, cervical dilation, and station of the fetal head were not differential factors (Table 3). In addition, cesarean delivery for nonreassuring fetal heart rate tracing was not different between the group with monitoring+fetal pulse oximetry (29%) and the group with monitoring alone (32%; relative risk, 0.95; 95% CI, 0.75, 1.22). Likewise, cesarean delivery for arrest disorder was similar between the group with monitoring+fetal pulse oximetry (22%) and the group with monitoring alone (23%; relative risk, 1.05; 95% CI, 0.79, 1.44). However, the decision-to-incision time was shorter for the group with monitoring+fetal pulse oximetry (17.8 ± 8.2 min) than for the group with monitoring alone (27.7 ± 13.9 min; $P < .0001$).

Conclusion.—The use of fetal pulse oximetry with electronic fetal heart rate monitoring does not decrease the rate of cesarean delivery, although it does alter the decision-to-incision time.

► Electronic fetal heart rate monitoring is almost universally used in tertiary care centers to assess fetal well-being. When the fetal heart rate trace is reassuring, there is a predictive value of 99% for confirming a nonacidotic fetus. Conversely, an abnormal fetal heart rate tracing has only a positive predictive

TABLE 3.—Delivery Factors

Factor	Electronic Fetal Monitoring + FPO (n = 150)	Electronic Fetal Monitoring Alone (n = 177)	P Value	RR (95% CI)
Cervical examination on admittance*				
Dilation (cm)	2.5 ± 1.8	2.5 ± 1.9	.853	
Station	-3.6 ± 1.4	-3.7 ± 1.3	.759	
Cervical examination on randomization*				
Dilation (cm)	5.8 ± 1.5	5.6 ± 1.4	.321	
Station	-1.6 ± 1.8	-1.5 ± 1.9	.790	
Cesarean delivery (n)	77 (51%)	98 (55%)		0.91 (0.72,1.16)
Dystocia (n)	34 (22%)	41 (23%)		1.05 (0.75,1.47)
Nonreassuring FHR tracing (n)	43 (29%)	57 (32%)		0.95 (0.68,1.33)
Decision-to-incision time for cesarean delivery				
Nonreassuring FHR tracing (min)*	17.8 ± 8.2	27.7 ± 13.9	< .0001	
Within 30 minutes (n/N)	39/43 (91%)	33/57 (58%)		3.79 (1.49,9.63)

*Data are given as mean ± SD.
Abbreviations: FPO, Fetal pulse oximetry; RR, relative risks; FHR, fetal heart rate.
(Courtesy of Klauser CK, Christensen EE, Chauhan SP, et al: Use of fetal pulse oximetry among high-risk women in labor: a randomized clinical trial. Am J Obstet Gynecol 192:1810-1819, 2005. Copyright 2005 by Elsevier. Reprinted by permission.)

value of 50% for fetal compromise. Although fetal heart rate monitoring is widely used, numerous studies show that such monitoring has failed to decrease perinatal morbidity and mortality rates in comparison with intermittent assessment during labor. Other interventions (fetal scalp monitoring) have been shown to be more predictive but are not used because of a variety of characteristics that make them not amenable to safe and widespread use. To this end, other modalities have been evaluated, and fetal pulse oximetry has been proposed as an adjunctive means of fetal assessment. Unfortunately, this trial from the University of Mississippi shows that the use of fetal pulse oximetry did not decrease the rate of cesarean section, although it did alter the decision-to-incision time. Accordingly, further studies are needed to develop other fetal evaluation paradigms to better assess the high-risk woman in labor and to better determine when to intervene in her pregnancy.

H. P. van Geijn, MD, PhD

Maternal Self-administered Fetal Heart Rate Monitoring and Transmission From Home in High-Risk Pregnancies
Kerner R, Yogev Y, Belkin A, et al (Rabin Med Ctr, Petah Tiqva, Israel; Tel Aviv Univ, Israel)
Int J Gynecol Obstet 84:33-39, 2004   11–2

Objectives.—To evaluate the feasibility of high-risk pregnancy surveillance by patient-directed fetal heart rate monitoring and transmission, and to assess patient satisfaction with this technology.

Methods.—Thirty-six women with high-risk pregnancies performed daily non-stress tests at home and transmitted the data to our perinatal care center by telephone. At each transmission, patients were asked by a physician about perceived fetal movements and uterine contractions and given the results. If the tracing was unsatisfactory, further evaluation was performed. In addition, patients completed a questionnaire on quality of life and anxiety state before and after the study.

Results.—All patients were able to perform the tests and transmissions. The quality of recorded data was significantly correlated with maternal body mass index, but not with gestational age at the time of monitoring or birth weight. Thirty-nine of the total 562 tracings (6.9%) were inconclusive or non-reassuring. After repeated testing, 32 of them (82%) were considered normal, and seven patients (18%) were referred for additional in-hospital evaluation. Of this group, four were discharged for further surveillance with routine home monitoring and the remaining three were hospitalized for continued evaluation. There were no significant immediate adverse maternal or neonatal outcomes as a result of the monitoring. Patient satisfaction was high.

Conclusions.—Daily home FHR monitoring in high-risk patients is safe and feasible at all gestational ages, based on this initial pilot evaluation. It is easily and reliably performed and accepted by patients with a high level of satisfaction.

▶ This study from the perinatal group at the Rabin Medical Center of Tel Aviv University sought to determine the feasibility of high-risk pregnancy surveillance by patient-directed fetal heart rate monitoring and to assess patient satisfaction with the technology. The authors found that daily home fetal heart rate monitoring in high-risk pregnancies was safe and feasible at all gestational ages and was associated with a high level of patient satisfaction. As the nonstress test is widely recognized to be a sensitive screening modality in identifying fetuses in immediate danger of deterioration and compromise, the incorporation of home monitoring could provide additional and important evaluations of pregnancies at increased risk for adverse outcomes. This study shows that home monitoring in well-counseled patients is not only feasible but is well accepted by women who are being evaluated and treated for a variety of fetal and maternal issues that could increase the risk of fetal demise and other adverse outcomes.

H. P. van Geijn, MD, PhD

Use of Umbilical-Cerebral Doppler Ratios in Predicting Fetal Growth Restriction in Near-Term Fetuses
To WWK, Chan AMY, Mok K-M (United Christian Hosp, Hong Kong)
Aust N Z J Obstet Gynaecol 45:130-136, 2005   11–3

Objective.—To compare the sensitivity and specificity of different umbilical-cerebral ratios in the prediction and detection of fetal growth restriction in near-term fetuses when the umbilical arterial waveform is within normal.

Methods.—A prospective cross-sectional observational study was carried out recruiting consecutive singleton pregnancies with clinically suspected fetal growth restriction after 34 weeks gestation. The umbilical-cerebral ratios were then calculated from the S/D, RI and PI values and correlated with immediate perinatal outcome.

Results.—A total of 187 patients were recruited. Twelve cases had abnormal UA Doppler flow velocity waveform studies. Of the 175 with normal UA Doppler findings, 92 (53.1%) were confirmed to have fetal growth restriction (FGR) with birth weights below the tenth centile for gestation. The detection rate of FGR by ultrasound biometry was 96.7%. The mean umbilical artery S/D, RI and PI values were higher in the fetal growth restriction group, while the middle cerebral artery values were lower as compared to fetuses with no growth restriction. A small but significant difference was seen in the umbilical-cerebral ratios of the different indices between the two groups. Receiver operator characteristic curves showed that there was little difference between the performances of the S/D, RI or PI ratios and all had limited power in predicting fetal growth restriction.

Conclusion.—In the presence of normal umbilical artery Doppler waveforms, umbilical-cerebral ratios have limited power to predict fetal growth restriction.

Fetal Cerebral Venous Doppler Velocimetry in Normal and High-Risk Pregnancy

Cheema R, Dubiel M, Breborowicz G, et al (Univ Hosp MAS, Malmö, Sweden; Univ School of Med Sciences, Poznan, Poland)
Ultrasound Obstet Gynecol 24:147-153, 2004   11–4

Objective.—In previous pilot studies, fetal vein of Galen (GV) blood velocity has been shown to be non-pulsatile in normal pregnancies. A pulsating pattern in high-risk pregnancies has been related to adverse outcome of pregnancy. The aim of this study was to establish reference ranges for fetal cerebral venous blood flow and compare them to the recordings in high-risk pregnancies in terms of predicting adverse perinatal outcome.

Methods.—The GV, straight sinus (SS) and transverse sinus (TS) were located by color Doppler ultrasound in 189 normal pregnancies between 23 and 43 weeks of gestation. Recordings were also made in 102 pregnancies complicated by pregnancy-induced hypertension and/or intrauterine growth restriction. The following parameters were measured: peak systolic velocity, minimum diastolic velocity, time-averaged maximum velocity, pulsatility index for veins (PIV) and preload index (PLI). GV pulsations were noted. In high-risk pregnancies, Doppler measurements were correlated to pregnancy outcome, including emergency operative intervention and/or neonatal distress. Umbilical vein and umbilical, uterine and middle cerebral artery blood velocities were also recorded at the same time.

Results.—In normal pregnancy, pulsating venous blood velocity was observed in GV in 8% of cases, in SS in 79% of cases and in TS in 100% of cases. GV and SS maximum velocity increased with gestational age and TS-PIV showed linear decreasing values and TS-PLI showed increasing values with gestational age. In high-risk pregnancies, pulsating blood velocity in the GV was found in 59 (58%) cases and was related to adverse outcome of pregnancy including mortality. Abnormal values for TS-PIV and PLI and SS maximum velocity were found in nine, six and five cases, respectively and were only related to perinatal mortality. GV pulsations were more frequent than umbilical venous pulsations.

Conclusions.—Of the fetal cerebral veins studied, the presence of pulsations in the GV seems to be the best predictor of adverse outcome of high-risk pregnancy. Pulsations in the GV are more frequent than in the umbilical vein and might therefore appear earlier during worsening fetal condition, and thus be of potential value for fetal surveillance in high-risk pregnancies.

▶ Doppler US technology has become a routine part of clinical surveillance of a wide variety of high-risk pregnancies. Recordings of the umbilical and uterine arteries have been shown to successfully detect increased vascular resistance and thus predict adverse outcomes of pregnancy. These 2 articles (Abstracts 11–3 and 11–4) show the utilization of Doppler technology to predict adverse outcomes in high-risk pregnancies. The article by To and colleagues (Abstract 11–3) demonstrates that the determination of umbilical-cerebral Doppler ratios was highly sensitive in predicting fetal growth restriction in near-term fetuses. Cheema and colleagues (Abstract 11–4) showed that the presence of pulsations in the fetal vein of Galen was a very good predictor of adverse outcomes in high-risk pregnancies. Further studies of the clinical relevance of Doppler waveforms will likely provide important approaches for the clinical evaluation and, hopefully, therapeutic interventions for high-risk pregnancies affected by abnormal blood flow patterns.

H. P. van Geijn, MD, PhD

Cervical Length in the Early Second Trimester for Detection of Triplet Pregnancies at Risk for Preterm Birth
Maslovitz S, Hartoov J, Wolman I, et al (Tel Aviv Univ, Israel)
J Ultrasound Med 23:1187-1191, 2004   11–5

Objective.—Preterm triplet delivery is common and has a tremendous impact on neonatal mortality and morbidity. We aimed at assessing early second-trimester cervical length as a means of detecting triplet pregnancies at risk for preterm birth.

Methods.—Cervical length was measured in triplet pregnancies during weeks 14 to 20. Cervical length of less than 25 mm was used as a cutoff to divide individuals into 2 groups. Perinatal outcome parameters were compared between the 2 groups and included gestational age at delivery, birth weights, and neonatal intensive care unit admission rates. Sensitivity, specificity, and positive and negative predictive values were calculated for cervical length as a screening method for preterm birth.

Results.—We evaluated 36 triplets during weeks 14 to 20. Cervical length of less than 25 mm was measured in 14 (group I), 12 of which were delivered before 32 weeks (mean ± SD, 28.4 ± 3.1 weeks). Four of 22 women with cer-

TABLE 2.—Comparison of Perinatal Parameters Between Women With Short (Group I) and Long (Group II) Cervices

Characteristic	Group I	Group II	P
Cervical length, mm	22.8 ± 1.8	36.4 ± 2.1	<.001
Gestational age at measurement, wk	16.75 ± 2.1	15.96 ± 2.1	NS
Gestational age at delivery, wk	28.4 ± 1.6	32.8 ± 2.1	<.001
Birth weight, g	981 ± 79	1864 ± 231	<.001
Mean 5-min Apgar score	4.5 ± 2.1	8.1 ± 1.5	<.001
NICU admission	42/42	33/66	<.001

Values except NICU admission are mean ± SD.
Abbreviations: NS, Not significant; *NICU*, neonatal ICU.
(Courtesy of Maslovitz S, Hartoov J, Wolman I, et al: Cervical length in the early second trimester for detection of triplet pregnancies at risk for preterm birth. *J Ultrasound Med* 23:1187-1191, 2004. Publisher AIUM.)

vical length of greater than 25 mm (group II) had delivery before 32 weeks (mean, 30.1 ± 1.8 weeks). The mean gestational age at delivery for all parturients from group II was 33.1 ± 2.1 weeks ($P < .05$). Group I neonates had lower birth weights (972 versus 1889 g; $P < .001$) and higher rates of low 5-minute Apgar scores and neonatal intensive care unit admissions compared with group II neonates (Table 2). The sensitivity of a shorter cervix as a predictor of preterm labor was 75%, with specificity of 90%, a positive predictive value of 83%, and a negative predictive value of 81%.

Conclusions.—Cervical length of less than 25 mm at 14 to 20 weeks' gestation is associated with preterm delivery and adverse perinatal outcome in triplet pregnancies.

Impact of Ultrasound Cervical Length Assessment on Duration of Hospital Stay in the Clinical Management of Threatened Preterm Labor
Sanin-Blair J, Palacio M, Delgado J, et al (Universitat Autònoma de Barcelona; Universitat de Barcelona)
Ultrasound Obstet Gynecol 24:756-760, 2004   11–6

Objective.—To evaluate the impact of ultrasound cervical length measurement on duration of hospital stay in patients admitted for threatened preterm labor.

Study Design.—This was a prospective, comparative study in 294 patients with threatened preterm labor in three hospitalization units (Units A, B and C). In the first phase of the study (observational), cervical length was measured by transvaginal ultrasound, but managing physicians were blinded to the results. In the second phase (interventional), physicians from Unit A remained blinded to cervical length information, but Units B and C incorporated these data into their clinical management protocols. Early discharge was contemplated if the cervix measured 25 mm or more on admission (Unit B) or no changes were observed over 48 h (Unit C). Duration of hospital stay and delivery rates within 7 days and before 37 weeks' gestation were recorded.

Results.—Hospital stay was significantly reduced in Units B and C in the interventional phase, while no changes were observed in Unit A. Delivery rates within 7 days and before 37 weeks' gestation were similar in the three units during the two stages of the study.

Conclusion.—Routine use of ultrasound cervical length assessment in patients admitted with threatened preterm labor may reduce the duration of hospital stay without increasing the rate of preterm births. These data should be confirmed by means of an appropriately designed randomized clinical trial.

Sonographic Cervical Length in Singleton Pregnancies With Intact Membranes Presenting With Threatened Preterm Labor

Fuchs IB, Henrich W, Osthues K, et al (Virchow Clinic Charité, Berlin)
Ultrasound Obstet Gynecol 24:554-557, 2004   11–7

Objective.—Less than 10% of women presenting with preterm contractions progress to active labor and delivery. This study investigates whether cervical length measurements by ultrasound can discriminate between true and false labor in women presenting with threatened preterm labor.

Methods.—Cervical length was measured by transvaginal ultrasound in 253 women with singleton pregnancies presenting with painful uterine contractions at a median age of 31 (range, 24-35) weeks of gestation. Women presenting in active labor, defined by the presence of cervical dilatation of ≥3 cm, those with ruptured membranes and those that underwent prior or subsequent cervical cerclage were excluded from the study. The clinical management was determined by the attending obstetrician without taking into account the cervical length. Primary outcome of the study was delivery within 7 days of presentation based on the results of randomized studies on the use of tocolytics in women with preterm labor that reported a prolongation of pregnancy by 7 days.

Results.—Delivery within 7 days of presentation occurred in 21/253 (8.3%) pregnancies and this was inversely related to cervical length. Receiver-operating characteristics (ROC) curves established a cervical length of 15 mm as the most relevant cut-off level for the prediction of preterm delivery within 7 days. In 217 cases the cervical length was ≥15 mm and only four of these (1.8%) delivered within 7 days. In the 36 women with cervical length <15 mm, delivery occurred in 17 (47.2%) within 7 days. Logistic regression analysis demonstrated that significant independent contribution in the prediction of delivery within 7 days was provided by cervical length, contraction frequency at presentation, previous history of preterm delivery and vaginal bleeding. There was no significant contribution from gestation at presentation, ethnic origin, maternal age, parity, cigarette smoking or the administration of tocolysis, antibiotics or steroids. Similar results were shown in a subanalysis of 162 patients presenting at a gestational age below 32 weeks: 9/19 patients (47.4%) with a cervical length below 15 mm delivered within 7 days compared to 3/143 (2.1%) with a cervical length ≥15 mm. Univariate as well as multivariate analyses confirmed cervical length to be a significant independent predictor of delivery within 7 days in this population.

Conclusions.—Sonographic measurement of cervical length helps to avoid overdiagnosis of preterm labor in women with preterm contractions and intact membranes.

▶ Preterm delivery still accounts for the vast majority of perinatal morbidity and mortality in children born without congenital anomalies. Unfortunately, there are still no reliable clinical criteria to discriminate between true cheap preterm labor and harmless early contractions. Accordingly, overdiagnosis and subsequent overtreatment is a common problem. Furthermore, the prevalence of multifetal pregnancies has increased considerably in the last decade, and in addition to the other maternal and fetal morbidities associated with multifetal pregnancies, the frequency of preterm labor is very high. These 3 articles (Abstracts 11–5, 11–6, and 11–7) review various diagnostic interventions to assess the risk for preterm delivery. The article by Maslovitz and colleagues (Abstract 11–5) demonstrated that a cervical length of less than 25 mm between 14 and 20 weeks' gestation was associated with a higher likelihood of preterm delivery and adverse perinatal outcome in triplet pregnancies. Fuchs and colleagues (Abstract 11–6) found that sonographic measurement of cervical length in singleton pregnancies was an important factor in avoiding overdiagnosis of preterm labor in women with preterm contractions and intact membranes. Sanin-Blair and colleagues (Abstract 11–7) found that the use of US to measure cervical length in women admitted with threatened preterm labor reduced the duration of hospital stay without increasing the rate of preterm births. These articles all demonstrate that the judicious use of US to assess cervical length in a variety of women at increased risk for preterm labor and preterm delivery provides considerable clinical benefit in predicting which women will go on to experience preterm delivery, thus providing both clinical and economic benefit in the management of these patients.

H. P. van Geijn, MD, PhD

Increased Cardiac Atrial-to-Ventricular Length Ratio in the Fetal Four-Chamber View: A New Marker for Atrioventricular Septal Defects
Machlitt A, Heling K-S, Chaoui R (Humboldt-Univ, Berlin)
Ultrasound Obstet Gynecol 24:618-622, 2004   11–8

Objectives.—Atrioventricular septal defects (AVSDs) are the most common cardiac abnormality in fetuses with numerical chromosomal aberrations, in particular trisomy 21. The majority of AVSDs are not detected by routine ultrasound examination in pregnancy. We report two simple cardiac measurements that may substantially improve antenatal detection of AVSDs.

Methods.—Cross-sectional ultrasound images through the fetal thorax demonstrating the four-chamber plane of the heart were obtained in 123 normal fetuses between 10 and 38 weeks of gestation. Heart length was measured at the level of interventricular septum by placing the calipers on the epicardium at the apex of the heart and on the endocardium at the top of the atrium. Ventricular length was measured by shifting the atrial caliper to the crossing point of the ventricular septum and mitral valve. Atrial length was calculated as the difference between the heart length and ventricular length. Based on these measurements, the atrial-to-ventricular length (AVL) ratio was calculated. Data were compared to measurements from 29 consecutive fetuses with AVSD between 13 and 39 weeks of gestation.

Results.—In normal fetuses, the AVL ratio did not change with gestation and the mean AVL ratio was 0.47 (95% prediction interval 0.35 to 0.63). In the AVSD group, the mean AVL ratio was 0.77 (range, 0.59–0.99). If a cut-off value for the AVL ratio of 0.6 was chosen, the detection rate of AVSD was 86.2% at a 5.7% false-positive rate. For a 100% detection rate, the false-positive rate was 7.3%.

Conclusions.—The AVL ratio can accurately discriminate between hearts with AVSDs and normal cardiac anatomy. Incorporation of the AVL ratio measurement into routine antenatal ultrasonography may substantially improve the ability to diagnose AVSDs antenatally.

▶ The improving ability of US to detect fetal anomalies has been an important part of the changes in obstetric care over the past 2 decades. This study from Humboldt University in Berlin reports on the use of the AVL ratio to identify fetuses with AVSDs more accurately. Accordingly, the use of such measurements may make for more accurate US examinations and improve our ability to provide accurate information to clinicians and patients.

P. P. van den Berg, MD, PhD

Threshold Values of Maternal Blood Glucose in Early Diabetic Pregnancy: Prediction of Fetal Malformations
Wender-Ożegowska E, Wróbewska K, Zawiejska A, et al (KM Univ, Poznañ, Poland)
Acta Obstet Gynecol Scand 84:17-25, 2005   11–9

Background.—The prevention of congenital malformations in the newborns of diabetic mothers still constitutes one of the main problems in this group of patients.

Aim.—The aim of this study was to analyze the prevalence of fetal malformations in diabetic pregnancies, as well as detection of the cut-off points for the first-trimester glycemia levels, relating to diabetes-induced fetal malformations.

Methods.—The data for analysis were collected retrospectively from the case histories of diabetic pregnant women and their newborns, treated in our departments. For the evaluation of maternal diabetes control, the whole-day glycemia profiles as well as glycated hemoglobin (HbA_{1C}) levels were registered. To establish the glucose cut-off values for malformations, we have used receiver operating characteristic (ROC) curves for fasting, 1-hr, and 2-hr postprandial glucose levels. To determine how metabolic control influences the risk of giving birth to a malformed infant, we followed 198 newborns of diabetic mothers and 4700 infants born of healthy mothers (control group).

Results.—We detected malformations in the infants of 8.6% ($n = 17$) of diabetic mothers and 3.8% of the control (odds ratio: 2.35, 95% CI = 1.40-3.96). We compared this group of diabetic patients to another diabetic pregnancy group, analyzed over a period of 1988-93 ($n = 209$), in which 13 newborns (6.2%) manifested congenital malformations (odds ratio: 1.41, 95% CI = 0.67-2.99) (the difference was statistically insignificant). HbA_{1C} level

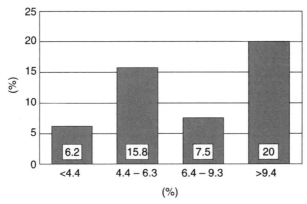

FIGURE 2.—Prevalence of fetal malformations, relating to maternal glycated hemoglobin levels measured up to 16th week of gestation ($n = 119$). (Courtesy of Wender-Ożegowska E, Wróbewska K, Zawiejska A, et al: Threshold values of maternal blood glucose in early diabetic pregnancy: Prediction of fetal malformations. *Acta Obstet Gynecol Scand* 84:17-25, 2005. Reprinted by permission of Blackwell Publishing.)

during organogenesis was not significantly higher in women whose infants were malformed. We proved, however, that the risk of malformations was higher, when HbA_{1C} value exceeded 9.3% (Fig 2). The malformation rate in diabetes classes D-H (according to White) was higher than in classes B and C, but the difference was not significant. A wide spectrum of anomalies has been observed in the newborns of diabetic mothers.

Conclusions.—Our results confirm the view that diabetic pregnancy, despite the improved metabolic control, is still a strong risk factor for alterations in fetal development, particularly in patients with a tendency to brittle

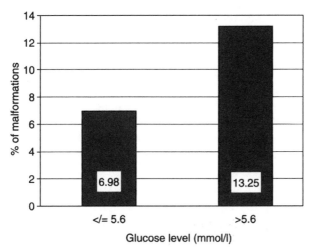

FIGURE 1.—The occurrence of fetal malformations in the study group related to mean diurnal glycemia levels measured up to 16th week of gestation ($n = 119$). (Courtesy of Wender-Ożegowska E, Wróbewska K, Zawiejska A, et al: Threshold values of maternal blood glucose in early diabetic pregnancy: Prediction of fetal malformations. *Acta Obstet Gynecol Scand* 84:17-25, 2005. Reprinted by permission of Blackwell Publishing.)

glycemia during first trimester of pregnancy. It seems that keeping fasting glucose levels in first trimester below 5.8 mmol/l and postprandial glucose levels below 9.1 mmol/l can contribute to decreasing number of fetal malformations in pregestational diabetes mellitus (PGDM) pregnancy (Fig 1). The ROC curves appear to be useful and adequate tool for the analysis of factors influencing fetal development in diabetic pregnancy.

▶ Despite improved evaluation and treatment of diabetic women, there seems to be no further decrease in the prevalence of congenital malformations in the newborns of these mothers. A large retrospective, hospital-based, case-control study of diabetic and control pregnancies was conducted by these authors. It revealed that more than twice as many congenital anomalies occurred in the newborns of diabetic mothers compared with controls. Clinical and epidemiologic studies suggest that metabolic disturbances in diabetic pregnancies detrimentally affect embryogenesis. This study showed clearly increased risks for congenital malformations in diabetic women with mean diurnal glycemia of greater than 5.5 mmol/L in early pregnancy. Additional ROC curve analysis showed that very strict glucose control during the whole day has to be achieved in order to avoid malformations. This is in line with other recent findings that in nonpregnant women, glucose levels, even in the normal through upper range, lead to a more than 4-fold increased risk of having an infant with spina bifida.[1,2] The HbA_{1c} concentration is a stable marker of the glucose status during the preceding 6 to 8 weeks. This study also showed an increased risk of congenital malformation when HbA_{1c} values were above 9.3%. Although the strength of the correlation between the HbA_{1c} concentrations in early pregnancy and the occurrence of congenital malformations in newborns has not been consistent, it should be stressed that glucose status, also by means of this biomarker, should be carefully controlled in early pregnancy. However, diabetic control before pregnancy should have intensive attention, as a large part of organogenesis has already taken place the moment a woman enters a prenatal care program. The most common malformations noted in diabetes mellitus are cardiovascular, followed by CNS, skeletal, and urogenital system malformations. These malformations are also sensitive to folate deficiency. Whether folic acid supplementation prevents malformations in diabetic pregnancies is not entirely clear but can be investigated in the United States where folic acid fortification has been carried out since 1998.

E. A. P. Steegers, MD, PhD

References

1. Groenen PMW, Klootwijk R, Schijvenaars MMVAP, et al: Spina bifida and genetic factors related to myoinositol, glucose and zinc. *Mol Genet Metab* 82:154-161, 2004.
2. Groenen PM, Van Rooij IA, Peer PG, et al: Low maternal dietary intakes of iron, magnesium, and niacin are associated with spina bifida in the offspring. *J Nutr* 134:1516-1522, 2004.

Pulmonary Hypoplasia: Prediction With Use of Ratio of MR Imaging-measured Fetal Lung Volume to US-estimated Fetal Body Weight

Tanigaki S, Miyakoshi K, Tanaka M, et al (Keio Univ, Tokyo)

Radiology 232:767-772, 2004   11–10

Purpose.—To determine the ratio of fetal lung volume (FLV) to fetal body weight (FBW) by using ultrasonography (US) and magnetic resonance (MR) imaging and to evaluate the usefulness of this ratio in predicting pulmonary hypoplasia (PH) in fetuses at high risk.

Materials and Methods.—MR imaging lung volumetry and US biometry were performed in 90 fetuses at 25-39 weeks gestation. In the control group of 73 fetuses, normal lung development was confirmed at neonatal follow-up and the normative ratio of MR imaging–measured FLV to US-estimated FBW (FLV/FBW) was determined. The high-risk group included 17 fetuses at risk for PH. The FLV/FBW was compared between the control and high-risk groups and with US parameters for predicting the development of PH in the high-risk group. Measurements 2 or more standard deviations below the mean control group measurement were considered abnormal. Comparisons of the FLV/FBW between groups were made by using the Student *t* test. The association between development of PH and measurement of each parameter was analyzed by using the Fisher exact probability test.

Results.—In the control group, the FLV/FBW decreased with gestational age during the third trimester and had a normal distribution (mean ratio, 0.028 mL/g; range, 0.015-0.444 mL/g) (Fig 3). The mean FLV/FBW for the nine fetuses with PH (0.012 mL/g ± 0.008) was significantly lower ($P < .001$)

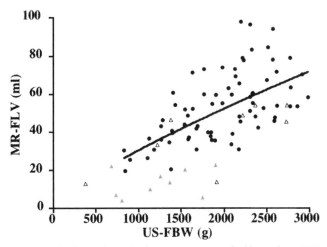

FIGURE 3.—Scatterplot shows relationship between MR imaging fetal lung volume (*FLV*) and US fetal body weight (*FBW*). *Dots* represent 73 fetuses at low risk for pulmonary hypoplasia; *open triangles*, 8 fetuses at high risk but without pulmonary hypoplasia; and *gray triangles*, 9 fetuses at high risk and with pulmonary hypoplasia. MR imaging FLV correlated with US FBW in fetuses at low risk ($r = 0.59$). (Courtesy of Tanigaki S, Miyakoshi K, Tanaka M, et al: Pulmonary hypoplasia: Prediction with use of ratio of MR imaging–measured fetal lung volume to US-estimated fetal body weight. *Radiology* 232:767-772, 2004. Copyright 2004, Radiological Society of North America.)

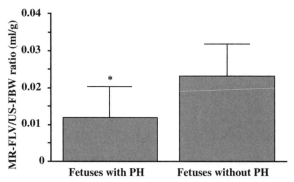

FIGURE 7.—Graph illustrates comparison of mean fetal lung volume/fetal body weight (*FLV/FBW*) values (±standard deviations) between fetuses in the high-risk group with and fetuses in the the high-risk group without pulmonary hypoplasia (*PH*). *Asterisk* = *P* < .05 for difference in FLV/FBW between the two groups. The FLV/FBW was significantly lower in the fetuses in the high-risk group with pulmonary hypoplasia than in those in the high-risk group without the abnormality. (Courtesy of Tanigaki S, Miyakoshi K, Tanaka M, et al: Pulmonary hypoplasia: Prediction with use of ratio of MR imaging–measured fetal lung volume to US-estimated fetal body weight. *Radiology* 232:767-772, 2004. Copyright 2004, Radiological Society of North America.)

than that for the control group (0.028 mL/g ± 0.007) (Fig 7). Fetuses with abnormal FLV/FBW values were at significantly greater risk (*P* < .05) for PH development. Abnormal FLV/FBW values had higher diagnostic accuracy than abnormal US parameters. Sensitivity of the FLV/FBW was 89% (eight of nine fetuses); specificity, 88% (seven of eight fetuses); positive predictive value, 89% (eight of nine fetuses); negative predictive value, 88% (seven of eight fetuses); and accuracy, 88% (15 of 17 fetuses).

Conclusion.—The FLV/FBW reflects the adequacy of intrauterine lung growth and can help predict PH.

▶ This article from multiple investigators at Keio University in Tokyo shows that the ratio of FLV to FBW was an accurate measurement of intrauterine lung growth and development and was a sensitive predictor of PH. The authors utilize MRI to assess FLV and applied it to a US-estimated measurement of FBW. The ability to detect the presence of development of fetal PH is an important part of perinatal management and parental counseling because neonates with PH require intensive therapy immediately after birth. In this regard, pregnancies at increased risk for fetal PH can now be more accurately evaluated by this imaging "cocktail." It is a universally held belief that the ability to obtain a more accurate assessment of at-risk fetuses for PH will lead to considerably improved perinatal outcomes.

H. P. van Geijn, MD, PhD

Ultrasonographic Evaluation of Lower Uterine Segment Thickness in Patients of Previous Cesarean Section
Sen S, Malik S, Salhan S (Vardhman Mahavir Med College, New Delhi, India)
Int J Gynaecol Obstet 87:215-219, 2004   11–11

Objective.—To evaluate by ultrasonography, the lower uterine segment thickness of women with a previous cesarean delivery and determine a critical thickness above which safe vaginal delivery is predictable.

Methods.—A prospective observational study of 71 antenatal women with previous cesarean delivery and 50 controls was carried out. Transabdominal and transvaginal ultrasonography were used in both groups to evaluate lower uterine segment thickness. The obstetric outcome in patients with successful vaginal birth and intraoperative findings in women undergoing cesarean delivery were correlated with lower segment thickness.

Results.—The overall vaginal birth after cesarean section (VBAC) was 46.5% and VBAC success rate was 63.5%, the incidence of dehiscence was 2.82%, and there were no uterine ruptures. There was a 96% correlation between transabdominal ultrasonography with magnification and transvaginal ultrasonography. The critical cutoff value for safe lower segment thickness, derived from the receiver operator characteristic curve, was 2.5 mm.

Conclusion.—Ultrasonographic evaluation permits better assessment of the risk of scar complication intrapartum, and could allow for safer management of delivery.

► In an effort to predict the chance of rupture of a uterine scar, it becomes more and more in use to measure uterine wall thickness. Sen et al showed that all control women and all women with no dehiscence at cesarean section had a lower uterine segment of more than 2 mm. This suggests that it is safe to offer women a trial of labor if the lower uterine segment after a cesarean section is 2.5 mm or more. One may question, however, if the study has the power to guarantee safety. Also, one may question just how unsafe it really is to attempt vaginal delivery if the uterine segment is 2 mm or less. The true added value of US in the prediction of dehiscence or rupture of a uterine scar remains to be determined.

F. K. Lotgering, MD, PhD

12 Maternal/Fetal Therapy

Efficacy of an Intervention to Prevent Excessive Gestational Weight Gain
Olson CM, Strawderman MS, Reed RG (Cornell Univ, Ithaca, NY; Research Inst Basset Healthcare, Cooperstown, NY)
Am J Obstet Gynecol 191:530-536, 2004   12–1

Objective.—This study was undertaken to evaluate the efficacy of an intervention directed at preventing excessive gestational weight gain.

Study Design.—Healthy pregnant women with normal and overweight early pregnancy body mass index were monitored from early pregnancy until 1-year postpartum. One hundred seventy-nine women in the intervention group had their gestational weight gains monitored by health care providers and also received by-mail patient education. Three hundred eighty-one women formed an historical control group. The proportions in each group gaining more weight in pregnancy than is recommended and retaining more than 2.27 kg at 1-year postpartum were compared using logistic regression analysis.

Results.—Low-income women who received the intervention had a significantly reduced risk of excessive gestational weight gain (odds ratio [OR] = 0.41, 95% CI = 0.20-0.81). Overweight women within this income subgroup were at significantly reduced risk of retaining more than 2.27 kg (OR = 0.24, 95% CI = 0.07-0.89).

Conclusion.—The intervention appeared to reduce the risk of excessive gestational weight gain only in the low-income subgroup.

▶ Excess gestational weight gain can lead to clinical morbidity. This study assessed the efficacy of an interventional approach to prevent excessive weight gain during pregnancy. The intervention included clinical counseling and patient education components, including reading materials. It was seen that low-income pregnant patients benefited the most from this intervention by reducing the likelihood of excessive maternal weight gain. Overweight women in this group also reduced their risk of gaining more weight. The social and psychological variables that factor into weight gain need to be further studied; this study is a good first step toward that goal.

S. H. Ural, MD

Association of Fish and Fish Liver Oil Intake in Pregnancy With Infant Size at Birth Among Women of Normal Weight Before Pregnancy in a Fishing Community

Thorsdottir I, Birgisdottir BE, Halldorsdottir S, et al (Univ of Iceland, Reykjavik, Iceland)

Am J Epidemiol 160:460-465, 2004   12–2

Abstract.—This 1998 study investigated the association between intake of fish and fish oil during pregnancy and full-term infants' size at birth in an Icelandic fishing community. Healthy women aged 20-40 years of normal weight before pregnancy (body mass index: 19.5-25.5 kg/m^2 and at 38-43 weeks of gestation were selected randomly. Information on infant size at birth was collected from maternity records. Intake of fish and fish oil in pregnancy was ascertained (n = 491, 80.1%) by using a validated, focused, food frequency questionnaire. Infants of women in the lowest quartile of fish consumption weighed less (p = 0.036), were shorter (p < 0.001), and had a smaller head circumference (p < 0.001) at birth than those of women consuming higher amounts of fish. Infants of women in the highest quartile of fish oil intake ($\geq$1 tablespoon (11 ml)/day), consuming threefold the recommended dietary allowance of vitamin A and twofold that of vitamin D, were shorter (p = 0.036) and had a smaller head circumference (p = 0.003) than those of women consuming less. Infant size at birth increased with fish consumption, especially for women in the lower quartiles of consumption. Smaller birth size was linked to the highest levels of fish oil intake. Constituents of fish and fish oil might affect birth size differently depending on the amount consumed.

▶ This interesting study focused on the association between fish and fish liver oil consumption and birthweight. A validated, focused, food frequency questionnaire was used. If women were in the lower quartile of consumption, their neonates appeared to have less birthweight, height, and head circumference. Frequency of fish consumption was positively associated with infant birth length and head circumference. Interestingly, a high consumption level of fish liver oil was associated with smaller babies. These data appear contradictory in comparison to previous data. This may be because multiple variables play into birthweight/height and head circumference, although food intake may also play a central role.

S. H. Ural, MD

Reproductive Outcomes After Pregnancy Complicated by Maternal-Fetal Surgery

Wilson RD, Johnson MP, Flake AW, et al (Children's Hosp of Philadelphia; Univ of Pennsylvania, Philadelphia)
Am J Obstet Gynecol 191:1430-1436, 2004   12–3

Objective.—The reproductive outcomes for women after the pregnancy complicated by maternal-fetal surgery were evaluated to obtain evidence-based information for prenatal risk counseling.

Study Design.—The retrospective review identified 83 women with maternal-fetal surgery from a single institution (1996-2002). These women were sent a consent form and a questionnaire to document postoperative problems, fertility, obstetric outcomes, and psychosocial concerns in pregnancy after the index fetal therapy. Institutional Review Board approval was obtained from Committee for Protection of Human Subjects.

Results.—The total return rate was 55 (66%). The pregnancy rate was 62% (18% spontaneous abortion, 24% preterm delivery, and 58% term delivery). Complications were reported in 12 of 34 pregnancies (35%), including uterine dehiscence/rupture (12%/6%), cesarean hysterectomy (3%), and antepartum hemorrhage requiring transfusion (9%) (Table 2).

Conclusion.—The reproductive outcome of uterine dehiscence, rupture, and hysterectomy was 12%, 6%, and 3%, respectively, after a pregnancy

---

TABLE 2.—Subsequent Pregnancy (After Maternal-Fetal Surgery): Total 34

No concerns	16 (47%)
Abnormal outcome (single	12 (35%)
entry per pregnancy)	
Uterine	7 (21%)
Rupture/dehiscence (6)*†‡§‖¶	(18%)
Cesarean hysterectomy (1)#	(3%)
Hemorrhage + transfusion§#**	3
PTL/D(35,* 33,‡ 35,§ 33,‖ 24,¶ 35,†† 33‡‡ wks)	7
(preterm labor/delivery)	
Hypertension (pre or postnatal)	2
Miscarriage	6 (18%)
Postlung maturity amniocentesis labor	1
Congenital anomalies	
Congenital heart disease	1

*35 wks with PTL/PTD and dehiscence at repeat cesarean section; recommend no further pregnancies.
†37 wks with dehiscence at repeat cesarean section.
‡33 wks with PTL/PTD and dehiscence at repeat cesarean section.
§35 wks with PTL/PTD and dehiscence at repeat cesarean section; placenta was adherent to fetal surgery scar.
‖33 wks with PTL/PTD with rupture at repeat cesarean section; recommend no further pregnancies.
¶24 wks with PTL/PTD and rupture at repeat cesarean section with neonatal death.
#37 wks with repeat cesarean section with hemorrhage and transfusion requiring hysterectomy.
**37 wks with abruptio placenta, hemorrhage, and transfusion for 2 assisted reproductive pregnancies in the same patient.
††35 wks with PTL/PTD, repeat cesarean section and twins.
‡‡33 wks with PTL and at 37 wks repeat cesarean section.
Abbreviations: PTL, Preterm labor; *PTD*, preterm delivery.
(Courtesy of Wilson RD, Johnson MP, Flake AW, et al: Reproductive outcomes after pregnancy complicated by maternal-fetal surgery. *Am J Obstet Gynecol* 191:1430-1436, 2004. Copyright 2004 by Elsevier. Reprinted by permission.)

complicated by maternal-fetal surgery. The uterine rupture rate is similar to the rupture rate after "classical" cesarean section (4%-9%).

▶ Intrauterine surgery with hysterotomy is controversial and generally available only in a research setting. Despite such settings, the evaluation of benefits and risks of fetal surgery is mostly limited to index pregnancies, while from a methodological point of view it would be preferable to assess lifetime reproductive performance after such an intervention. As shown in Table 2, the main risks in a subsequent pregnancy are related to preterm labor and uterine dehiscence (12%) or rupture (6%). These figures should be included in the counseling of potential candidates for fetal surgery.

F. K. Lotgering, MD, PhD

Fetal Head Biometry Following *in-utero* Repair of Myelomeningocele
Danzer E, Johnson MP, Wilson RD, et al (Univ of Pennsylvania, Philadelphia)
Ultrasound Obstet Gynecol 24:606-611, 2004   12–4

Objective.—To evaluate the impact of prenatal myelomeningocele repair on fetal head biometry.

Methods.—Fifty fetuses underwent open fetal myelomeningocele repair at our institution between January 1998 and July 2002. All had serial head circumference (HC) and lateral ventricular diameter (VD) measurements taken preoperatively and weekly for 8 weeks after repair. Cortical index (CI) was defined as HC/VD. Measurements were compared with gestational age-matched values from nomograms. One-sample t-test, ANOVA and repeated measures analysis were used to assess HC, VD and CI after fetal repair.

Results.—Preoperatively, the HC in fetuses with myelomeningocele was smaller than control values (186.4 vs. 198.8 mm, $P = 0.0004$). Eight weeks' postoperatively this difference had resolved (293 vs. 301.6 mm, $P = 0.76$). The mean increase in CI after repair was 20% ($P = 0.02$) compared with the predicted 51% in normal cases. The average increase in VD was 3.9 mm (38.8%, $P < 0.001$).

Conclusions.—Mid-gestational repair of myelomeningocele alters fetal head growth. Increased CI suggests HC changes are not due to ventriculomegaly alone.

Balloon Dilation of Severe Aortic Stenosis in the Fetus: Potential for Prevention of Hypoplastic Left Heart Syndrome Candidate Selection, Technique, and Results of Successful Intervention
Tworetzky W, Wilkins-Haug L, Jennings RW, et al (Harvard Med School, Boston)
Circulation 110:2125-2131, 2004   12–5

Background.—Preventing the progression of fetal aortic stenosis (AS) to hypoplastic left heart syndrome (HLHS) requires identification of fetuses with salvageable left hearts who would progress to HLHS if left untreated, a successful in utero valvotomy, and demonstration that a successful valvotomy promotes left heart growth in utero. Fetuses meeting the first criterion are undefined, and previous reports of fetal AS dilation have not evaluated the impact of intervention on in utero growth of left heart structures.

Method and Results.—We offered fetal AS dilation to 24 mothers whose fetuses had AS. At least 3 echocardiographers assigned a high probability that all 24 fetuses would progress to HLHS if left untreated. Twenty (21 to 29 weeks' gestation) underwent attempted AS dilation, with technical success in 14. Ideal fetal positioning for cannula puncture site and course of the needle (with or without laparotomy) proved to be necessary for procedural success. Serial fetal echocardiograms after intervention demonstrated growth arrest of the left heart structures in unsuccessful cases and in those who declined the procedure, while ongoing left heart growth was seen in successful cases. Resumed left heart growth led to a 2-ventricle circulation at birth in 3 babies.

Conclusions.—Fetal echocardiography can identify midgestation fetuses with AS who are at high risk for developing HLHS. Timely and successful aortic valve dilation requires ideal fetal and cannula positioning, prevents left heart growth arrest, and may result in normal ventricular anatomy and function at birth.

Creation of an Atrial Septal Defect in Utero for Fetuses With Hypoplastic Left Heart Syndrome and Intact or Highly Restrictive Atrial Septum
Marshall AC, van der Velde ME, Tworetzky W, et al (Harvard Med School, Boston; CS Mott Children's Hosp, Ann Arbor, Mich)
Circulation 110:253-258, 2004   12–6

Background.—Infants born with hypoplastic left heart syndrome and an intact or highly restrictive atrial septum face a neonatal mortality of at least 48% despite early postnatal left atrial decompression and palliative surgery. Prenatal left atrial decompression has been suggested as a means of improving these outcomes. This study reports the feasibility of fetal catheterization to create an interatrial communication and describes technical considerations.

Method and Results.—Seven fetuses at 26 to 34 weeks' gestation with hypoplastic left heart syndrome and intact or highly restrictive atrial septum underwent attempted prenatal intervention. Under ultrasound guidance, the atrial septum was approached with a needle introduced percutaneously from the maternal abdominal surface. In 6 of 7 fetuses, the atrial septum was successfully perforated, with balloon dilation of this iatrogenic defect resulting in a small but persistent interatrial communication. There were no maternal complications. One fetus died after the procedure. The remaining fetuses were liveborn at term, although 4 died as neonates.

Conclusions.—Ultrasound-guided fetal atrial septoplasty consisting of septal puncture and balloon dilation is feasible and can be performed percutaneously to minimize maternal risk. Although we have not demonstrated any positive clinical impact to date, it is our hope that further technical evolution will ultimately enable prenatal left atrial decompression and improvement of outcomes in fetuses with hypoplastic left heart syndrome and intact atrial septum.

▶ The use of in utero surgery to treat a wide variety of fetal abnormalities has gained popularity in the past decade. In general, such approaches have been characterized by high rates of fetal loss with little to no benefit observed for many of the conditions chosen for treatment. However, improvements in maternal and fetal surgical techniques have begun to result in better outcomes for some fetal conditions. These 3 studies report on in utero surgical approaches to specific fetal anomalies. Danzer et al from Children's Hospital of Philadelphia found that mid-gestational repair of myelomeningocele altered fetal head growth, thus suggesting that HC changes in such cases are not due to ventriculomegaly alone. Tworetzky et al reported on the use of fetal echocardiography to prospectively identify fetuses at high risk for developing HLHS so that balloon dilation of the aortic valve could be considered. This group was able to successfully perform balloon dilation in 14 of 20 cases with ongoing left heart growth observed in the successful cases with 2-ventricle circulation observed at birth for 3 babies. Marshall et al reported on the use of an in utero US-guided fetal atrial septoplasty in fetuses with HLHS. Although the authors were unable to report a positive clinical effect of this procedure, they did find the procedure was able to be accomplished in a percutaneous fashion to minimize maternal risk.

These reports present continuing updates on the use of in utero surgical techniques for fetuses with structural abnormalities. Unfortunately, the considerable limitations of these techniques are well documented. Randomized studies such as the Management of Myelomeningocele Study trial will provide stronger evidence concerning the impact of these procedures; however, it is clear that such procedures will not likely be a part of routine care for the foreseeable future.

P. P. van den Berg, MD, PhD

13 Operative Obstetrics

The Impact of Occiput Posterior Fetal Head Position on the Risk of Anal Sphincter Injury in Forceps-Assisted Vaginal Deliveries
Benavides L, Wu JM, Hundley AF, et al (Univ of North Carolina at Chapel Hill)
Am J Obstet Gynecol 192:1702-1706, 2005   13–1

Objective.—A forceps-assisted vaginal delivery is a well-recognized risk factor for anal sphincter injury. Some studies have shown that occiput posterior (OP) fetal head position is also associated with an increased risk for third- or fourth-degree lacerations. The objective of this study was to assess whether OP position confers an incrementally increased risk for anal sphincter injury above that present with forceps deliveries.

Study Design.—This was a retrospective cohort study of 588 singleton, cephalic, forceps-assisted vaginal deliveries performed at our institution between January 1996 and October 2003. Maternal demographics, labor and delivery characteristics, and neonatal factors were examined. Statistical analysis consisted of univariate statistics, Student t test, χ^2, and logistic regression.

Results.—The prevalence of occiput anterior (OA) and OP positions was 88.4% and 11.6%, respectively. The groups were similar in age, marital status, body mass index, use of epidural, frequency of inductions, episiotomies, and shoulder dystocias. The OA group had a higher frequency of rotational forceps (16.2% vs 5.9%, $P = .03$), greater birth weights (3304 ± 526 g vs 3092 ± 777 g, $P = .004$), and a larger percentage of white women (48.8% vs 34.3%, $P = .04$). Overall, 35% of forceps deliveries resulted in a third- or fourth-degree laceration. Anal sphincter injury occurred significantly more often in the OP group compared with the OA group (51.5% vs 32.9%, $P = .003$), giving an odds ratio of 2.2 (CI: 1.3-3.6) (Table 3). In a logistic regression model that controlled for occiput posterior position, maternal body mass index, race, length of second stage, episiotomy, birth weight, and rotational forceps, OP head position was 3.1 (CI: 1.6-6.2) times more likely to be associated with anal sphincter injury than OA head position.

Conclusion.—Forceps-assisted vaginal deliveries have been associated with a greater risk for anal sphincter injury. Within this population of forceps deliveries, an OP position further increases the risk of third- or fourth-degree lacerations when compared with an OA position.

TABLE 3.—Odds Ratio for Severe Anal Sphincter Laceration

Characteristic	Unadjusted OR (95% CI)	Adjusted OR (95% CI)
OP position	2.2 (1.3-3.6)	3.1 (1.6-6.2)
BMI	1.0 (0.98-1.03)	1.0 (0.97-1.04)
Race*		
White	1.3 (0.93-1.8)	2.3 (1.1-4.5)
Hispanic	1.0 (0.7-1.5)	0.6 (0.3-1.4)
Other	1.3 (.91-1.9)	4.0 (1.6-9.8)
Length of second stage (h)	1.3 (1.2-1.5)	1.3 (1.1-1.5)
Episiotomy	2.4 (1.5-3.8)	3.1 (1.6-5.8)
Rotational forceps	0.8 (0.5-1.4)	0.96 (0.5-1.9)
Birth weight (kg)	1.8 (1.3-2.6)	1.3 (0.8-2.1)
Neonatal head circumference (cm)	1.2 (1.1-1.3)	1.1 (.99-1.3)

* Reference group is African American.
(Courtesy of Benavides L, Wu JM, Hundley AF, et al: The impact of occiput posterior fetal head position on the risk of anal sphincter injury in forceps-assisted vaginal deliveries. *Am J Obstet Gynecol* 192:1702-1706. Copyright 2005 by Elsevier.)

▶ The association of vaginal delivery with a variety of urogenital problems is becoming better understood by obstetricians as well as gynecologists. In this study from the University of North Carolina at Chapel Hill, investigators found that although forceps-assisted vaginal deliveries have always been associated with a greater risk for anal sphincter injury, the performance of this operative maneuver with the fetus presenting in an OP position further increased the risk of a third- or fourth-degree laceration when compared with a fetus presenting in an OA position. Such studies provide important information that can be used by obstetricians in assessing proper management of labor and delivery and facilitating optimal care for this pregnancy and for the patient's future life.

L. P. Shulman, MD

The Effect of Placental Removal Method and Site of Uterine Repair on Postcesarean Endometritis and Operative Blood Loss

Baksu A, Kalan A, Ozkan A, et al (Şişli Etfal Training and Research Hosp, Istanbul, Turkey)
Acta Obstet Gynecol Scand 84:266-269, 2005   13–2

Background.—Our purpose was to determine whether blood loss during cesarean section and postoperative endometritis rate were associated with the method of placental removal and site of uterine repair.

Methods.—This prospective randomized study involved 840 women who underwent cesarean section. The patients were grouped into four: (1) manual placental delivery + exteriorized uterine repair; (2) spontaneous placental delivery + exteriorized uterine repair; (3) manual placental delivery + *in situ* uterine repair; (4) spontaneous placental delivery + *in situ* uterine repair. Patients were excluded if they had received intrapartum antibiotics, had chorioamnionitis, required an emergency cesarean hysterectomy, had rupture of membranes for more than 12 hr, had bleeding diathesis, and had abnormal placentation or prior postpartum hemorrhage. The main outcome measures were postoperative hemoglobin and hematocrit values, and postcesarean endometritis.

Results.—There were no statistically significant differences in mean maternal age, parity, gestational age, presence and duration of membrane rupture and number of vaginal examinations between the four groups. The decrease in postoperative hemoglobin ($P < 0.05$) and hematocrit ($P < 0.001$) was significantly greater in the manual removal groups (groups 1 and 3) than in the spontaneous expulsion groups (groups 2 and 4) at 48 hr postoperatively. The incidence of postoperative endometritis was significantly higher in manual removal groups (15.2%) (groups 1 and 3) than in spontaneous groups (5.7%) (groups 2 and 4) ($P < 0.05$).

Conclusions.—Manual removal of the placenta at cesarean delivery results in more operative blood loss and a higher incidence of postcesarean endometritis.

▶ Historically, obstetricians were taught to manually remove the placenta to shorten the time the placenta remained in situ and in so doing, decrease blood loss. Interestingly, more recent data suggest just the opposite. By allowing the placental bed vessels to spasm before placental separation rather than manually removing the placenta and with the vessels still dilated, blood loss may be decreased. This study is the largest prospective study to date on this topic. Patients were roughly divided into those with manual placental removal versus spontaneous placental delivery, with each group further divided into in situ versus exteriorization of the uterus for repair. The results confirm previous studies that have shown a greater blood loss with manual placental removal[1,2], as well as higher endometritis rate.

V. A. M. Givens, MD

References

1. Wilkinson C, Enkin MW: Manual removal of placenta at caesarean section. *Cochrane Database Syst Rev* 2:CD00130, 2000.
2. Morales M, Ceysens G, Jastrow N, et al: Spontaneous delivery or manual removal of the placenta during caesarean section: A randomised controlled trial. *BJOG* 111:908-912, 2004.

Neonatal Impact of Elective Repeat Cesarean Delivery at Term: A Comment on Patient Choice Cesarean Delivery
Fogelson NS, Menard MK, Hulsey T, et al (Med Univ of South Carolina, Charleston)
Am J Obstet Gynecol 192:1433-1436, 2005   13–3

Background.—In clinical reasoning regarding the benefits of patient-choice cesarean section, the risks and benefits for both mother and child must be considered. The potential maternal benefits of patient-choice cesarean delivery have been described, but there have been no direct comparisons of neonatal outcomes of elective cesarean to outcomes of uncomplicated pregnancies intending to deliver vaginally. It has been reported that infants delivered to scheduled repeat cesarean have an increased risk of pulmonary hypertension, transient tachypnea of the newborn, and respiratory distress. The purpose of this study was to compare neonatal outcomes of pregnancies delivered by elective repeat cesarean delivery with the outcomes of uncomplicated pregnancies of mothers intending to delivery vaginally.

Methods.—A retrospective cohort study was conducted to describe the neonatal outcomes of term uncomplicated pregnancies. Neonates of mothers intending to deliver vaginally (3134 neonates) were compared with neonates born by elective repeat cesarean delivery before labor (117 neonates).

Results.—Infants born by elective repeat cesarean were more frequently admitted to advanced-care units than infants born to mothers who intended to deliver vaginally. The rate of admission to an advanced care nursery was 14.5% in the elective cesarean group versus 4.1% in the intended vaginal group. Neonatal admissions to the intensive care unit occurred at a rate of 3.4% in the elective cesarean group versus 1.2% in the intended vaginal group. Surfactant use and need for intubation in the nursery were statistically similar for the two groups, as were Apgar scores at 1 and 5 minutes. The need for intravenous medications and volume expanders were also similar between groups, but oxygen was used at resuscitation more frequently in the cesarean group.

Conclusions.—The decision to undergo elective cesarean delivery appeared to have a negative effect on immediate neonatal outcomes. Patients considering elective cesarean delivery should be counseled as to the potential adverse effects on the neonate as well as potential adverse maternal effects.

▶ Elective repeat cesarean section is an obstetrical management issue that affects almost every obstetrician. Although much has been written concerning its impact on maternal health and well being, there is little information concerning neonatal outcomes in neonates born to women undergoing elective cesarean section. In this study from the Medical University of South Carolina, the authors found that neonates born by elective repeat cesarean section were more likely to be admitted to advanced care nurseries than children born to mothers intending to deliver vaginally. Such information is critical for the counseling of women who are considering obstetrical management options after undergoing a prior cesarean section.

H. N. Lafeber, MD, PhD

Umbilical Arterial pH <7.00 in Newborns Delivered by Nonelective Cesarean Delivery: Risk Factors and Peripartum Outcomes

Chauhan SP, Magann EF, Bufin L, et al (Spartanburg Regional Med Ctr, SC; Univ of Western Australia, Perth; Univ of Mississippi, Jackson)
Am J Perinatol 21:281-287, 2004   13–4

Background.—Umbilical arterial pH <7.00 is associated with increased neonatal morbidity and mortality. The prevalence of pathological acidosis is 0.3% to 1.9%, and acidosis has been linked to stillbirth, unexplained seizures, hypoxic ischemic encephalopathy, other end-organ failure, and neonatal death. Previous studies have reported an increased rate of cesarean delivery among patients with low pH, but there have been few studies of antecedent risk factors and peripartum complications associated with cesarean delivery and abnormal pH. The purposes of this study were to identify the antepartum complications and intrapartum factors associated with nonelective cesarean delivery and pathologic acidosis and to describe the neonatal course among women with pH <7.00.

Methods.—In this case-control study, parturients who delivered by nonelective cesarean delivery and had a neonate with a pH <7.00 were compared with the next 4 patients who delivered abdominally but had a newborn with a normal pH.

Results.—Among 45 newborns with pH <7.00, the rate of cesarean delivery for nonreassuring fetal heart rate was significantly more common among the cases (56%) than in the control group (16%). The rates of end-organ failure and neonatal death were similar for both groups. Although newborns with pH <7.00 were significantly more likely to have cesarean delivery for nonreassuring fetal heart rate patterns and to be admitted to the neonatal intensive care unit, there was no method for identification of these patients until the abnormalities were manifest in tracing.

Conclusions.—At present there are no clinically useful predictors of patients who will require cesarean delivery and will deliver a newborn with umbilical arterial pH <7.00. Most newborns with pathological acidosis who had cesarean delivery will survive and will not show evidence of end-organ damage.

▶ Umbilical artery pH values less than 7.00 are associated with increased neonatal morbidity and mortality. pH values less than 7.00 have also been associated with an increased frequency of nonelective cesarean delivery. The authors of this paper sought to identify antepartum complications and intrapartum factors associated with nonelective cesarean delivery and fetal acidosis. This study shows that there are no clinically useful predictors of patients who will require cesarean section and deliver a newborn with an umbilical artery pH of less than 7.00. Further studies are needed to better identify women at increased risk for adverse neonatal outcomes and develop more effective approaches to prevent neonatal compromise.

H. N. Lafeber, MD, PhD

Systematic Review of the Incidence and Consequences of Uterine Rupture in Women With Previous Caesarean Section

Guise J-M, McDonagh MS, Osterweil P, et al (Oregon Health & Science Univ, Portland)

BMJ 329:1-7, 2004   13–5

Background.—Over the past 2 decades labor has been encouraged for women who have had a previous cesarean delivery. However, recent studies showing that both mother and fetus may be a greater risk than previously thought, largely because of the risk of uterine rupture, have renewed controversy regarding the safety of vaginal birth after cesarean section. The incidence and consequences of uterine rupture in women who have previously delivered by cesarean section were evaluated.

Methods.—A systematic review was conducted using MEDLINE, HealthSTAR, Cochrane Database of Systematic Reviews, Cochrane Controlled Trials Register, National Centre for Reviews and Dissemination, reference lists, and national experts.

Results.—The review included 568 full-text articles to identify 71 potentially eligible studies, 21 of which were rated at least fair in quality. Compared with elective repeat cesarean delivery, trial of labor increased the risk of uterine rupture by 2.7 per 1000 cases. No maternal deaths were related to rupture. For women attempting vaginal delivery, the additional risk of perinatal death from rupture of a uterine scar was 1.4 per 10,000, and the additional risk of hysterectomy was 3.4 per 10,000. The rates of asymptomatic uterine rupture in trial of labor and elective repeat cesarean section were not significantly different.

Conclusions.—The literature is somewhat imprecise and inconsistent regarding uterine rupture. However, the indication from existing studies is that 370 elective cesarean deliveries would need to be performed to prevent 1 symptomatic uterine rupture.

▶ This systematic review by Guise et al is important from a medicolegal point of view. It confirms that symptoms of uterine rupture are more common in women undergoing trial of labor compared with planned cesarean delivery, but the additional risk is less than previously perceived. For every 1000 women attempting trial of labor, there would be 2.7 additional symptomatic uterine ruptures, 0.14 perinatal deaths related to rupture, and 0.34 hysterectomies related to rupture. Guise et al excluded from the review the high-impact study of Lydon-Rochelle et al[1] because of its methodologic limitations. Lydon-Rochelle et al reported a particularly high risk of uterine rupture associated with the use of prostaglandins (relative risk, 15.6; 95% confidence interval, 8.1-30). In contrast, Guise et al conclude that the question whether prostaglandins really increase the risk of uterine rupture is still open to debate.

F. K. Lotgering, MD, PhD

Reference

1. Lydon-Rochelle M, Holt VL, Easterling TR, et al: Risk of uterine rupture during labor among women with a prior cesarean delivery. *N Engl J Med* 345:3-8, 2001.

Successful Conservative Management of Placenta Previa Accreta During Cesarean Section

Lam H, Pun TC, Lam PW (Queen Mary Hosp, HKSAR, China)
Int J Gynecol Obstet 86:31-32, 2004   13–6

Background.—Conservative management of accreta has been reported with success after vaginal delivery. This case report described a successful use of conservative management in a patient with placenta previa accreta. This approach should be an option at the time of cesarean section for patients at risk for placenta previa, particularly when the patient wants to retain the uterus.

Case Report.—A 39-year-old gravida 5 para 3 woman with 2 previous lower segment cesarean deliveries was diagnosed with anterior placenta previa accreta. US examination showed the absence of a normal subplacental sonulucent layer, and the anterior lower uterine wall was deeply invaded by the placenta. The patient was strongly motivated to keep the uterus, so an anecdotal approach was selected. The placenta was left in situ with the cord tied close to its insertion during emergency lower segment cesarean section at 36 weeks, and a healthy infant weighing 2.9 kg was delivered. The patient received 3 U of blood and prophylactic broad-spectrum antibiotics. An MRI

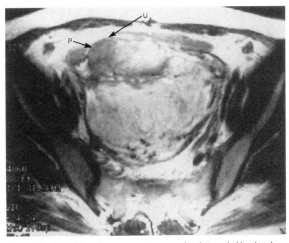

FIGURE 2.—T2-weighted MRI showing myometrium was deeply invaded by the placenta leaving a very thin serosal layer (U, uterine serosa; P, placenta). (Courtesy of Lam H, Pun TC, Lam PW: Successful conservative management of placenta previa accreta during cesarean section. *Int J Gynecol Obstet* 86:31-32, 2004.)

performed at day 10 showed that the accreta also involved part of the posterior myometrium (Fig 2). Follow-up scan showed gradual shrinkage of the placenta with reduced vascularity. A section of gray-white tissue was expelled with fresh vaginal bleeding on day 56. Menstruation resumed at 5 months after delivery.

Conclusions.—Conservative management can be successful in managing placenta previa accreta during cesarean section.

▶ From anecdotal reports of obstetricians working in Third World countries, we know that conservative management of an abnormally attached placenta may be safer than surgical removal. This case report shows the natural history of a placenta that is left in place to disappear gradually but completely (except for some calcifications) in the course of 6 months. It remains to be determined which is better or worse, the conservative approach of placenta accreta, surgery, or treatment with methotrexate.

F. K. Lotgering, MD, PhD

Self-inflicted Cesarean Section With Maternal and Fetal Survival
Molina-Sosa A, Galvan-Espinosa H, Gabriel-Guzman J, et al (Hosp Gen Dr Manuel Velasco Suarez, San Pablo, Huixtepec, Zimatlan, Oaxaca, Mexico; Northwestern Univ, Chicago)
Int J Gynecol Obstet 84:287-290, 2004   13–7

Abstract.—An unusual case of self-inflicted cesarean section with maternal and child survival is presented. No similar event was found in an Internet literature search. Because of a lack of medical assistance and a history of fetal death in utero, a 40-year-old multiparous woman unable to deliver herself

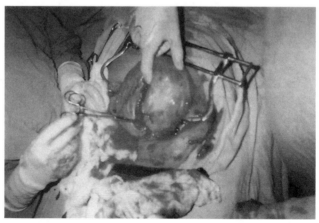

FIGURE 1.—Uterine incision at the time of abdominal exploration and uterine repair. (Courtesy of Molina-Sosa A, Galvan-Espinosa H, Gabriel-Guzman J, et al: Self-inflicted cesarean section with maternal and fetal survival. *Int J Gynecol Obstet* 84:287-290, 2004.)

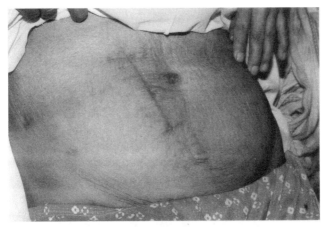

FIGURE 4.—Incision healed, observed 4 weeks after surgery. (Courtesy of Molina-Sosa A, Galvan-Espinosa H, Gabriel-Guzman J, et al: Self-inflicted cesarean section with maternal and fetal survival. *Int J Gynecol Obstet* 84:287-290, 2004.)

alone vaginally sliced her abdomen and uterus and delivered her child. She was transferred to a hospital where she underwent repair of the incisions and had to remain hospitalized (Figs 1 and 4). Mother and child survived the event. Unusual and extraordinary measures to preserve their offspring sometimes moves women to extreme decisions endangering their own lives. Social, educational, and health measures should be instituted all over the world, particularly in rural areas of developing countries, to avoid such extreme events.

▶ This is the first detailed report on a self-inflicted cesarean section. It demonstrates just how far a mother's desire to preserve her offspring can go under unusual circumstances.

F. K. Lotgering, MD, PhD

Anterior Placenta Percreta: Surgical Approach, Hemostasis and Uterine Repair

Palacios Jaraquemada JM, Pesaresi M, Nassif JC, et al (Univ of Buenos Aires, Argentina)
Acta Obstet Gynecol Scand 83:738-744, 2004   13–8

Background.—To describe an accurate approach, hemostatic procedures and uterine repair in patients with anterior placenta percreta.

Methods.—A total of 68 patients with anterior placenta percreta were included. A large retrovesical and parametrial dissection was performed in all cases (Fig 3). Hemostasis was achieved with selective vascular ligature or with surgical myometrial compression. The anterior wall defect was repaired using a myometrial suture, fibrin glue and polyglycolic mesh (Fig 6). Finally, a nonadherent cellulose layer was applied over this reconstruction.

Superior

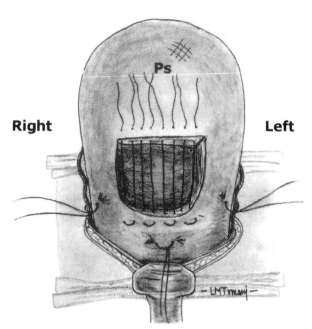

Right   **Left**

Inferior

FIGURE 3.—Placement of myometrial pulley sutures (Ps). (Courtesy of Palacios Jaraquemada JM, Pesaresi M, Nassif JC, et al: Anterior placenta percreta: Surgical approach, hemostasis and uterine repair. *Acta Obstet Gynecol Scand* 83:738-744, 2004. Reprinted by permission of Blackwell Publishing.)

Hysteroscopy and T2 magnetic resonance imaging (MRI) were performed as a reconstruction control at 90 days after discharge.

Results.—Elective surgery was performed in 49 patients and emergency surgery in 19. In 59 midline incisions were performed and in nine lower transverse incisions. Forty-nine patients underwent fundal hysterotomy and 19 transplacental segmental uterine approaches. The uteri of 50 patients with anterior placenta percreta were repaired. Of the 18 hysterectomies performed in this series, 16 were indicated due to massive destruction and two were secondary to coagulopathies. The following surgical complications developed: pelvic hemorrhage (one), coagulopathies (two), uterine infection (three), low ureteral ligations (two), iatrogenic foreign bodies (two) and collection (three). Uterine conservation was highly significant between the upper and lower invasion areas. Ten pregnancies were reported after the repair, resulting in uncomplicated cesarean delivery.

Conclusion.—This approach has allowed an adequate uterine repair in patients with anterior placenta percreta. Based on these results it is valid to assume that a functional and anatomic uterine repair has been successfully performed.

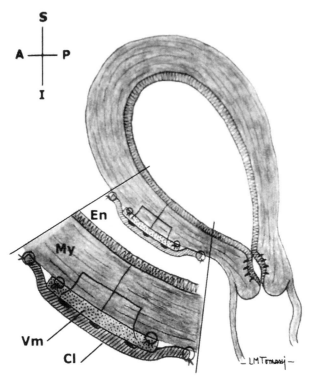

FIGURE 6.—Midline-sagittal view of the uterus. In detail, the layers of myometrial repair: *En*, endometrium; *My*, myometrium; *Vm*, polyglycolic Vicryl™ mesh; *Cl*, cellulose layer. (Courtesy of Palacios Jaraquemada JM, Pesaresi M, Nassif JC, et al: Anterior placenta percreta: Surgical approach, hemostasis and uterine repair. *Acta Obstet Gynecol Scand* 83:738-744, 2004. Reprinted by permission of Blackwell Publishing.)

▶ A large uterine defect, as may result from placenta percreta, may be hard to repair. In many cases, hysterectomy may be the only solution. However, in selective cases, repair may be possible and preferable. The authors report that MRI was performed in most cases to allow for optimal preparation. Repair of the uterus, by the method shown in the illustrations, resulted in conservation of the uterus in 50 patients. As 10 of these women became pregnant again and were delivered by elective cesarean section without complications, it seems warranted to attempt to preserve the uterus in case of a large defect.

F. K. Lotgering, MD, PhD

Use of Sengstaken–Blakemore Tube in Massive Postpartum Hemorrhage: A Series of 17 Cases

Seror J, Allouche C, Elhaik S (Hôpital d'Évreux, France)

Acta Obstet Gynecol Scand 84:660-664, 2005   13–9

Background.—To evaluate the efficacy and identify the indications of intrauterine tamponade with a Sengstaken-Blakemore tube in acute postpartum hemorrhage.

Methods.—Retrospective study was performed in 17 female patients with massive postpartum hemorrhage despite appropriate medical treatment, and requiring surgery (embolization techniques were not available in our hospital). Patients were treated by inserting a Sengstaken–Blakemore tube in the uterus through the vagina in case of vaginal delivery or through the hysterotomy incision in case of cesarean section. The esophageal balloon was inflated with 250 ml of isotonic saline solution. Patients underwent regional or general anesthesia. A preventive treatment with broad-spectrum antibiotics was systematically administered.

Results.—Tamponade treatment prevented surgery in 88% of patients, hemorrhage was controlled in 71% of cases (reducing the need for embolization by 80%), and waiting for a transfer for embolization was made possible for 18% of patients.

Conclusion.—Intrauterine tamponade with a Sengstaken–Blakemore tube appears as a simple, low-cost, readily available and effective means of treating life-threatening postpartum hemorrhage. The only apparent contraindication is the discovery of an infection during delivery.

▶ Postpartum hemorrhage remains a major cause of maternal morbidity and mortality; indeed, it is the primary cause of maternal mortality in France, where the authors of this study are from. This report presents data concerning the use of a Sengstaken–Blakemore tube in providing an intrauterine tamponade to reduce and hopefully halt the excessive blood loss. Use of the tube was successful in the majority of cases, with control of the hemorrhage achieved in approximately 70% of cases. Obstetric services should consider having this tube available in labor and delivery as a first-line therapeutic option for postpartum hemorrhage.

L. P. Shulman MD

14 Multifetal Pregnancy

Twins and Triplets: The Effect of Plurality and Growth on Neonatal Outcome Compared With Singleton Infants
Garite TJ, for the Pediatrix/Obstetrix Perinatal Research Group (Univ of California, Irvine; et al)
Am J Obstet Gynecol 191:700-707, 2004   14–1

Objective.—Information on outcome by gestational age from large numbers of twins and triplets is limited and is important for counseling and decision-making in obstetric practice. We reviewed one of the largest available neonatal databases to describe mortality and morbidity rates and growth in newborn infants from multiple gestations and compared these data with data for singletons.

Study Design.—Data from a large prospectively recorded neonatal database that incorporated neonatal records from January 1997 to July 2002 were reviewed. We evaluated birth weight and neonatal mortality and morbidity rates that affected long-term outcome for each week of gestational age from 23 to 35 weeks of gestation for all nonanomolous inborn twins and triplets who were admitted to the neonatal intensive care unit and compared these data to all singletons who met similar criteria during the same time period.

Results.—There were 12,302 twin and 2155 triplet births that met the entry criteria. The data for these newborn infants were compared with 36,931 singletons. Average birth weights at each gestational week were similar for all gestational ages until 29 weeks of gestation for triplets and 32 weeks of gestation for twins. After these gestational ages, the entire difference between twins and singletons was due to the weight of the smaller twin; the larger twins' mean weights were similar to singletons at all weeks that were studied. Birth order at each week also did not affect neonatal mortality rates, even when corrected for route of delivery and antenatal steroids. Neonatal morbidities associated with adverse long-term outcomes (intraventricular hemorrhage, retinopathy of prematurity, necrotizing enterocolitis) were also not different between multiple infants and singletons. Intrauterine growth restriction (IUGR) was associated with increased mortality rates at all gestational ages, but in the absences of IUGR, discordance was not.

Conclusion.—Data on a large number of twins and triplets provide reassurance that neonatal outcome at all viable premature weeks of gestation are similar to singletons. Intrauterine growth restriction and prematurity are therefore the principal issues that drive neonatal mortality and morbidity rates in multiple gestations. These data are important for obstetric decision-making and patient counseling.

▶ With prematurity being a major determinant of neonatal outcome, the increased likelihood of preterm birth in multiple gestations makes the management of women carrying multiple gestations difficult and challenging. Conventional wisdom concerning the preterm birth of multifetal pregnancies has been that clinical outcomes were worse than in comparable singleton pregnancies. In this study, the authors found that neonatal outcomes of viable preterm infants of multifetal pregnancies were similar to those of singleton pregnancies. Although multifetal pregnancy does increase the likelihood of preterm birth, patients and clinicians can be reassured that neonatal outcomes of multifetal pregnancies will likely be similar to those of singleton pregnancies of similar gestational ages.

H. N. Lafeber, MD, PhD

Neurological Sequelae in Twins Born After Assisted Conception: Controlled National Cohort Study

Pinborg A, Loft A, Schmidt L, et al (Copenhagen Univ Hosp; Univ of Copenhagen; Natl Board of Health, Copenhagen)
BMJ 329:311-314, 2004   14–2

Objective.—To compare neurological sequelae in twins born after assisted conception with singletons after assisted conception and naturally conceived twins and to assess neurological sequelae in children conceived after in vitro fertilisation (IVF) compared with intracytoplasmic sperm injection (ICSI).

Design.—Controlled, national register based, cohort study.

Participants.—Twins (n = 3393) and singletons (n = 5130) conceived by using assisted reproductive technologies and naturally conceived twins (n = 10,239) born in Denmark between 1995 and 2000. The children's age at time of follow up was 2-7 years.

Data Sources.—Children were identified by cross linkage of the national medical birth registry and the national registry for in vitro fertilisation. Neurological and psychiatric diagnoses were retrieved from the national patients' registry and the Danish psychiatric central registry.

Main Outcome Measures.—Neurological sequelae, defined as cerebral palsy, mental retardation, severe mental developmental disturbances, and retarded psychomotor development. Further we made separate analyses on the specific cerebral palsy diagnosis.

Results.—The crude prevalence rates per 1000 of neurological sequelae in twins and singletons after assisted conception and in naturally conceived twins were 8.8, 8.2, and 9.6, and of cerebral palsy 3.2, 2.5, and 4.0, respectively. In twins after assisted conception compared with control twins, the odds ratios of neurological sequelae and specifically of cerebral palsy, ad-

TABLE 2.—Multiple Logistic Regression Analysis Showing Independent Effects of Being a Twin Infant, Assisted Conception (IVF and ICSI), Maternal Age ≥35 Years, Male Sex, and Low Birth Weight (<2500 g) (**Upper Panel**) or Low Gestational Age (≤37 weeks) (**Lower Panel**) on the Risk of Neurological Sequelae and Cerebral Palsy. Results are Presented as Odds Ratios (95% Confidence Intervals), Adjusted for Child Sex and Year of Birth

	Neurological Sequelae		Cerebral Palsy	
	All Cases	Twins	All Cases	Twins
Effects of birth weight				
Twin	0.7 (0.4 to 1.2)	—	0.6 (0.2 to 1.4)	—
Assisted conception	0.9 (0.6 to 1.4)	0.9 (0.6 to 1.4)	0.8 (0.4 to 1.5)	0.8 (0.4 to 1.5)
Low birth weight	2.3 (1.6 to 3.2)	1.9 (1.4 to 2.8)	4.4 (2.5 to 7.8)	3.0 (1.7 to 5.4)
Male sex	2.0 (1.4 to 2.8)	1.9 (1.3 to 2.8)	1.9 (1.1 to 3.2)	2.0 (1.1 to 3.5)
Maternal age ≥35 years	0.8 (0.6 to 1.2)	0.8 (0.5 to 1.4)	0.8 (0.4 to 1.5)	0.8 (0.4 to 1.7)
Effects of gestational age				
Twin	0.8 (0.5 to 1.3)	—	0.6 (0.2 to 1.4)	—
Assisted conception	0.9 (0.6 to 1.4)	0.9 (0.6 to 1.4)	0.8 (0.4 to 1.6)	0.8 (0.4 to 1.6)
Low gestational age	2.0 (1.4 to 2.8)	1.8 (1.2 to 2.6)	4.5 (2.5 to 8.1)	3.1 (1.7 to 5.7)
Male sex	1.9 (1.3 to 2.6)	1.8 (1.2 to 2.6)	1.8 (1.0 to 3.0)	1.9 (1.0 to 3.4)
Maternal age ≥35 years	0.8 (0.6 to 1.2)	0.8 (0.5 to 1.4)	0.8 (0.4 to 1.5)	0.8 (0.4 to 1.8)

Abbreviations: IVF, In vitro fertilization; *ICSI*, intracytoplasmic sperm injection.
(Courtesy of Pinborg A, Loft A, Schmidt L, et al: Neurological sequelae in twins born after assisted conception: Controlled national cohort study. *BMJ* 329:311-314, 2004. With permission from the BMJ Publishing Group.)

justed for child sex and year of birth, were 0.9 (95% confidence interval 0.6 to 1.4) and 0.8 (0.4 to 1.6), respectively (Table 2). The corresponding odds ratios for twins after assisted conception compared with singletons after assisted conception were 1.1 (0.7 to 1.7) for neurological sequelae and 1.3 (0.6 to 2.9) for cerebral palsy. The odds ratio of neurological sequelae in children conceived by ICSI was 0.9 (0.5 to 1.7) *v* children conceived by IVF.

Conclusions.—Twins from assisted conception have a similar risk of neurological sequelae as their naturally conceived peers and singletons from assisted conception. Children born after ICSI have the same risk of neurological sequelae as children born after IVF.

▶ Debate continues regarding whether pregnancies conceived through assisted technologies face an inherently higher risk of maternal and neonatal complications than naturally conceived pregnancies. Denmark has both the highest per capita IVF utilization and one of the most detailed national neonatal health registries in Europe. These facts, in addition to a substantial number of cases with appropriately lengthy follow-up, have permitted the authors to impart power to their conclusions. The authors' conclusions that IVF-conceived twins face no increased risk of serious neurologic sequelae compared with their naturally conceived counterparts are further supported by the findings of another retrospective cohort study from Hungary reaching similar conclusions for both singleton and twin pregnancies, published in 2003.[1] However, numerous previous investigations have reached opposing conclusions to the present study, and this issue is likely to remain unresolved for some time to come.

M. R. Drews, MD

Reference

1. Kozinszky Z, Zadori J, Orvos H, et al: Obstetric and neonatal risk of pregnancies after assisted reproductive technology: A matched control study. *Acta Obstet Gynecol Scand* 82:850-856, 2003.

The Cost of Twin Pregnancy: Maternal and Neonatal Factors
Luke B, Brown MB, Alexandre PK, et al (Univ of Miami, Fla; Univ of Michigan, Ann Arbor; Jackson Mem Hosp, Miami, Fla; et al)
Am J Obstet Gynecol 192:909-915, 2005   14–3

Objective.—The purpose of this study was to evaluate factors affecting birth charges in twin pregnancies.

Study Design.—Clinical and financial data were obtained on 1486 twin pregnancies delivered between 1995 to 2002 at medical centers in Maryland, Florida, Michigan, and South Carolina. Maternal and neonatal length of stay (LOS) and charges were modeled by gestational age and other risk factors using a general linear model.

Results.—Maternal and infant birth admission LOS and charges increased significantly with a decline in gestational age. Maternal LOS and charges were also significantly increased by cesarean delivery and preeclampsia. Newborn LOS and charges increased significantly by monochorionicity and slowed growth between 20 to 28 weeks. For mother and infants, the shortest LOS and lowest birth charges were at 37 to 38 weeks.

Conclusion.—These findings reflect the substantial maternal and neonatal morbidity associated with twin pregnancies, and demonstrate that 37 to 38 weeks is their optimal gestation.

▶ Data from 1486 twin gestations were obtained. This study demonstrated that as gestational age decreased, LOS and charges increased. Other factors leading to increased charges were cesarean delivery, preeclampsia, and monochorionicity. This is a very relevant study because economical factors are affecting management decisions in all medical specialties. One must also take into consideration that delivering twins at 37 to 38 weeks of pregnancy is the most optimal period to decrease morbidity or mortality or both and the associated charges and costs.

S. H. Ural, MD

Quality of Intrapartum Cardiotocography in Twin Deliveries
Bakker PCAM, Colenbrander GJ, Verstraeten AA, et al (Vrije Universiteit, Amsterdam)
Am J Obstet Gynecol 191:2114-2119, 2004   14–4

Objective.—Intrapartum fetal heart rate (FHR) recordings in twins were compared for fetal signal loss during both stages of labor to assess the quality

TABLE 3.—Percentages of Fetal Signal Loss (Medians ± Interquartile Ranges) and Number of Recordings Exceeding FIGO Criteria (Percentage) During the First and Second Stages of Labor

	First Stage		Second Stage		P Value*
Recording technique	US 1	US 2	US 1	US 2	
Number	104	104	33	33	
Fetal signal loss	12 (27)	11 (25)	23 (21)	21 (23)	<.05
Exceeding FIGO criteria[23]	36 (35%)	36 (35%)	18 (55%)	21 (63%)	
Recording technique	DI 1	US 2	DI 1	US 2	
Number	140	140	150	150	
Fetal signal loss	0.4 (2)	9 (17)	9 (12)	16 (16)	<.01
Exceeding FIGO criteria[23]	3 (2%)	36 (26%)	25 (17%)	62 (41%)	

*Wilcoxon signed ranks test used to compare fetal signal loss in the first stage with fetal signal loss in the second stage for all groups.
Abbreviations: FIGO, International Federation of Gynecology and Obstetrics; *US 1*, ultrasound twin 1; *US 2*, ultrasound twin 2; *DI 1*, direct registration twin 1.
(Courtesy of Bakker PCAM, Colenbrander GJ, Verstraeten AA, et al: Quality of intrapartum cardiotocography in twin deliveries. *Am J Obstet Gynecol* 191:2114-2119, 2004. Copyright 2004 by Elsevier. Reprinted by permission.)

of these recordings by the method that had been used: external ultrasound or directly via a scalp electrode.

Study Design.—Analysis of recordings collected between January 1, 1994, and January 1, 2002, from consecutive twin deliveries at the Vrije Universiteit Medical Center in Amsterdam. One hundred seventy-two twins that delivered via the vaginal route were included in the study. FHR recordings had a duration of at least 1 hour before the birth of the second twin. Subdivision took place on the basis of the recording technique, ie, ultrasound or scalp electrode. FHR data was obtained with HP-M1350 cardiotocographs. The status (pen on, pen off, maternal signal) and the mode of the signals were acquired. The duration of pen lifts and maternal signals was divided by the total duration of the recording. Statistical analyses were performed with the Mann-Whitney U test and the Wilcoxon signed ranks test.

Results.—Recordings obtained via ultrasound demonstrated significantly more fetal signal loss than those obtained via the direct mode, particularly in the second stage. Approximately 26% to 33% of first stage and 41% to 63% of second stage ultrasound intrapartum FHR recordings in twins exceeded the International Federation of Gynecology and Obstetrics (FIGO) criteria for fetal signal loss (Table 3).

Conclusion.—Intrapartum FHR monitoring via ultrasound provides far poorer quality FHR signals than the direct mode. The direct mode deserves a more prominent position in fetal surveillance than it currently has.

▶ As the number of twin and higher-order multiple pregnancies increases, the obstetric complications associated with prenatal and perinatal management will invariably increase. The objective of this study from Vrije Universiteit Medical Center in Amsterdam was to compare the assessment of intrapartum FHR at recordings obtained by either external US or directly via a scalp electrode. The authors found that intrapartum FHR monitoring by external US provided a far poorer quality signal than the direct mode, and thus, direct surveillance warrants a more serious consideration in fetal surveillance of twins and possibly other high-risk pregnancies. If the ability to deliver babies in a relatively rapid fashion at many medical centers is a critical aspect of improving neonatal outcomes, then the ability to detect alterations or deteriorations in FHR patterns may play an important role in determining perinatal outcomes in twin pregnancies and other high-risk situations.

H. P. van Geijn, MD, PhD

Delayed Interval Delivery and Infant Survival: A Population-Based Study
Zhang J, Hamilton B, Martin J, et al (NIH, Bethesda, Md; Ctrs for Disease Control and Prevention, Bethesda, Md)
Am J Obstet Gynecol 191:470-476, 2004   14–5

Objective.—Delaying delivery of the remaining fetus(es) in a multifetal pregnancy is feasible in some cases. However, the impact of this procedure on infant survival is unclear.

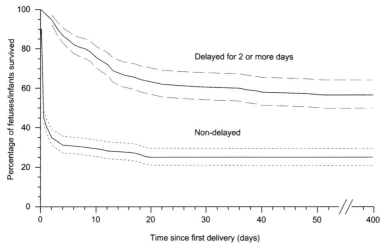

FIGURE 2.—The feto-infant survival curves adjusting for maternal age, education, marital status, prenatal care, fetal sex of the second twin, and 95% confidence limits in delayed and nondelayed second born twins. The delayed group includes fetal death, which was counted as an event as an infant death. The nondelayed group had no fetal death. (Courtesy of Zhang J, Hamilton B, Martin J, et al: Delayed interval delivery and infant survival: A population-based study. *Am J Obstet Gynecol* 191:470-476, 2004. Copyright 2004 by Elsevier. Reprinted by permission.)

Study Design.—We used the US 1995-1998 Matched Multiple Birth File. We identified 200 twin pregnancies in which the first twin was delivered between 17 and 29 weeks of gestation and the second twin was delivered 2 or more days later. We individually matched the delayed deliveries with 374 twin pregnancies in which the second twin was delivered on the same or next calendar day. Perinatal outcomes and infant survival were compared between the delayed and nondelayed twins.

Results.—Among the 200 pregnancies with delayed delivery, the mean gestational age at first delivery was 23 weeks and the median duration of delay was 6 days (ranging from 2-107 days). One week of delay in delivery was associated with an increase in infant birth weight of 131 g on average (95% CI: 115-147 g). Moreover, 56% of the delayed second twins survived to 1 year of age, whereas only 24% of the nondelayed second twins survived to 1 year of age ($P < .001$). However, 11% of the second twin in delayed delivery (95% CI: 6%-16%) experienced fetal death before 24 weeks.

Conclusion.—Delayed delivery of the remaining fetus(es) before 30 weeks of gestation for 2 or more days was associated with improved infant survival (Fig 2).

▶ As even a few days' delay may help to improve lung maturity, theoretically it makes sense to attempt delayed delivery of the second twin. Since case reports of delayed delivery are criticized for publication bias, and randomized studies are absent and probably unfeasible, at present this matched control study may best approach the truth. As shown by Figure 2, a delay of 2 days or more is associated with improved survival. The survival rate of the second twin increased by delay at 17 to 24 weeks from 12% to 33%, and at 24 to 30 weeks from 58% to 82%. From the second twin's point of view, an attempt at delayed delivery would seem beneficial. Unfortunately, the study did not provide information on maternal and neonatal morbidity, including maternal sepsis, which should be part of the equation of benefits and risks.

F. K. Lotgering, MD, PhD

15 Postpartum

The Immediate Management of Fresh Obstetric Fistulas
Waaldijk K (Babbar Ruga Fistula Hosp, Katsina, Nigeria)
Am J Obstet Gynecol 191:795-799, 2004   15–1

Objective.—It has been a general rule to wait with the repair of an obstetric fistula for a minimum period of 3 months allowing the patient to become an outcast. In a prospective way an immediate management was studied and antibiotics were not used, all according to basic surgical principles.

Methods.—A total of 1716 patients with a fistula duration of 3 to 75 days after delivery were treated immediately on presentation by catheter and/or early closure. Instead of antibiotics, a high oral fluid regimen was instituted. The fistulas were classified according to anatomic and physiologic location in types I, IIAa, IIAb, IIBa, and IIBb, and according to size in small, medium, large, and extensive. The operation became progressively more complicated from type I through type IIBb and from small through extensive.

Results.—At first attempt 1633 fistulas (95.2%) were closed and another 57 could be closed at further attempt(s), accounting for a final closure in 1690 patients (98.5%) (Table 6); 264 patients (15.4%) were healed by catheter only. Of these 1690 patients with a closed fistula, 1575 (93.2%) were continent and 115 (6.8%) were incontinent. The results as to closure and to continence became progressively worse from type I through type IIBb and from small through extensive. Postoperative wound infection was not noted; postoperative mortality was encountered in 6 patients (0.4%).

TABLE 6.—Results as to Size of Fistula

Size	No.	Closed First Attempt	Finally Closed	Incontinent	Mortality
Small	685	676 (98.7%)	684 (99.9%)	3 (0.4%)	—
Medium	481	460 (95.6%)	473 (98.3%)	35 (7.4%)	4
Large	168	158 (94.0%)	167 (99.4%)	14 (8.4%)	—
Extensive	382	346 (90.6%)	366 (95.8%)	63 (17.2%)	3

(Courtesy of Waaldijk K: The immediate management of fresh obstetric fistulas. *Am J Obstet Gynecol* 191:795-799, 2004. Copyright 2004 by Elsevier. Reprinted by permission.)

Conclusion.—This immediate management proves highly effective in terms of closure and continence and will prevent the patient from becoming an outcast with progressive downgrading medically, socially, and mentally.

▶ A woman with an obstetric fistula is likely to become an outcast. Traditional dogma told us to delay surgical repair for at least 3 months. Waaldijk, however, shows us that, in experienced hands, such delay is unnecessary, as the soonest possible repair has an overall 95% success rate. As Table 6 shows, more than 90% of even extensive fistulas were successfully repaired at first attempt. The advantages of immediate repair of obstetric fistulas seem to outweigh the presumed benefits of delayed repair.

F. K. Lotgering, MD, PhD

Management of Severe Postpartum Haemorrhage by Uterine Artery Embolization

Wee L, Barron J, Toye R (Middlesex Hosp, London; Kings College, London; Medway Maritime Hosp, Kent, England)
Br J Anaesth 93:591-594, 2004   15–2

Background.—Obstetric hemorrhage is a significant cause of maternal mortality and morbidity. Arterial embolization is an alternative management approach to hysterectomy or bilateral uterine or hypogastric artery ligation. A case is presented in which arterial embolization was used to manage a patient with severe postpartum hemorrhage.

Case Report.—A 33-year-old prima gravida American Society of Anesthesiologists class I woman was admitted in early labor at 39 weeks' gestation. After 16 hours an epidural provided good pain relief, and a Syntocinon infusion was started. Caesarean delivery was planned 4 hours later for failure to progress. A live male infant was delivered, and Syntocinon 10 U was given as a bolus, followed by an infusion of 40 U in 500 mL 0.9% saline over a 4-hour period. The operation was completed without incident. Blood loss was estimated at 500 mL. The patient was initially stable but later reported lightheadedness. Her blood pressure dropped, pulse and breathing rate rose, and she became very pale and sweaty. Gelofusine and blood were administered with good results. However, 1 hour later the patient again had the same symptoms as well as hypertension. Two more units of blood were administered. Examination of the patient's abdomen showed some distension, but the abdomen was soft and not tender to palpation. Intraabdominal bleeding was assumed, and the patient underwent laparotomy. Her blood pressure dropped while awaiting transfer to the ICU after laparotomy, and the heart rate increased. Heavy bleeding from the vagina was evident, and the uterus was atonic. A large blood clot was expelled after vigorous external massage, but uterine atony returned when massage was

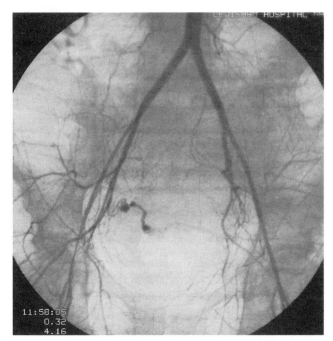

FIGURE 1.—Angiogram showing bleeding right uterine artery. (Courtesy of Wee L, Barron J, Toye R: Management of severe postpartum haemorrhage by uterine artery embolization. *Br J Anaesth* 93:591-594, 2004, by permission of Oxford University Press.)

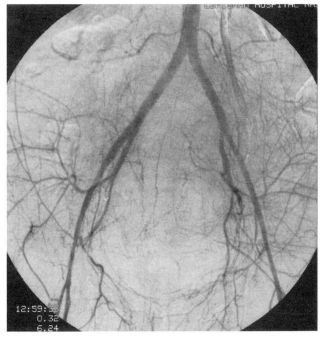

FIGURE 3.—Cessation of bleeding after embolization. (Courtesy of Wee L, Barron J, Toye R: Management of severe postpartum haemorrhage by uterine artery embolization. *Br J Anaesth* 93:591-594, 2004, by permission of Oxford University Press.)

halted. An angiogram showed active bleeding from the right uterine artery (Fig 1). A Sims I catheter was positioned with its tip in the right uterine artery, which resulted in near cessation of bleeding. Embolization was performed successfully. A repeat angiogram showed no further bleeding (Fig 3). Her hematologic variables had returned to normal the next day. The patient was discharged after 7 days.

Conclusions.—Selective uterine arterial embolization was effective in controlling postpartum bleeding and avoiding the need for hysterectomy.

▶ Arterial embolization is an elegant technique for controlling obstetric hemorrhage. If local measures and uterine drugs fail to control the bleeding, one may have the choice of arterial embolization or surgical intervention. Since even bilateral hypogastric or uterine artery ligation is successful in only about 60% of cases, surgical intervention may eventually result in hysterectomy. If an experienced interventional radiologist is available and the patient can temporarily be stabilized for the intervention, uterine artery embolization would seem to be the treatment of choice.

F. K. Lotgering, MD, PhD

16 Newborn

Premature Infants Are Less Capable of Maintaining Thermal Balance of Head and Body With Increases of Thermal Environment Than With Decreases

Simbruner G, Ruttner E-M, Schulze A, et al (Leopold Franzens Univ, Innsbruck, Tyrol, Austria; Klinikum Schwabing, Munich; Ludwig-Maximilian Univ, Munich)
Am J Perinatol 22:25-33, 2005
16–1

Background.—After oxygen and nutrition, an adequate thermal environment is important for the survival, morbidity, and growth of newborn infants, particularly those that are premature. The detrimental effects of moderate or severe hypothermia on premature infants have been well-known for many years. The thermal environment for preterm infants has been more closely adapted to intrauterine conditions, and target rectal temperatures between 37.0°C and 37.5°C have been suggested. In recent years, new concepts, such as a comfort temperature, have been proposed. Some premature infants at comfort temperature exhibited a rectal temperature close to 39°C. Mild to moderate increases in brain temperature are considered to be high risk for neurological damage, and mild to moderate hypothermia may be neuroprotective. The purpose of this study was to investigate whether premature infants nursed at the upper range of normal body temperature are better able to maintain their nasopharyngeal and rectal temperature when exposed to a 1°C increase or a 1°C decrease of incubator temperature.

Methods.—A randomized controlled trial was conducted in which premature infants were exposed to 1°C increase (10 infants) or a 1°C decrease (10 infants) in incubator temperature. Nasopharyngeal, rectal, and skin temperatures were measured over 6 hours, as were heat flux at various sites, heart rate, and activity.

Results.—Absolute changes in core temperatures were significantly greater in the infants exposed to a 1°C increase in incubator temperature compared with those exposed to a 1°C decrease in incubator temperature.

Conclusions.—Premature infants with a relatively high rectal temperature (from 37.0°C to 37.4°C) are less capable of coping with small increases in incubator temperature than with small decreases in temperature. Rapid increases and high levels of head core temperature may place the premature infant at risk for increased rate of apnea and possible increased risk of neuronal injury because higher body core or brain temperatures may be associated with hypoxic conditions such as oxygen desaturations and bradycardias.

▶ Maintaining suitable thermal environment is critical for survival and proper organic and neurological development. This is especially true for preterm infants who may be more prone to the adverse effects of thermal abnormalities than full-term infants. In particular, mild to moderate increases in brain temperature are associated with increased risk for neurological damage, thus demonstrating the critical importance of thermoregulation in clinical outcomes of preterm infants. This study found that preterm infants were less able to cope with increases in incubator temperature and that this may be an important cause of adverse clinical outcomes in preterm infants.

H. N. Lafeber, MD, PhD

Proactive Management Promotes Outcome in Extremely Preterm Infants: A Population-Based Comparison of Two Perinatal Management Strategies
Håkansson S, Farooqi A, Holmgren PA, et al (Inst of Clinical Science, Umeå, Sweden)
Pediatrics 114:58-64, 2004   16–2

Objective.—There is a need for evidence-based knowledge regarding perinatal management in extreme prematurity. The benefit of a proactive attitude versus a more selective one is controversial. The objective of the present study was to analyze perinatal practices and infant outcome in extreme prematurity in relation to different management policies in the North (proactive) and South of Sweden.

Methods.—A population-based, retrospective, cohort study design was used. Data in the Swedish Medical Birth Register (MBR) from 1985 to 1999 were analyzed according to region of birth and gestational age (22 weeks + 0 days to 27 weeks + 6 days). A total of 3 602 live-born infants were included (North = 1040, South = 2562). Survival was defined as being alive at 1 year. Morbidity in survivors, based on discharge diagnoses of major morbidity during the first year of life, was described by linking the MBR to the Hospital Discharge Register.

Results.—In infants with a gestational age of 22 to 25 weeks, the proactive policy was significantly associated with 1) increased incidence of live births, 2) higher degree of centralized management, 3) higher frequency of caesarean section, 4) fewer infants with low Apgar score (<4) at 1 and 5 minutes, 5) fewer infants dead within 24 hours, and 6) increased number of infants alive at 1 year. There were no indications of increased morbidity in survivors of the proactive management during the first year of life, and the proportion of survivors without denoted morbidity was larger.

Conclusion.—In infants with a gestational age of 22 to 25 weeks, a proactive perinatal strategy increases the number of live births and improves the infant's postnatal condition and survival without evidence of increasing morbidity in survivors up to 1 year of age.

▶ The extreme preterm infant poses a great challenge for the neonatologist and pediatrician, given the profound morbidity and mortality rates associated with delivery between 22 and 25 weeks' gestation. In this study from the University Hospital in Umeå, Sweden, the authors found that a proactive perinatal strategy increased the number of live births and improved the infant's postnatal condition and survival without increasing morbidity up to 1 year of age. As the identification of women who will be delivered of their children between 22 and 25 weeks' gestation cannot always be predicted, such deliveries should occur, whenever possible, at tertiary care centers that have developed coordinated protocols with obstetrics and neonatology.

P. P. van den Berg, MD, PhD

Outcome of Extremely-Low-Birth-Weight Infants at Highest Risk: Gestational Age ≤24 Weeks, Birth Weight ≤750 g, and 1-Minute Apgar ≤3
Shankaran S, Johnson Y, Langer JC, et al (Wayne State Univ, Detroit; Research Triangle Inst, Research Triangle Park, NC; Women and Infants Hosp, Providence, RI; et al)
Am J Obstet Gynecol 191:1084-1091, 2004   16–3

Objective.—The purpose of this study was to evaluate neurodevelopmental outcome in extremely-low-birth-weight (ELBW) infants, all of whom had 3 characteristics: gestational age (GA) ≤24 weeks, birth weight ≤750 g, and 1-minute Apgar score ≤3.

Study Design.—Surviving infants were evaluated at 18 to 22 months' corrected age with a neurologic examination and the Bayley II Mental and Psychomotor Developmental Index (MDI and PDI).

Results.—Between 1993 and 1999, 1016 infants had GA ≤24 weeks, birth weight ≤750 g, and 1-minute Apgar score ≤3. Of 246 survivors, 30% had cerebral palsy (CP), 5% had hearing impairment, and 2% were blind. MDI was ≥85 in 33% and <70 in 46% of infants, while PDI was ≥85 in 41% and <70 in 36% infants. Predictors of MDI <70 were grade III-IV ICH, cystic periventricular leukomalacia (PVL), male gender, black race, and Medicaid insurance. Two-parent household was associated with an MDI >70. Predictors of PDI <70 were grade III-IV ICH, PVL, steroids for bronchopulmonary dysplasia (BPD), and Medicaid insurance. CP was associated with grade III-IV ICH and PVL.

Conclusion.—Perinatologists and neonatologists should be aware of the risk of morbidity and mortality in this high-risk ELBW group.

Neurologic and Developmental Disability at Six Years of Age After Extremely Preterm Birth

Marlow N, for the EPICure Study Group (Univ of Nottingham, England; et al)

N Engl J Med 352:9-19, 2005   16–4

Background.—Birth before 26 weeks of gestation is associated with a high prevalence of neurologic and developmental disabilities in the infant during the first two years of life.

Methods.—We studied at the time of early school age children who had been born at 25 or fewer completed weeks of gestation in the United Kingdom and Ireland in 1995. Each child had been evaluated at 30 months of age. The children underwent standardized cognitive and neurologic assessments at six years of age. Disability was defined as severe (indicating dependence on caregivers), moderate, or mild according to predetermined criteria.

Results.—Of 308 surviving children, 241 (78 percent) were assessed at a median age of six years and four months; 160 classmates delivered at full term served as a comparison group. Although the use of test reference norms showed that cognitive impairment (defined as results more than 2 SD below the mean) was present in 21 percent of the children born extremely preterm (as compared with 1 percent in the standardized data), this value rose to 41 percent when the results were compared with those for their classmates. The rates of severe, moderate, and mild disability were 22 percent, 24 percent, and 34 percent, respectively; disabling cerebral palsy was present in 30 children (12 percent). Among children with severe disability at 30 months of age, 86 percent still had moderate-to-severe disability at 6 years of age. In contrast, other disabilities at the age of 30 months were poorly predictive of developmental problems at 6 years of age.

Conclusions.—Among extremely preterm children, cognitive and neurologic impairment is common at school age. A comparison with their classroom peers indicates a level of impairment that is greater than is recognized with the use of standardized norms.

▶ The care of the woman who is threatening to deliver an ELBW infant presents great challenges for obstetricians and neonatologists. A critical part of the care provided to these women includes counseling concerning potential newborn outcomes. Especially important to such counseling is the ability to provide information concerning short- and long-term prognoses for the child. In the study by Shankaran et al, the authors found that among more than 1000 infants with a variety of demographic characteristics indicative of ELBW (<750 g), considerable morbidities were present in the approximately 25% of infants who survived. Those problems included CP (30%), hearing impairment (5%), and deafness (2%). Marlow et al similarly found considerable impairment at 6 years of age in children who were extremely preterm. In this study, severe cognitive impairment was noted for 41% of these children when compared with their peers. Clinicians who care for women in preterm labor and the neonatologists who care for the ELBW child must be able to provide accurate and evidence-based information when decisions concerning the management, especially decisions concerning delivery, of these high-risk pregnancies need to be made.

P. P. van den Berg, MD, PhD

Comparison of Early-Onset Neonatal Sepsis Caused by *Escherichia coli* **and Group B** *Streptococcus*
Mayor-Lynn K, González-Quintero VH, O'Sullivan MJ, et al (Univ of Miami, Fla; Jackson Health System, Miami, Fla)
Am J Obstet Gynecol 192:1437-1439, 2005   16–5

Objective.—The purpose of this study was to compare maternal characteristics and neonatal morbidity and mortality rates that are associated with early-onset neonatal sepsis that is caused by group B *Streptococcus* and *Escherichia coli.*

Study Design.—This was a retrospective review of newborn infants with a positive blood culture (and/or cerebrospinal fluid) that was positive for either *E coli* or group B *Streptococcus* during the first week of life. Data were abstracted from maternal and neonatal medical records.

Results.—Among 28,659 deliveries during the study period, 102 episodes of early-onset neonatal sepsis were identified, 61 of which were caused by group B *Streptococcus* and 41 of which were caused by *E coli. E coli* sepsis cases had a lower birth weight, a higher percentage with 5-minute Apgar score <7, and a longer stay in the hospital neonatal intensive care unit and required mechanical ventilation more frequently. Death after early-onset neonatal sepsis with *E coli* was also more frequent.

Conclusion.—Early-onset sepsis with *E coli* is associated with more morbidity and a higher mortality rate compared with early-onset group B *Streptococcus.*

▶ Bacterial sepsis plays an increasing role in morbidity and mortality in patients of all ages, although it is an infrequent complication of the very low birth weight infant. This study from the School of Medicine at the University of Miami sought to compare maternal characteristics and neonatal outcomes in cases of early-onset neonatal sepsis caused by group B *Streptococcus* and *E coli.* The authors found that neonatal *E coli* sepsis was associated with greater morbidity and mortality rates than found with group B *Streptococcus*, including lower birth weights, lower Apgar scores, and longer hospital stays. Regardless of the causative organism, prompt diagnosis and intervention remains a key factor in reducing adverse outcomes with neonatal sepsis.

H. N. Lafeber, MD, PhD

Maternal Age and Other Predictors of Newborn Blood Pressure

Gillman MW, Rich-Edwards JW, Rifas-Shiman SL, et al (Harvard Med School, Boston; Univ of Rochester, NY)

J Pediatr 144:240-245, 2004   16–6

Objective.—To investigate perinatal predictors of newborn blood pressure.

Study Design.—Among 1059 mothers and their newborn infants participating in Project Viva, a US cohort study of pregnant women and their offspring, we obtained five systolic blood pressure readings on a single occasion in the first few days of life. Using multivariate linear regression models, we examined the extent to which maternal age and other pre- and perinatal factors predicted newborn blood pressure level.

Results.—Mean (SD) maternal age was 32.0 (5.2) years, and mean (SD) newborn systolic blood pressure was 72.6 (9.0) mm Hg. A multivariate model showed that for each 5-year increase in maternal age, newborn systolic blood pressure was 0.8 mm Hg higher (95% CI, 0.2, 1.4). In addition to maternal age, independent predictors of newborn blood pressure included maternal third trimester blood pressure (0.9 mm Hg [95% CI, 0.2, 1.6] for each increment in maternal blood pressure); infant age at which we measured blood pressure (2.4 mm Hg [95% CI 1.7, 3.0] for each additional day of life); and birth weight (2.9 mm Hg [95% CI, 1.6, 4.2] per kg).

Conclusions.—Higher maternal age, maternal blood pressure, and birth weight were associated with higher newborn systolic blood pressure. Whereas blood pressure later in childhood predicts adult hypertension and its consequences, newborn blood pressure may represent different phenomena, such as pre- and perinatal influences on cardiac structure and function.

▶ Recent studies have shown that risk for adult cardiovascular disease begins early in life, with prenatal events possibly affecting this risk. The authors found that greater maternal age and higher blood pressures and higher birth weights were associated with higher newborn systolic pressures. Although the authors are unable to associate their findings with an increased risk of hypertension in adults, the findings do suggest that newborn blood pressures may provide clues to fetal cardiac development that can have implications for later development of cardiovascular disease.

H. N. Lafeber, MD, PhD

Neonatal Brachial Plexus Palsy: Outcome of Absent Biceps Function at Three Months of Age
Smith NC, Rowan P, Benson LJ, et al (Children's Hosp at Westmead, Sydney; Brisbane Orthopaedics and Sports Medicine, Australia; Denver Children's Hosp; et al)
J Bone Joint Surg Am 86-A:2163-2170, 2004   16–7

Background.—An important prognostic factor in neonatal brachial plexus palsy is the time interval to biceps muscle recovery. Although the natural history is not clear, biceps muscle recovery after more than three months of age has been used to predict poor long-term shoulder function. The absence of biceps muscle function at three months of age has been adopted as an indication for early brachial plexus microsurgery, in an attempt to improve recovery. To provide a benchmark for outcome comparison, the long-term outcome of patients with absent biceps muscle function at three months of age was studied.

Methods.—Between 1980 and 1992, 170 patients with neonatal brachial plexus palsy were entered into a prospective study in which details of the birth and serial clinical examinations were recorded. Patients were grouped according to the level of injury and the time interval to biceps muscle recovery. Twenty-nine patients were observed to have absent biceps muscle function at three months of age. Twenty-eight of those patients were available for long-term followup at a mean age of eleven years and one month. At the time of follow-up, patients answered a questionnaire and underwent manual muscle strength testing, sensory evaluation, and grading of their shoulder function according to Gilbert's modification of the Mallet score, in which the function was graded as II, III, or IV with class I (no function) and V (normal) eliminated. The level of injury and the time that biceps muscle function returned were compared with the final outcomes.

Results.—The level of injury was C5-C6 in thirteen (46%) of our twenty-eight patients with absent biceps muscle function at three months of age, C5-C7 in five (18%), and pan-plexus (C5-T1) in ten (36%). Biceps contraction was observed by six months of age in twenty patients (71%), including all thirteen patients with a C5-C6 level of injury. Twenty-two patients did not have surgery on the brachial plexus, but nine of those patients had subsequent orthopaedic procedures. At the time of follow-up, twenty-seven of the twenty-eight patients had at least antigravity biceps muscle function. Patients who regained biceps muscle function between three and six months of age had better scores for abduction (p = 0.04) and for hand-to-neck (p = 0.05) and hand-to-back (p < 0.001) function than did patients who regained biceps muscle function after six months of age. Patients with a C5-C6 lesion had better scores for external rotation (p = 0.04) and for hand-to-neck (p = 0.05), hand-to-mouth (p < 0.01), and hand-to-back (p < 0.001) function than did patients with a pan-plexus lesion. Twelve (55%) of the twenty-two patients who did not have brachial plexus surgery had a class-IV shoulder (good function) according to the modified Mallet score. Of the twelve patients with a C5-C6 level of injury who did not have brachial plexus surgery, eight had a class-IV shoulder.

Conclusions.—This study indicated associations between prolonged neurological recovery and a more extensive level of injury and worse long-term shoulder function. Patients with a C5-C6 injury and absent biceps muscle function at three months of age often have good long-term shoulder function without brachial plexus surgery.

► Most neonates with brachial plexus palsy have spontaneous recovery of arm function, with normal function expected if recovery occurs within the first 4 weeks after birth. However, some patients with persistent neurologic defects at 3 months will demonstrate permanent disability. An important prognostic factor for these individuals is the time interval to biceps muscle recovery. This study found that children with a C5-C6 level injury and absent biceps muscle function at 3 months often have good long-term shoulder function without brachial plexus surgery. Reduction of brachial plexus injuries at birth should be a primary goal of obstetric management.

H. N. Lafeber, MD, PhD

End-of-Life After Birth: Death and Dying in a Neonatal Intensive Care Unit
Singh J, Lantos J, Meadow W (Univ of Chicago; MacLean Ctr for Clinical Med Ethics, Chicago)
Pediatrics 114:1620-1626, 2004   16–8

Objective.—In canonical modern bioethics, withholding and withdrawing medical interventions for dying patients are considered morally equivalent. However, electing not to administer cardiopulmonary resuscitation (CPR) struck us as easily distinguishable from withdrawing mechanical ventilation. Moreover, withdrawing mechanical ventilation from a moribund infant "feels" different from withdrawing mechanical ventilation from a hemodynamically stable child with a severe neurologic insult. Most previous descriptions of withdrawing and withholding intervention in the neonatal intensive care unit (NICU) have blurred many of these distinctions. We hypothesized that clarifying them would more accurately portray the process of end-of-life decision-making in the NICU.

Methods.—We reviewed the charts of all newborn infants who had birth weight >400 g and died in our hospital in 1988, 1993, and 1998 and extracted potential ethical issues (resuscitation, withdrawal, withholding, CPR, do-not-resuscitate orders, neurologic prognosis, ethics consult) surrounding each infant's death.

Results.—Using traditional definitions, roughly half of all deaths in our NICU in 1993 and 1998 were associated with "withholding or withdrawing." In addition, by 1998, >40% of our NICU deaths could be labeled "active withdrawal," reflecting the extubation of infants regardless of their physiologic instability. This practice is growing over time. However, 2 important conclusions arise from our more richly elaborated descriptions of death in the NICU. First, when CPR was withheld, it most commonly occurred in the context of moribund infants who were already receiving ventilation and dopamine. Physiologically stable infants who were removed from mechanical ventilation for quality-of-life reasons accounted for only 3% of NICU deaths in 1988, 16% of NICU deaths in 1993, and 13% of NICU deaths in 1998. Moreover, virtually none of these active withdrawals took place in premature infants. Second, by 1998 infants, who died without CPR almost always had mechanical ventilation withdrawn. Finally, the median and average day of death for 100 nonsurvivors who received full intervention did not differ significantly from the 78 nonsurvivors for whom intervention was withheld.

Conclusions.—In our unit, a greater and greater percentage of doomed infants die without ever receiving chest compressions or epinephrine boluses. Rather, we have adopted a nuanced approach to withdrawing/withholding NICU intervention, providing what we hope is a humane approach to end-of-life decisions for doomed NICU infants. We suggest that ethical descriptions that reflect these nuances, distinguishing between withholding and withdrawing interventions from physiologically moribund infants or physiologically stable infants with morbid neurologic prognoses, provide a more accurate reflection of the circumstances of dying in the NICU.

▶ Despite the considerable improvements in neonatal resuscitation over the past 3 decades, the unfortunate reality of working in neonatology is the all-too-frequent requirement of dealing with end-of-life issues in the nursery. The authors present their experience with a nuanced approach to the interventions provided to compromised and doomed infants, recognizing that a rigid approach to the process of intervening with critically ill neonates does not and cannot exist and that individualization of care is required to provide humane and effective care for these critically ill children.

H. N. Lafeber, MD, PhD

Refining the Apgar Score Cut-Off Point for Newborns at Risk
Chong DSY, Karlberg J (Univ of Hong Kong)
Acta Paediatr 93:53-59, 2004   16–9

Aim.—To evaluate the Apgar score predictive power for mortality during different periods in the first year of life in a population with a very low mortality rate.

Methods.—The records of all singleton live births without severe congenital malformations and length of gestation >25 wk ($n = 976635$) were collected from the Swedish Medical Birth Registry, 1990 to 1998. Receiver operating characteristic (ROC) analysis was utilized.

Results.—Both the 1-min and the 5-min Apgar scores were shown to be good discriminators for early mortality, with the area under the ROC curve >0.85. For babies at risk of early death, the selected cut-off values for the 1-min Apgar score was <8 for preterm (true-positive (TP) rate: 83.9%; false-positive (FP) rate: 17.7%) and term babies (TP rate: 69.4%; FP rate: 6.7%). At 5 min, the analysis revealed that newborns with an Apgar score <9 were at risk for early death (preterm babies: TP rate: 79.8%; FP rate: 13.3%; term babies: TP rate: 73.8%; FP rate: 3.4%).

Conclusions.—Our analysis did not support the common practice in the clinic or in research of grouping infants at risk in Apgar score groups, i.e. a score below 4 or a score below 7. However, the data presented here allow the clinicians and researchers to identify and define a suitable cut-off point in relation to the quality of neonatal care and resources available, rather than adhering to a historical cut-off value that has not been studied in depth.

▶ The Apgar score has been the mainstay of newborn evaluation since Virginia Apgar published her first study in 1953. The Apgar score remains an important component of our overall evaluation of the ill newborn. In the continuing research to develop more effective screening protocols for adverse neonatal outcomes, Dr Apgar and others have recommended the use of certain cut-off scores to identify newborns at increased or decreased risk for adverse outcomes. This current study from the University of Hong Kong does not support the practice of using Apgar cut-offs of less than 4 or less than 7 to predetermine the degree of intervention needed for resuscitation; rather, the authors suggest that the determination of Apgar score cut-offs be individualized to each center so as to optimize newborn outcomes in each program and center. As newborn concerns will vary from center to center, this study presents compelling information that should hopefully help improve neonatal outcomes worldwide.

H. N. Lafeber, MD, PhD

Is It Safer to Intubate Premature Infants in the Delivery Room?
Aly H, Massaro AN, Patel K, et al (George Washington Univ, Washington, DC; Children's Natl Med Ctr, Washington, DC)
Pediatrics 115:1660-1665, 2005   16–10

Objectives.—Early nasal continuous positive airway pressure (ENCPAP) has recently emerged in neonatal units as an acceptable alternative to routine intubation and mandatory ventilation. The risks and benefits of ENCPAP have yet to be established. In this study, we aimed to examine variables that influenced the decision to initiate ENCPAP in the delivery room (DR). We also explored potential harmful effects of early intubation and examined whether unsuccessful ENCPAP attempts might subject infants to any unforeseen morbidity.

Methods.—All inborn very low birth weight (VLBW) infants admitted to the NICU since the implementation of the ENCPAP policy were included in this retrospective study. Infants were stratified initially into 2 cohorts according to whether they were intubated in the DR or began ENCPAP. Infants were then stratified into 4 groups according to the respiratory management during their first week of life. Infants in group 1 were supported with ENCPAP in the DR and continued to receive continuous positive airway pressure (CPAP) at least for the entire first week. Infants in group 2 began ENCPAP treatment in the DR but required intubation during the first week of life. Infants in group 3 were intubated in the DR but transitioned successfully to CPAP within the first 48 hours and were treated with CPAP for the first week of life or longer. Infants in group 4 were intubated in the DR and treated with intermittent mandatory ventilation for >48 hours. Univariate analyses compared different groups with the Wilcoxon nonparametric test, Kruskal-Wallis test, and analysis of variance. A multivariate regression model adjusted for differences in birth weights (BWs), gestational ages (GAs), race, and Apgar scores between the groups.

Results.—A total of 234 VLBW infants (weight of <1500 g) were admitted to the NICU during the period from August 1997 to December 2003. The mean BW was 977.1 ± 305.8 g, and the mean GA was 27.7 ± 2.7 weeks. The overall mortality rate was 11.1%, and the incidence of bronchopulmonary dysplasia among survivors was 17.4%. ENCPAP was implemented successfully in the DR for 151 (64.5%) infants, whereas 83 (35.5%) infants required intubation. Infants who required intubation had significantly lower GAs, BWs, and 1-minute Apgar scores. The use of ENCPAP in the DR increased significantly over time. The chance of successful maintenance with ENCPAP for >48 hours was not demonstrable at <24 weeks of gestation (10% success). Use of ENCPAP improved significantly by 25 weeks of gestation (45% success). Infants in group 1 required a shorter duration of oxygen use than did infants in group 3 (7.9 ± 18.3 vs 39 ± 32.7 days; regression coefficient $[b]$ = 19 ± 5.3). None of the infants in group 1 developed intraventricular hemorrhage of grade III or IV or retinopathy of prematurity of stage 3 or 4. Infants in group 3 did not show improved outcomes, compared with group 1. Compared with group 4, infants in group 2 had a higher incidence of necrotizing enterocolitis (15.6% vs 7.3%; b = 2.5 ± 1.2).

Conclusions.—The success of ENCPAP improved with increased GA and with staff experience over time. Infants treated successfully with ENCPAP were unlikely to develop intraventricular hemorrhage of grade III or IV. Infants who experienced ENCPAP failure were at increased risk for the development of necrotizing enterocolitis. Infants who were intubated briefly in the DR were at increased risk for prolonged oxygen requirement. An individualized approach should be considered for respiratory support of VLBW infants.

▶ The initial airway management for preterm and premature infants continues to be a subject of considerable debate among neonatologists and pediatricians. This debate is usually centered around the benefits and risk of intubations and a nonintubating procedure known as ENCPAP. The authors found that those infants treated successfully with ENCPAP were unlikely to develop advanced intraventricular hemorrhages; however, those infants who had a failed ENCPAP were at increased risk for developing necrotizing enterocolitis.

The authors concluded that ENCPAP is an important and valued addition to the resuscitative measures available for preterm infant resuscitation after birth but that an individualized approach in deciding which techniques to use must be utilized, as risks and benefits for both techniques exist and success and failure of either technique depends on the presentation of the preterm infant.

L. P. Shulman, MD

17 Therapy

Amnioinfusion for the Prevention of the Meconium Aspiration Syndrome
Fraser WD, for the Amnioinfusion Trial Group (Université de Montréal; et al)
N Engl J Med 353:909-917, 2005   17–1

Background.—It is uncertain whether amnioinfusion (infusion of saline into the amniotic cavity) in women who have thick meconium staining of the amniotic fluid reduces the risk of perinatal death, moderate or severe meconium aspiration syndrome, or both.

Methods.—We performed a multicenter trial in which 1998 pregnant women in labor at 36 or more weeks of gestation who had thick meconium staining of the amniotic fluid were stratified according to the presence or ab-

TABLE 4.—Distribution of Maternal Disorders and Indicators of Complications, According to Study Group*

Disorder or Indicator	Amnioinfusion (N = 986)	Control (N = 989)	Relative Risk (95% CI)
	No. (%)		
Cesarean delivery†	314 (31.8)	287 (29.0)	1.10 (0.96-1.25)
Fetal distress	133 (13.5)	114 (11.5)	—
Dystocia	162 (16.4)	164 (16.6)	—
Other	19 (1.9)	9 (0.9)	—
Peripartum fever‡	31 (3.1)	33 (3.3)	0.94 (0.58-1.53)
Maternal death or serious morbidity§	15 (1.5)	15 (1.5)	1.00 (0.49-2.04)
Uterine rupture	2 (0.2)	1 (0.1)	2.00 (0.18-22.09)
Antepartum hemorrhage¶	3 (0.3)	1 (0.1)	3.01 (0.31-28.85)
Hysterectomy	2 (0.2)	0	
Admission to the intensive care unit	3 (0.3)	1 (0.1)	3.01 (0.31-28.88)
Maternal death	0	1 (0.1)	
Disseminated intravascular coagulation	3 (0.3)	1 (0.1)	3.01 (0.31-28.91)
Postpartum hemorrhage‖	11 (1.1)	11 (1.1)	1.00 (0.44-2.30)

*CI denotes confidence interval, and dashes not assessed.
†Indications for cesarean delivery included suspected fetal compromise, which was determined on the basis of an abnormal fetal heart-rate tracing or an abnormal fetal-scalp pH, and dystocia, which was defined as failure to progress, cephalopelvic disproportion, or failed forceps or vacuum delivery.
‡Peripartum fever was defined as intrapartum fever (≥38.5°C on at least one reading between randomization and delivery), postpartum fever (≥38.5°C on at least two readings more than 24 hours apart, excluding the first 24 hours after delivery) or both.
§Maternal death or serious morbidity was defined as death or at least one maternal complication. In the case of missing values, the mother was considered to be negative for the disorder or indicator.
¶Antepartum hemorrhage (without uterine rupture) was defined as that requiring urgent delivery.
‖Postpartum hemorrhage was defined as blood loss of at least 500 ml requiring blood transfusion.
(Courtesy of Fraser WD, for the Amnioinfusion Trial Group: Amnioinfusion for the prevention of the meconium aspiration syndrome. *N Engl J Med* 353:909-917, 2005. Copyright Massachusetts Medical Society, all rights reserved.)

sence of variable decelerations in fetal heart rate and then randomly assigned to amnioinfusion or to standard care. The composite primary outcome measure was perinatal death, moderate or severe meconium aspiration syndrome, or both.

Results.—Perinatal death, moderate or severe meconium aspiration syndrome, or both occurred in 44 infants (4.5 percent) of women in the amnioinfusion group and 35 infants (3.5 percent) of women in the control group (relative risk, 1.26; 95 percent confidence interval, 0.82 to 1.95). Five perinatal deaths occurred in the amnioinfusion group and five in the control group. The rate of cesarean delivery was 31.8 percent in the amnioinfusion group and 29.0 percent in the control group (relative risk, 1.10; 95 percent confidence interval, 0.96 to 1.25) (Table 4).

Conclusions.—For women in labor who have thick meconium staining of the amniotic fluid, amnioinfusion did not reduce the risk of moderate or severe meconium aspiration syndrome, perinatal death, or other major maternal or neonatal disorders.

▶ The staining of amniotic fluid by the fetal meconium is a relatively common occurrence; however, the aspiration of meconium-stained fluid can lead to considerable fetal morbidity and complicates the management of anywhere from 5% to 30% of newborns. As with newborns with meconium aspiration syndrome, a similar range (5%-40% mortality rate) has been observed. Meconium aspiration syndrome results from aspirating meconium during intrauterine gasping or at the time of the initial breath. Unfortunately, prophylactic suctioning and tracheal aspiration have not been shown to reduce the risk of meconium aspiration syndrome. To this end, amnioinfusion has been proposed as a method to reduce the risk of meconium aspiration syndrome. The authors sought to determine through a multicenter trial whether amnioinfusion, or the infusion of saline into the amniotic cavity by a transcervical route, would reduce the frequency of meconium aspiration syndrome and the morbidity and mortality associated with it. Unfortunately, this study found that amnioinfusion did not reduce the risk of moderate or severe meconium aspiration syndrome in women who have thick meconium staining of the amniotic fluid. In addition, perinatal death or other major maternal or neonatal disorders were not affected by amnioinfusion. Despite the potential theoretical benefits of amnioinfusion, this study provides important information as to the lack of clinical benefit of amnioinfusion for the prevention of meconium aspiration syndrome.

L. P. Shulman, MD

Oral Zinc Supplementation in Pregnant Women and Its Effect on Birth Weight: A Randomised Controlled Trial

Hafeez A, Mehmood G, Mazhar F (KRL Hosp, Islamabad, Pakistan; Pakistan Inst of Med Sciences, Islamabad)

Arch Dis Child Fetal Neonatal Ed 90:F170-F171, 2005   17–2

Background.—Previous trials of zinc supplementation have produced conflicting results on various pregnancy outcomes. Pakistan is in a part of the world in which the soil is deficient in zinc. The few studies conducted on the zinc status of women and children living in this region have shown an alarming prevalence of zinc deficiency. Oral supplementation is one measure to prevent the birth of low birth weight babies and thus avert the morbidity and mortality of newborns associated with this condition. The effects of oral zinc supplementation on the birth weight of newborns were evaluated.

Methods.—A double-blind, randomized, controlled trial was conducted for 1 year at 2 large urban hospitals and in 1 rural community. All pregnant women at 10 to 16 weeks' gestation were offered the opportunity to enter the study at the booking visit. Women with known systemic disease were excluded. The patients were randomly assigned to test and control groups and given either elemental zinc or placebo in capsule form.

Results.—A total of 242 participants were enrolled. The mean (SD) age of the patients was 25.7 (4.8) years (range, 16 to 40 years). Birth weights and other anthropometric data did not differ significantly between the zinc supplemented group and the placebo group.

Conclusions.—Oral supplementation of pregnant women with 20 mg elemental zinc did not provide a significant increase in the birth weight of this study population. Supplementation trials with larger doses of zinc should be performed.

▶ Zinc is a cofactor for several metalloenzymes and a constituent of proteins, hormones, and neuropeptides. It is crucial for embryonic development as a component of cellular multiplication, differentiation, and apoptosis as well as for the integrity of cellular membranes. Zinc is also of importance because of its role in the absorption of natural folate. An important issue in developing countries such as Pakistan is the high prevalence of zinc deficiency; therefore, high-risk groups such as pregnant women and children need zinc supplementation. The literature on the association between zinc supplementation during pregnancy and birth weight is controversial. This is often due to small samples and nonrandomized study designs. This study seems to be optimally designed as a randomized, controlled trial and therefore is relevant. The dosage of 20 mg elementary zinc (in addition to the supplementation with folic acid and iron) seems to be adequate though in the upper level of the recommended daily allowance. A higher dose often gives gastrointestinal side effects and could therefore interact with other nutrients. The results, however, are negative although smaller differences than 250 g in birth weight cannot be ruled out. This may be due to the exclusion of women with systemic diseases who potentially may gain the most benefit from zinc supplementation. For example, zinc status is often compromised in women with diabetes. Ideally, supplementation studies should start before pregnancy as the most important stages of placentation, an important determinant of birth weight, take place during the first trimester of pregnancy. Finally, as birth weight is only a surrogate marker for the quality of intrauterine development, a study of parameters concerning postnatal growth and development may provide more important information.

E. A. P. Steegers, MD, PhD

Perinatal Risk Factors of Adverse Outcome in Very Preterm Children: A Role of Initial Treatment of Respiratory Insufficiency?
Hansen BM, for the Danish ETFOL Group (Rigshospitalet, Copenhagen)
Acta Paediatr 93:185-189, 2004 17–3

Aim.—To investigate risk factors of adverse outcome in a cohort of very preterm children treated mainly with nasal continuous positive airway pressure (CPAP) during the neonatal course.

Methods.—In Denmark, preterm children are treated with nasal CPAP as a first approach to respiratory support. A national prospective study of all infants with a birthweight below 1000 g or a gestational age below 28 wk born in 1994-1995 was initiated to evaluate this approach. Of the 269 surviving children 164 (61%) were not treated with mechanical ventilation in the neonatal period. A follow-up of the children at 5 y of age was conducted. Data from the neonatal period and the 5-y follow-up were analysed.

Results.—In multivariate analyses including 250 children, a severely abnormal neonatal brain ultrasound scan was predictive of cerebral palsy (OR = 19.9, CI 95%: 6.1–64.8) and intellectual disability (OR = 6.2, CI 95%: 2.3–16.5). A high Clinical Risk Index for Babies (CRIB) score (OR = 2.4, CI 95%: 1.1–5.5) and chronic lung disease (OR = 2.8, CI 95%: 1.2–6.9) were predictive of intellectual disability. In univariate analyses mechanical ventilation was associated with cerebral palsy (OR = 4.3, CI 95%: 1.7–10.8) and intellectual disability (OR = 2.2, CI 95%: 1.2–4.2), but the associations became insignificant in multivariate analyses including chronic lung disease and a severely abnormal ultrasound scan.

Conclusion.—The associations between neonatal risk factors and adverse outcome in our cohort were very similar to those found in other cohorts with another initial treatment of respiratory insufficiency. We found no significant adverse effects of mechanical ventilation beyond what could be explained by associations with chronic lung disease and IVH 3–4/PVL.

▶ Prematurity remains a major determinant of perinatal morbidity and mortality. Treatment of very preterm infants with CPAP may be a more effective approach to resolving pulmonary insufficiency than mechanical ventilation. In this 5-year follow-up study from Rigshospitalet in Copenhagen, where CPAP is almost universally used, the authors found an increased risk of cerebral palsy and intellectual disability in children who had been exposed to mechanical ventilation after preterm birth, although the findings became nonsignificant when evaluated in a multivariate analysis adding chronic lung disease and severely abnormal US findings. In this well-followed cohort, mechanical ventilation appeared to play no beneficial or adverse role in the care of the extremely preterm infant. However, readers are cautioned to recognize that this cohort was almost uniformly treated with CPAP, a practice that may not occur at many centers.

P. P. van den Berg, MD, PhD

REPRODUCTIVE ENDOCRINOLOGY AND INFERTILITY

18 Endocrinology

Oestrogen Treatment to Reduce the Adult Height of Tall Girls: Long-term Effects on Fertility
Venn A, Bruinsma F, Werther G, et al (Univ of Tasmania, Hobart, Australia; La Trobe Univ, Victoria, Australia; Murdoch Childrens Research Inst, Melbourne, Australia)
Lancet 364:1513-1518, 2004   18–1

Background.—Treatment with oestrogen to reduce the adult height of tall girls has been available since the 1950s. We undertook a retrospective cohort study to assess the long-term effects of this treatment on fertility.

Methods.—Eligible participants were identified from the records of Australian paediatric endocrinologists who assessed tall girls from 1959 to 1993, and from self-referrals. Individuals included girls who had received oestrogen treatment (diethylstilboestrol or ethinyl oestradiol) (treated group) and those who were assessed but not treated (untreated group). Information about reproductive history was sought by telephone interview.

Findings.—1432 eligible individuals were identified, of whom 1243 (87%) could be traced. Of these, 780 (63%) completed interviews: 651 were identified from endocrinologists' records, 129 were self-referred. Treated (n=371) and untreated (n=409) women were similar in socioeconomic and other characteristics. After adjustment for age, treated women were more likely to have ever tried for 12 months or more to become pregnant without

TABLE 2.—History of Fertility Problems by Treatment Status

	Treated n=371	Untreated n=409	Adjusted RR* (95% CI)
Ever tried for ≥12 months to become pregnant without succeeding	133 (35·9%)	76 (18·6%)	1·80 (1·40-2·30)
Ever seen a doctor because of trouble becoming pregnant	127 (34·2%)	73 (17·9%)	1·80 (1·39-2·32)
Ever taken fertility drugs	68 (18·3%)	34 (8·3%)	2·05 (1·39-3·04)
Ever been pregnant	287 (77·4%)	313 (76·5%)	0·93 (0·87-0·99)
Ever had livebirth	248 (66·9%)	267 (65·3%)	0·87 (0·79-0·95)

*Adjusted for current age. Data are n (%) unless otherwise indicated.
(Courtesy of Venn A, Bruinsma F, Werther G, et al: Oestrogen treatment to reduce the adult height of tall girls: Long-term effects on fertility. *Lancet* 364:1513-1518, 2004. Reprinted with permission from Elsevier.)

success (relative risk [RR] 1.80, 95% CI 1.40-2.30); more likely to have seen a doctor because they were having difficulty becoming pregnant (RR 1.80, 1.39-2.32); and more likely to have ever taken fertility drugs (RR 2.05, 1.39-3.04) (Table 2). Time to first pregnancy analysis showed that the treated group was 40% less likely to conceive in any given menstrual cycle of unprotected intercourse (age-adjusted fecundability ratio 0.59, 95% CI 0.46-0.76). These associations persisted when self-referred women were excluded.

Interpretation.—High-dose oestrogen treatment in adolescence seems to reduce female fertility in later life. This finding has implications for current treatment practices and for our understanding of reproductive biology.

▶ This is another cautionary tale regarding the use of unproven therapies for questionable indications. In this Australian study of 780 women evaluated in adolescence for tall stature, 371 were treated with estrogen and 409 were untreated. The treated subjects were almost twice as likely as the untreated to have a history of infertility, to have seen a doctor for infertility, or to have taken infertility drugs. The fecundity rate was also significantly lower in the treated women compared with the untreated (0.59). However, the risk of ever having a live birth was not affected by treatment. There were no differences between the 2 groups with regard to infertility diagnoses. I find this interesting, because I would suspect that if premenarcheal estrogen therapy were to affect fertility, it would be most likely to do so by altering the hypothalamic-pituitary-ovarian axis and increasing the likelihood of anovulation. However, the rate of ovulatory problems as an infertility diagnosis was the same in the treated (28%) and untreated (30%) groups.

Although it is likely that tall stature in women is more socially acceptable now than in the past, the authors point out that a study of US pediatric endocrinologists published in 2002 found that 22% had treated tall girls with estrogen in the preceding 5 years, though most had treated fewer than 5.[1] The sixth edition (1999) of *Clinical Gynecologic Endocrinology and Infertility* (p 409) states that "A predicted height of greater than 6 feet probably deserves treatment." Anyone considering estrogen therapy for tall girls must be aware of its possible effect on fertility in adulthood.

R. Barnes, MD

Reference

1. Barnard ND, Scialli AR, Bobela S: The current use of estrogens for growth-suppressant therapy in adolescent girls. *J Pediatr Adolesc Gynecol* 15:23-26, 2002.

Metformin Treatment in Patients With Polycystic Ovary Syndrome Undergoing in Vitro Fertilization: A Prospective Randomized Trial

Önalan G, Pabuçcu R, Goktolga U, et al (Centrum Clinic, Ankara, Turkey; Gulhane School of Medicine, Ankara, Turkey)
Fertil Steril 84:798-801, 2005   18–2

Background.—Polycystic ovary syndrome (PCOS) is the most common cause of anovulatory female infertility. The presence of insulin resistance in women with PCOS undergoing infertility treatment may result in higher doses of gonadotropins administered to these patients, higher cancellation rates from risk of ovarian hyperstimulation, and lower fertilization rates. A hypothesis was investigated that the insulin-sensitizing drug metformin, which reduces hyperinsulinemia, insulin resistance, and secretion by increasing insulin sensitivity, might improve the results of in vitro fertilization (IVF) or intracytoplasmic sperm injection (ICSI).

Methods.—The study group was composed of 110 infertile women with PCOS who were referred to 1 IVF clinic after failure to conceive by conventional therapies. All the patients were undergoing their first IVF/ISI attempts. The patients received a standard long protocol of pituitary suppression with gonadotropin-releasing hormone agonist (triptorelin 0.1 mg), followed by administration of recombinant follicle-stimulating hormone with a standard initial dose of 2 to 4 ampules/day. Human chorionic gonadotropin was administered with the detection of a minimum of 3 leading follicles of 18 mm or more mean diameter and serum levels of prostaglandin E_2 less than 5500 pg/mL. All the patients were offered ICSI because of the poor fertilization rate experienced with IVF in patients with PCOS. Two patients abandoned the treatment cycles. The remaining 108 patients were divided into placebo (55 patients) and metformin (53 patients) groups.

Results.—In the metformin group, patients with a glucose/insulin ratio less than 4.5 had lower day-3 serum levels of luteinizing hormone and prostaglandin E_2 and lower number of follicles (17 mm in diameter) compared with the placebo group. Patients with a body mass index less than 28 had similar outcomes in both groups. Patients with a body mass index of 28 or greater in the metformin group had lower serum levels of luteinizing hormone, increased numbers of antral follicles, and increased numbers of follicles (17 mm in diameter) compared with patients in the placebo group. No failure of fertilization was observed. Four cases of mild ovarian hyperstimulation syndrome occurred in the placebo group and 3 cases in the metformin group.

Conclusions.—Metformin did not contribute to any improvement in IVF/ICSI outcomes in women with PCOS.

▶ Although metformin is effective in inducing ovulation in women with PCOS either as a single agent or in combination with clomiphene in clomiphene-resistant women,[1] its role in ovarian stimulation protocols for IVF is less clear. A retrospective study found a favorable effect of metformin treatment on both follicular development and pregnancy rate. Metformin decreased the total number of follicles on the day of human chorionic gonadotropin treatment while significantly increasing the mean number of mature oocytes, fertilization rate, and clinical pregnancy rate (70% vs 30%) compared with follicle-stimulating hormone treatment alone.[2] A randomized trial of metformin in 73 PCOS patients stimulated with follicle-stimulating hormone after gonadotropin-releasing hormone agonist downregulation found no difference in ovarian stimulation or clinical pregnancy rate between metformin and placebo. However, in women with a body mass index (BMI) less than 28 there was an increased clinical pregnancy rate that did not reach statistical significance.[3]

This study included 108 women randomized to metformin 1700 mg (BMI less than 28) or 2550 mg (BMI less than 28). They underwent gonadotropin-releasing hormone agonist downregulation followed by follicle-stimulating hormone stimulation. Metformin increased the number of antral follicles in the high BMI subcategory, but otherwise there was no significant effect of metformin on follicle number, number of mature oocytes, fertilization rate, or clinical pregnancy rate overall or within the 2 BMI subcategories. Considering the findings of the 2 published randomized trials, one would have to conclude that there is at present no clear role for its use in PCOS patients undergoing IVF.

R. Barnes, MD

References

1. Lord JM, Flight IH, Norman RJ: Metformin in polycystic ovary syndrome: Systematic review and meta-analysis. *BMJ* 327:951-953, 2003.
2. Stadtmauer LA, Toma SK, Riehl RM, et al: Metformin treatment of patients with polycystic ovary syndrome undergoing in vitro fertilization improves outcomes and is associated with modulation of the insulin-like growth factors. *Fertil Steril* 75:505-509, 2001.
3. Kjotrod SB, von During V, Carlsen SM: Metformin treatment before IVF/ICSI in women with polycystic ovary syndrome: A prospective, randomized, double blind study. *Hum Reprod* 19:1315-1322, 2004.

Does Metformin Induced Ovulation in Normoandrogenic Anovulatory Women?

Carmina E, Lobo RA (Univ of Palermo, Italy; Columbia Univ, New York)
Am J Obstet Gynecol 191:1580-1584, 2004   18–3

Objective.—This study was undertaken to evaluate the efficacy of metformin in women with anovulation who do not have evidence for hyperandrogenism and classic polycystic ovary syndrome.

Study Design.—A randomized trial of metformin (1500 mg daily) and placebo in 24 anovulatory women was undertaken for 3 months. Assessments of changes in hormone levels and insulin sensitivity were carried out. Abnormal hormonal values were defined by levels exceeding the range in normal ovulatory controls.

Results.—Anovulatory women had normal androgen levels and luteinizing hormone but had higher serum insulin and lower insulin sensitivity compared with controls. Over 3 months, there were 16 ovulatory cycles with metformin and only 4 with placebo ($P < 05$). Success of ovulation did not correlate with changes in androgen, insulin, or insulin sensitivity parameters.

Conclusion.—Metformin may be useful for inducing ovulation in anovulatory women who do not have hyperandrogenism. This effect may be independent of a lowering of androgen or insulin levels.

▶ The uses of metformin for a wide variety of patients continue to expand as the beneficial effects of this drug are better delineated. One application involves the induction of ovulation in women with polycystic ovary syndrome. This study shows that metformin was useful for inducing ovulation in anovulatory women without hyperandrogenism and that the beneficial impact was likely independent of lowered androgen or insulin levels. Such studies provide valuable information that can improve clinical outcomes for infertile couples seeking to become pregnant.

L. P. Shulman, MD

Prospective Parallel Randomized, Double-Blind, Double-Dummy Controlled Clinical Trial Comparing Clomiphene Citrate and Metformin as the First-line Treatment for Ovulation Induction in Nonobese Anovulatory Women With Polycystic Ovary Syndrome
Palomba S, Orio F Jr, Falbo A, et al (Univ "Magna Graecia" of Catanzaro, Naples, Italy; Univ "Federico II" of Naples, Italy; Univ of Palermo, Italy)
J Clin Endocrinol Metab 90:4068-4074, 2005   18–4

Context.—Although metformin has been shown to be effective in the treatment of anovulation in women with polycystic ovary syndrome (PCOS), clomiphene citrate (CC) is still considered to be the first-line drug to induce ovulation in these patients.

Objective.—The goal of this study was to compare the effectiveness of metformin and CC administration as a first-line treatment in anovulatory women with PCOS.

Design.—We describe a prospective parallel randomized, double-blind, double-dummy controlled clinical trial.

Setting.—The study was conducted at the University "Magna Graecia" of Catanzaro, Catanzaro, Italy.

Patients.—One hundred nonobese primary infertile anovulatory women with PCOS participated.

Interventions.—We administered metformin cloridrate (850 mg twice daily) plus placebo (group A) or placebo plus CC (150 mg for 5 d from the third day of a progesterone withdrawal bleeding) (group B) for 6 months each.

Mean Outcome Measures.—The main outcome measures were ovulation, pregnancy, abortion, and live-birth rates.

TABLE 2.—Ovulation and Pregnancy Rates in PCOS Women Treated With Metformin Cloridrate (group A) or CC (group B) During Each Cycle of Treatment

Cycle	Ovulation Rate [No. Ovulatory Cycles/No. Cycles (%)]			Pregnancy Rate [No. Pregnancies/No. Cycles (%)]		
	Group A	Group B	P	Group A	Group B	P[a]
1	19/45 (42.2)	39/47 (83.0)	<0.001	3/45 (6.7)	6/47 (12.8)	0.49
2	24/42 (57.1)	33/41 (80.5)	0.02	4/42 (9.5)	5/41 (12.2)	0.74
3	25/38 (65.8)	25/36 (69.4)	0.74	6/38 (15.8)	2/36 (5.6)	0.26
4	22/32 (68.8)	19/34 (55.9)	0.28	5/32 (15.6)	2/34 (5.9)	0.25
5	21/27 (77.8)	17/32 (53.1)	0.049	6/27 (22.2)	1/32 (3.1)	0.04
6	18/21 (85.7)	15/31 (48.4)	0.006	7/21 (33.3)	0/31 (0.0)	0.001

Data were analyzed using χ^2 test unless otherwise specified.
[a]Fisher's exact test.
Abbreviations: PCOS, Polycystic ovary syndrome; CC, clomiphene citrate.
(Courtesy of Palomba S, Orio F Jr, Falbo A, et al: Prospective parallel randomized, double-blind, double-dummy controlled clinical trial comparing clomiphene citrate and metformin as the first-line treatment for ovulation induction in nonobese anovulatory women with polycystic ovary syndrome. *J Clin Endocrinol Metab* 90[7]:4068-4074, 2005. Copyright The Endocrine Society.)

Results.—The subjects of groups A (n = 45) and B (n = 47) were studied for a total of 205 and 221 cycles, respectively. The ovulation rate was not statistically different between either treatment group (62.9 vs. 67.0%, $P = 0.38$), whereas the pregnancy rate was significantly higher in group A than group B (15.1 vs. 7.2%, $P = 0.009$) (Table 2). The difference found between groups A and B regarding the abortion rate was significant (9.7 vs. 37.5%, $P = 0.045$), whereas a positive trend was observed for the live-birth rate (83.9 vs. 56.3%, $P = 0.07$). The cumulative pregnancy rate was significantly higher in group A than group B (68.9 vs. 34.0%, $P < 0.001$).

Conclusions.—Six-month metformin administration is significantly more effective than six-cycle CC treatment in improving fertility in anovulatory nonobese PCOS women.

▶ At first glance, this randomized trial of metformin versus CC as first-line treatment for ovulation induction is an impressive endorsement of metformin. The ovulation rate per cycle was equal between the 2 treatments; however, the cumulative pregnancy rate was significantly higher (69% vs 34%) and the spontaneous abortion rate was significantly lower (10% vs 37%) in the metformin group. I believe the differences in cumulative birth rate and abortion rate are due at least in part to the authors' nonstandard use of CC. All subjects were treated with 150 mg of CC from the onset instead of incremental doses of 50 to 100 to 150 mg. About 50% of World Health Organization group 2 women will ovulate on 50 mg of CC, and of the anovulatory 50%, almost 50% will ovulate on 100 mg. Of subjects who ovulate on CC, only 8% will require 150 mg.[1] Thus, about 90% of the clomiphene-treated subjects in this study were given a higher dose than necessary to induce ovulation and, perhaps, were adversely affected by an antiestrogenic dose effect that was much greater than necessary for ovulation induction.

Another recent trial of CC in ovulation induction that used the standard stepwise increment of CC found a cumulative pregnancy rate of 42% and a spontaneous abortion rate of only 11% in 259 women.[2] These values compare much more favorably to the metformin cumulative pregnancy rate of 69% and abortion rate of 10% in this study. Metformin may yet prove to be a better first choice for ovulation induction in women with PCOS, but this fatally flawed randomized trial is not that proof.

R. Barnes, MD

References

1. Imani B, Eijkemans MJ, te Velde ER, et al: Predictors of patients remaining anovulatory during clomiphene citrate induction of ovulation in normogonadotropic oligoamenorrheic infertility. *J Clin Endocrinol Metab* 83:2361-2365, 1998.
2. Imani B, Eijkemans MJ, te Velde ER, et al: A nomogram to predict the probability of live birth after clomiphene citrate induction of ovulation in normogonadotropic oligoamenorrheic infertility. *Fertil Steril* 77:91-97, 2002.

19 Infertility

Histological Dating of Timed Endometrial Biopsy Tissue Is Not Related to Fertility Status
Coutifaris C, for the NICHD National Cooperative Reproductive Medicine Network (Univ of Pennsylvania, Philadelphia; et al)
Fertil Steril 82:1264-1272, 2004   19–1

Objective.—To assess the ability of histological dating to discriminate between women of fertile and infertile couples. The utility of histological dating of endometrium in the evaluation of infertile couples is uncertain.

Design.—Prospective multicenter study, with subjects randomly assigned to biopsy timing. Criterion standard for infertility was 12 months of unprotected, regular intercourse without conception and for fertility at least one live birth within 2 years.

Setting.—University-based infertility practices.

Patient(s).—Volunteer subjects (847) recruited at 12 clinical sites participating in the National Institutes of Health-funded Reproductive Medicine Network. Inclusion criteria included ages 20-39 years, regular menstrual cycles, and no hormonal treatment or contraceptive use for 1 month before the study. Fertile controls were excluded if they had a history of infertility, recurrent pregnancy loss, or recent breastfeeding.

Intervention(s).—Subjects underwent daily urinary LH testing. After detection of the LH surge, subjects were randomized to biopsy in the mid (days 21-22) or the late (days 26-27) luteal phase. Pathologists at each site estimated the cycle day based on standard criteria. For the primary analysis, an out-of-phase biopsy was defined as a greater than 2-day delay in the histological maturation of the endometrium.

Main Outcome Measure(s).—The proportion of out-of-phase biopsies in fertile and infertile women was compared using logistic regression models with age at randomization as a covariate. Comparisons were also made between fertile vs. infertile at the midluteal or late luteal phase time points.

Result(s).—Biopsies were evaluated (301 mid and 318 late; N = 619). Out-of-phase biopsy results poorly discriminated between women from fertile and infertile couples in either the midluteal (fertile: 49.4%, infertile: 43.2%) or late luteal phase (fertile: 35.3%, infertile 23.0%). Results did not substantially differ using alternative definitions of "out-of-phase" or standardized cycle day (Table 2).

TABLE 2.—Prevalence of an Out-of-Phase Endometrial Biopsy in Fertile Women and in Women of Infertile Couples at Either the Midluteal or Late Luteal Phase

Variables	Women of Fertile Couples (n = 332)	Women of Infertile Couples (n = 287)	Odds Ratio Point Estimate	Odds Ratio Estimates 95% Wald CL	P Value
OOP>2	42.2%	32.7%	0.68	0.49-0.95	.0248
OOP>3	33.2%	20.9%	0.54	0.37-0.78	.0011[a]
OOP>4	19.9%	11.2%	0.49	0.31-0.78	.0027[a]

Note: *P* value for logistic regression, adjusting for age.
[a]OOP>2, OOP>3, and OOP>4 denotes more than 2, more than 3, and more than 4 days difference between the postovulatory day and the histological dating using the Noyes criteria. To adjust for preplanned multiple comparisons, fertility group differences were considered significant if $P \leq .0125$.
Abbreviations: CL, Confidence limit; *OOP*, out of phase.
(Courtesy of Coutifaris C, for the NICHD National Cooperative Reproductive Medicine Network: Histological dating of timed endometrial biopsy tissue is not related to fertility status. *Fertil Steril* 82:1264-1272, 2004. Reprinted by permission from the American College of Surgeons.)

Conclusion(s).—Histological dating of the endometrium does not discriminate between women of fertile and infertile couples and should not be used in the routine evaluation of infertility.

▶ Probably the oldest and perhaps most rancorous controversy in the history of infertility evaluation is the value of the endometrial biopsy. This article and its companion on observer variability in histologic dating of the endometrium[1] argue convincingly that an endometrial biopsy is of no value, primarily because out-of-phase biopsies are more common in fertile than in infertile subjects. The authors are careful to point out that this study does not address the issue of whether a luteal phase defect exists or is a cause of infertility, but it does convincingly argue that an endometrial biopsy for histologic dating is not useful to diagnose a luteal phase defect. This is because of the high prevalence of an abnormal biopsy in fertile women and the relatively poor agreement among expert pathologists as to the diagnosis of an out-of-phase biopsy. Most experts agree that this large, well-designed study of more than 600 biopsies in normal and infertile women provides convincing evidence of the lack of value of a luteal phase biopsy for histologic dating in the evaluation of infertility.[2-6] It is an expensive, often painful test with no discriminatory value.

R. Barnes, MD

References

1. Myers ER, Silva S, Barnhart K, et al: Interobserver and intraobserver variability in the histological dating of the endometrium in fertile and infertile women. *Fertil Steril* 82:1278-1282, 2004.
2. Garcia JE: Endometrial biopsy: A test whose time has come. *Fertil Steril* 82:1293-1294, 2004.
3. Haney AF: Endometrial biopsy: A test whose time has come and gone. *Fertil Steril* 82:1295-1296, 2004.
4. Kazer RR: Endometrial biopsy should be abandoned as a routine component of the infertility evaluation. *Fertil Steril* 82:1297-1298, 2004.
5. Lamb EJ: Looking at the endometrial biopsy with evidence-based medicine. *Fertil Steril* 82:1283-1285, 2004.

6. McDonough PG: Grading a developmental continuum: Elegy on the rise and fall of the endometrial biopsy. *Fertil Steril* 82:1286-1292, 2004.

Heparin and Aspirin Attenuate Placental Apoptosis In Vitro: Implications for Early Pregnancy Failure
Bose P, Black S, Kadyrov M, et al (Univ Hosp RWTH, Aachen, Germany; Imperial College, London)
Am J Obstet Gynecol 192:23-30, 2005   19–2

Objective.—Live birth rates are increased by treatment with heparin and aspirin in cases of poor pregnancy outcome such as antiphospholipid syndrome. Both drugs may attenuate miscarriage by inhibiting aberrant coagulation or by modulating trophoblast apoptosis. Here we assessed their roles in trophoblast apoptosis in vitro.

Study Design.—BeWo cells and placental villi were cultured in sera from women with successful or failing in vitro fertilization, with and without heparin or aspirin. Apoptosis was assessed by using DNA laddering, cytokeratin 18 neoepitope formation, Bcl-2, and caspase 7 expression.

Results.—In BeWo cells, sera from in vitro fertilization failure increased trophoblast apoptosis, whereas heparin and aspirin reversed these effects. In villous trophoblast, heparin increased Bcl-2 and cytokeratin 18 protein expression. Heparin and aspirin inhibited DNA laddering.

Conclusion.—Heparin and aspirin modulate trophoblast apoptosis suggesting a direct impact on trophoblast biology, thus providing an additional mechanism to explain the clinical benefits of heparin and aspirin on recurrent pregnancy loss.

▶ In addition to anticoagulation activity, heparin appears to bind antiphospholipid antibodies, with resultant attenuation of circulating antiphospholipid antibody titers. Chamley et al[1] have previously shown reduced trophoblast proliferation in the presence of anti-β_2-glycoprotein. Bose et al previously reported that heparin can improve trophoblast proliferation and decrease trophoblast apoptosis in vitro.

In this study, sera from subjects with success or failure of in vitro fertilization (IVF) were used for culturing of BeWo cells and placental villi. Apoptosis was assessed by DNA laddering, cytokeratin-18 neoepitope formation, Bcl-2, and caspase 7 expression. Heparin and aspirin appeared to decrease trophoblast apoptosis in cultures containing sera from subjects who had failed IVF cycles. This study suggests a direct role of heparin and aspirin on trophoblast and placental biology. Clinical applications for recurrent miscarriage and IVF failure require evaluation through well-designed effectiveness trials.

M. D. Stephenson, MD, MSc

Reference

1. Chamley LW, Duncalf AM, Mitchell MD, et al: Action of anticardiolipin and antibodies to beta2-glycoprotein-I on trophoblast proliferation as a mechanism for fetal death. *Lancet* 26:1037-1038, 1998.

Heparin Prevents Antiphospholipid Antibody–Induced Fetal Loss by Inhibiting Complement Activation

Girardi G, Redecha P, Salmon JE (Cornell Univ, New York)
Nature Med 10:1222-1226, 2004   19–3

Background.—Antiphospholipid syndrome (APS) is characterized by thrombosis and pregnancy loss that occur in the presence of aPL antibodies. In vivo and in vitro studies have shown that aPL antibodies trigger activation of endothelial cells, monocytes, neutrophils, and platelets and produce inflammation, thrombosis, and tissue damage. However, the pathogenic inter-

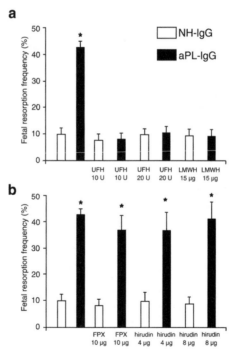

FIGURE 1.—Heparins protect mice from aPL-IgG induced pregnancy loss. (a) Pregnant BALB/c mice were treated with aPL-IgG or NH-IgG, and some mice also received UFH or LMWH (*n* = 6-8 mice per group). *aPL-IgG versus NH-IgG, *P* < 0.001. (b) Pregnant BALB/c mice were treated with aPL-IgG or NH-IgG, and some mice in each group were also treated with fondaparinux or hirudin (*n* = 6-8 mice per group). *NH-IgG + fondaparinux versus aPL-IgG + fondaparinux, *P* < 0.001; *NH-IgG + hirudin versus aPL-IgG + hirudin, *P* < 0.001. FPX, fondaparinux. (Courtesy of Girardi G, Redecha P, Salmon JE: Heparin prevents antiphospholipid antibody–induced fetal loss by inhibiting complement activation. *Nature Med* 10:1222-1226, 2004.)

TABLE 2.—Heparins Inhibit Complement Activation Initiated by aPL-IgG *in Vitro*

	Mouse Serum		Human Serum	
Treatment	C3 Positive Cells (%)	C3a desArg (ng/ml)	C3 Positive Cells (%)	C3a desArg (ng/ml)
NH-IgG	11 ± 4*	112 ± 35*	17 ± 6*	252 ± 66*
aPL-IgG	31 ± 11[a]	680 ± 30	43 ± 3[b]	1,209 ± 193
aPL-IgG + UFH (5 U/ml)	9 ± 5*	120 ± 20*	5 ± 1*	286 ± 30*
aPL-IgG + UFH (10 U/ml)	6 ± 4*	107 ± 22*	8 ± 1*	254 ± 60*
aPL-IgG + LMWH (8 mg/ml)	5 ± 3*	88 ± 31*	7 ± 3*	309 ± 72*
aPL-IgG + fondaparinux (5 mg/ml)	20 ± 6	745 ± 38	41 ± 4	1,335 ± 239
aPL-IgG + hirudin (2 mg/ml)	26 ± 7	580 ± 145	ND	ND
aPL-IgG + hirudin (4 mg/ml)	25 ± 6	720 ± 140	ND	ND

We treated BeWo cells with aPL-IgG or NH-IgG, followed by incubation with mouse or human serum in the presence or absence of UFH, LMWH, hirudin, or fondaparinux. To study aPL-IgG-mediated C3 activation *in vitro*, we measured the generation of C3a and cell-bound C3b. Results represent 4-8 experiments per treatment.

*$P < 0.001$ versus aPL-IgG.

[a]BeWo cells incubated with aPL-IgG and analyzed by flow cytometry were 56 ± 10% positive for human IgG. In the two-color experiments staining for human IgG and C3, 64 ± 8% of cells positive for human IgG were mouse C3-positive, whereas only 6 ± 2% of human IgG -negative cells were C3 positive.

[b]In the two-color experiments staining for human IgG and C3, 79 ± 7% of cells positive for human IgG were human C3-positive, whereas only 7 ± 2% of human IgG-negative cells were C3-positive. ND, not done.

(Courtesy of Girardi G, Redecha P, Salmon JE: Heparin prevents antiphospholipid antibody–induced fetal loss by inhibiting complement activation. *Nature Med* 10:1222-1226, 2004.)

mediates of injury are incompletely understood. A hypothesis was investigated that aPL antibodies, preferentially targeted at decidua and placenta, activate complement through the classical pathway, leading to the generation of potent anaphylatoxins and mediators of effector-cell activation.

Methods.—Pregnant mice were injected with human immunoglobulin G (IgG) containing aPL antibodies (aPL-IgG) or IgG from healthy individuals (NH-IgG). A comparison was made of the consequences of treating pregnant mice with aPL-IgG in the presence or absence of unfractionated heparin (UFH) or low-molecular-weight heparin (LMWH) (enoxaparin). To determine whether anticoagulation itself can prevent aPL antibody–associated fetal injury, mice were treated with the anticoagulants fondaparinux or hirudin.

Results.—Treatment with either UFH or LMWH reduced the frequency of fetal absorption to that of mice treated with IgG from healthy controls (Fig 1). Neither fondaparinux nor hirudin inhibited the generation of complement split products or prevented pregnancy loss (Table 2).

Conclusions.—Anticoagulant therapy does not provide sufficient protection against APS-associated miscarriage. Heparins were found to prevent obstetric complications in women with APS, not by their anticoagulant effects but because they block activation of complement-induced aPL antibodies targeted to decidual tissues.

▶ This group of investigators previously proposed that aPL antibodies target the decidua and placenta through the classic complement pathway, leading to the generation of anaphylatoxins and mediators of effector-cell activation. This, in turn, accelerates local alternative pathway activation and creates a proinflammatory amplification loop than enhances C3 activation and deposition, generates C3a and C5a, resulting in the further influx of inflammatory cells.[1] Depending on the extent of damage, intrauterine death or growth restriction ensues. In this study, Girardi et al tested the hypothesis that heparin protects mice from fetal loss caused by aPL antibodies by preventing complement activation on trophoblasts, in addition to its anticoagulant activity.

A case-control model was used in which human IgG containing aPL antibodies was injected into pregnant mice and compared with controls. Some of the aPL-IgG mice were treated with UFH or LMWH.

Passive transfer of aPL-IgG caused increased fetal resorption, which was abated with either UFH or LMWH, similar to the controls. In addition, some of the aPL-IgG mice were treated with fondaparinux sodium or hirudin, which are anticoagulants without complement activity. The fetal resorption was comparable to untreated aPL-IgG mice, thereby implying that the anticoagulant activity was not sufficient to prevent pregnancy loss.

The evidence supporting aPL antibody–induced pregnancy loss through activation of complement is mounting. Heparin appears to have several mechanisms of action, including inhibition of complement activation, which may be paramount in obstetric antiphospholipid syndrome.

M. D. Stephenson, MD, MSc

Reference

1. Girardi G, Berman J, Redecha P et al: Complement C5a receptors and neutrophils mediate fetal injury in the antiphospholipid syndrome. *J Clin Invest* 112:1644-1654, 2003.

20 Assisted Reproductive Technology

Endometrial Polyps and Their Implication in the Pregnancy Rates of Patients Undergoing Intrauterine Insemination: A Prospective, Randomized Study
Pérez-Medina T, Bajo-Arenas J, Salazar F, et al (Universidad Autónoma de Madrid)
Hum Reprod 20:1632-1635, 2005   20–1

Background.—It was our intention to determine whether hysteroscopic polypectomy before intrauterine insemination (IUI) achieved better pregnancy outcomes than no intervention.

Methods.—A total of 215 infertile women from the infertility unit of a university tertiary hospital with ultrasonographically diagnosed endometrial polyps (EP) undergoing IUI were randomly allocated to one of two pretreatment groups using an opaque envelope technique with assignment determined by a random number table. Hysteroscopic polypectomy was performed in the study group. Diagnostic hysteroscopy and polyp biopsy was performed in the control group.

Results.—Total pregnancy rates and time for success in both groups after four IUI cycles were compared by means of contingency tables and life-table analysis. A total of 93 pregnancies occurred, 64 in the study group and 29 in

TABLE 2.—Number and Percentage of Pregnancies After Hysteroscopic Polypectomy (*n* = 204)

	Polypectomy		*P*-Value
	Study (*n* = 101)	Control (*n* = 103)	
Pregnancy (%)			<0.001
Yes	64 (63.4)	29 (28.2)	
No	37 (36.6)	74 (71.8)	

Relative risk (RR) 2.1 (95% confidence interval [CI] 1.5-2.9).
(Courtesy of Pérez-Medina T, Bajo-Arenas J, Salazar F, et al: Endometrial polyps and their implication in the pregnancy rates of patients undergoing intrauterine insemination: A prospective, randomized study. *Hum Reprod* 20:1632-1635, 2005. Copyright European Society for Human Reproduction and Embryology, by permission of Oxford University Press/Human Reproduction.)

the control group. Women in the study group had a better possibility of becoming pregnant after polypectomy, with a relative risk of 2.1 (95% confidence interval 1.5-2.9) (Table 2). Pregnancies in the study group were obtained before the first IUI in 65% of cases.

Conclusions.—These data suggest that hysteroscopic polypectomy before IUI is an effective measure.

▶ With the increasing frequency of diagnosis of EP that occurs with expanded use of vaginal US, the clinician is often faced with the question of how to manage an incidental EP in infertile women. This study is the first randomized trial of polypectomy in infertility patients. All subjects (n = 204) were younger than 40 years, had been infertile for at least 2 years, and were candidates for treatment with follicle-stimulating hormone (FSH)/IUI. The authors found that women who had a polypectomy were more than twice as likely to achieve a pregnancy as those who had only a diagnostic hysteroscopy and polyp biopsy. There was no effect of polyp size on outcome. The benefit in patients with polyps of less than 5 mm was the same as in those with polyps of greater than 20 mm. Interestingly, 65% of the pregnancies in the polypectomy group occurred in the 3-month waiting period before treatment with FSH/IUI, suggesting that the polypectomy itself was a valid therapy. The great majority of patients in this study were treated with office hysteroscopy. This relatively large, well-designed study suggests that all EPs should be removed in infertile women.

R. Barnes, MD

Taskforce 8: Ethics of Medically Assisted Fertility Treatment for HIV Positive Men and Women
Shenfield F, for the ESHRE ETHICS and LAW Task Force (Univ College Hosp, London)
Hum Reprod 19:2454-2456, 2004   20–2

Abstract.—In this 8th statement of the ESHRE Taskforce on Ethics and Law, the focus is on the ethical issues raised by (assisted) reproduction for HIV positive men and women. Due to treatment improvements, their life expectancy has increased substantially. This, in combination with the reduction of perinatal transmission to the child, makes the creation of a family more acceptable. Recommendations are made concerning methods of avoiding HIV transmission in the couple and to their offspring. It is concluded that, if certain precautions are taken, medical assistance to reproduction of HIV positive people is ethically acceptable. For the time being, only cases of serodiscordant couples should be considered.

The Effect of Human Immunodeficiency Virus on Sperm Parameters and the Outcome of Intrauterine Insemination Following Sperm Washing

Nicopoullos JDM, Almeida PA, Ramsay JWA, et al (Chelsea & Westminster Hosp, London; Charring Cross Hosp, London)
Hum Reprod 19:2289-2297, 2004   20–3

Background.—This is the first study to assess the outcome of sperm washing and intrauterine insemination (IUI) cycles in human immunodeficiency virus-positive (HIV+) men to determine any predictors of success, as well as evaluating the effect of HIV on sperm parameters.

Methods.—Semen characteristics were evaluated in 106 HIV+ men and a control group of 234 HIV− men, and the effect of markers of HIV disease assessed. Age, stimulation regime, sperm parameters, markers of HIV disease and the use of anti-retrovirals were assessed as predictors of the outcome of sperm washing/IUI cycles in the HIV+ men.

Results.—Ejaculate volume, sperm concentration, total count, progressive motility and normal morphology were all significantly higher in the control group compared to the HIV+ men ($P < 0.05$). A significant positive correlation was observed between CD4 count and sperm concentration, total count, motility, progressive motility type 'a' + 'b' and post-preparation concentration and a significant negative correlation with normal sperm morphology of both raw and post-preparation samples. No correlation was observed between viral load (VL), years since diagnosis, use of anti-retrovirals or duration of use and any sperm parameter. The only factors that significantly improved IUI outcome were a VL <1000 copies/ml and the use of anti-retrovirals.

Conclusions.—These data demonstrate that sperm parameters are significantly impaired by the presence of HIV infection and in particular correlate with CD4 count. Undetectable VL and the use of anti-retrovirals improve the outcome of IUI/sperm washing in HIV+ men.

▶ HIV disease has become a controllable, albeit not curable, disease entity. The life expectancy of infected individuals now extends beyond 2 decades. As the outlook improves for HIV-infected men and women, it is only natural that they should want to seek parenthood. In addition, with the reduction in the risk of mother to child HIV transmission to less than 1% with highly active antiretroviral therapy (HAART) and elective cesarean delivery, the active choice to seek pregnancy on the part of infected women is a reasonable one. The question for discordantly infected couples has become how to achieve biological parenthood while not exposing their partner to the risk of transmission. For HIV-infected women, this merely amounts to insemination with their HIV− partner-donated semen. For HIV-infected men, however, assisted reproduction is necessary to achieve conception and not expose their HIV− female partners to the risk of transmission.

The Reproductive Endocrinology and Infertility (REI) community, with few notable exceptions, has been slow to respond to this need. The ESHRE Taskforce on Ethics and Law (Abstract 20–2) validated the desires of discordantly infected couples and concluded that medically assisted reproduction for discordantly infected couples is ethically acceptable. Many published reports have documented that sperm washing can safely accomplish conception for discordantly infected couples where the male partner is HIV⁺. In their report, Nicopoullos and colleagues (Abstract 20–3) add to this growing body of data. They report on the semen characteristics of 106 HIV⁺ men and show that HIV infection impairs sperm parameters. Semen samples from HIV⁺ men were processed with a combination of density gradient centrifugation/washing/swim-up techniques and used in 133 insemination cycles after undergoing HIV testing. Twenty-five clinical pregnancies resulted (18.8% per insemination). The clinical pregnancy rate was significantly higher in those samples from men with VLs less than 1000 copies/mL and who were on antiretroviral therapy. While the absolute safety of this technique cannot be addressed in this small study, it must be acknowledged that these assisted reproductive techniques are much more desirable than unprotected intercourse between discordantly infected couples.

P. M. Garcia, MD, MPH

Multiple-Birth Risk Associates With IVF and Extended Embryo Culture: USA, 2001
Kissin DM, Schieve LA, Reynolds MA (Ctrs for Disease Control and Prevention, Atlanta, Ga)
Hum Reprod 20:2215-2223, 2005   20–4

Background.—Multiple births are associated with serious adverse infant and maternal outcomes. The objective of this study was to assess the multiple-birth risk (MBR) associated with IVF and determine whether the risk is impacted by stage of embryo development at transfer.

Methods.—A population-based sample of 50 819 IVF transfers utilizing day 3 or day 5 embryos performed in the USA in 2001 on women aged 20–40 years was used to assess MBR and live-birth rate (LBR), stratified by patient age, supernumerary embryo availability, and number of embryos transferred.

Results.—Although significantly more day 5 than day 3 transfers used ≤2 embryos (69.2 versus 27.7%), the former were not associated with decreased MBR. MBR was high when >1 embryo was transferred, irrespective of embryo development stage. LBR were generally maximized with 2 embryos transferred, and for some (day 5 transfers, patients aged 35–37 years) with one embryo. Electing to transfer a single day 5 embryo appeared efficacious for some patients: women aged 20–37 years with supernumerary embryos cryopreserved had LBR of 31.6–39.5%.

Conclusions.—MBR is high when ≥2 embryos are transferred. Single embryo transfer is the only way to prevent many multiple births and associated adverse health outcomes.

▶ Multiple births are not only associated with serious adverse maternal outcomes but are increasing in numbers with the expanding utilization of assisted reproductive technologies by women throughout the world. There seems to be considerable debate concerning the optimal number of embryos to transfer back into women who are undergoing IVF. The authors of this study found that the risk for multiple births was considerably elevated when 2 or more embryos were transferred. According to these authors, single-embryo transfer is the only way to prevent many multiple births but may also be associated with reduced pregnancy outcomes in women undergoing IVF. Although our technology has advanced so that many centers are finding excellent clinical outcomes with reduced numbers of transferred embryos, this debate will likely continue in the years ahead to improve the technology that allows for better clinical outcomes while reducing the risks associated with IVF, including those risks associated with multiple births.

L. P. Shulman, MD

Elective Single-Embryo Transfer Versus Double-Embryo Transfer in In Vitro Fertilization
Thurin A, Hausken J, Hillensjö T, et al (Sahlgrenska Univ, Göteborg, Sweden; Haugesund Hosp, Norway; Carlanderska Hosp, Göteborg, Sweden; et al)
N Engl J Med 351:2392-2402, 2004   20–5

Background.—The risks of premature birth and perinatal death are increased after in vitro fertilization. These risks are mainly due to the high incidence of multiple births, which relates to the number of embryos transferred.

Methods.—We performed a randomized, multicenter trial to assess the equivalence of two approaches to in vitro fertilization with respect to the rates of pregnancy that result in at least one live birth and to compare associated rates of multiple gestation. Women less than 36 years of age who had at least two good-quality embryos were randomly assigned either to undergo transfer of a single fresh embryo and, if there was no live birth, subsequent transfer of a single frozen-and-thawed embryo, or to undergo a single transfer of two fresh embryos (Table 1). Equivalence was defined as a difference of no more than 10 percentage points in the rates of pregnancy resulting in at least one live birth.

Results.—Pregnancy resulting in at least one live birth occurred in 142 of 331 women (42.9 percent) in the double-embryo-transfer group as compared with 128 of 330 women (38.8 percent) in the single-embryo-transfer group (difference, 4.1 percentage points; 95 percent confidence interval, −3.4 to 11.6 percentage points); rates of multiple births were 33.1 percent and 0.8 percent, respectively ($P<0.001$) (Table 2). These results do not demonstrate equivalence of the two approaches in rates of live births, but they do indicate that any reduction in the rate of live births with the transfer of single embryos is unlikely to exceed 11.6 percentage points.

TABLE 1.—Characteristics of the Patients

Characteristic	Elective Single-Embryo Transfer (N = 330)	Double-Embryo Transfer (N = 331)	P Value
Age at fresh-embryo transfer — yr			0.70
Mean ±SD	30.9±3.0	30.8±3.0	
Range	22.6–35.9	21.6–35.9	
Body-mass index*			0.84
Mean ±SD	24.5±4.6	24.5±4.4	
Range	17.2–49.2	16.9–40.6	
Duration of infertility — yr			0.29
Mean ±SD	3.6±1.7	3.8±3.9	
Range	0–12	1–12	
Cause of infertility — no. (%)†			
Tubal factor	70 (21.2)	60 (18.1)	0.33
Endometriosis	58 (17.6)	38 (11.5)	0.03
Hormonal factor	64 (19.4)	80 (24.2)	0.16
Male factor	164 (49.7)	155 (46.8)	0.48
Other, including unknown	55 (16.7)	71 (21.5)	0.14
History of previous pregnancies — no. (%)	90 (27.3)	105 (31.7)	0.23
Live birth	27 (8.2)	36 (10.9)	0.29
Miscarriage	36 (10.9)	57 (17.2)	0.03
Ectopic pregnancy	8 (2.4)	15 (4.5)	0.20
Termination of pregnancy	35 (10.6)	20 (6.0)	0.04
History of previous treatment with in vitro fertilization — no. (%)	75 (22.7)	70 (21.1)	0.64
Pregnancy	9 (2.7)	16 (4.8)	
Live birth	2 (0.6)	4 (1.2)	

*The body-mass index is the weight in kilograms divided by the square of the height in meters.
†More than one diagnosis per couple was possible; 513 couples had one, 140 had two, and 8 had three diagnoses.

Conclusions.—In women under 36 years of age, transferring one fresh embryo and then, if needed, one frozen-and-thawed embryo dramatically reduces the rate of multiple births while achieving a rate of live births that is not substantially lower than the rate that is achievable with a double-embryo transfer.

▶ This Swedish study is one of the first to endeavor to address the issue of appropriate patient selection for single-embryo transfer (SET) and the outcomes such decisions lead to in a prospective, randomized fashion. Nordic and European nations continue to lead the United States in advancement and promotion of the concept of the SET, largely secondary to the economic pressures of nationalized health care and the astronomic costs associated with ART-conceived preterm multiple births. Thurin et al show that a workable paradigm for selecting patients for SET can be put into clinical practice without suffering a dramatic reduction in overall pregnancy and live birth rates, here not exceeding an 11.6% decline at most according to their statistical analysis.

It has long been argued that the high expectations for a successful in vitro fertilization (IVF) cycle, and the limited concern held by the vast majority of IVF patients regarding risks associated with conception and delivery of twin pregnancies, will likely conspire to make widespread acceptance of SET in the United States very unlikely. It is interesting to note that of 2698 IVF cycles that were eligible for enrollment in this study, patients refused participation in 2037 cases. The authors acknowledge that this very limited degree of elective participation may stem from some of these very same issues. State-mandated limitations on the number of embryos that may be transferred, as has been seen in many European nations, may prove to be the ultimate motivating force driving the move toward SET both abroad and here in the United States.

M. R. Drews, MD

TABLE 2.—Outcomes According to Treatment Group in the Intention-to-Treat Analysis*

Variable	Elective Single-Embryo Transfer (N = 330)	Double-Embryo Transfer (N = 331)	P Value	95% CI for the Difference in Percentage Between Groups
Treatment of patients — no. (%)†				
With IVF	178 (53.9)	189 (57.1)	0.43	
With ICSI	137 (41.5)	121 (36.6)	0.20	
With mixed IVF and ICSI‡	15 (4.5)	21 (6.3)	0.39	
Aspirated oocytes — no.				
Mean ±SD	13.0±5.7	12.6±5.4	0.37	
Range	2 to 31	3 to 44		
Fertilized oocytes — no.				
Mean ±SD	8.5±3.8	8.3±3.7	0.47	
Range	2 to 21	2 to 31		
Available good-quality embryos — no.				
Mean ±SD	4.6±2.4	4.6±2.4	0.98	
Range	2 to 16	2 to 17		
Day of transfer — no. (%)§				
Day 2	305 (92.4)	306 (92.4)		
Day 3	16 (4.8)	16 (4.8)		
Day 5	8 (2.4)	8 (2.4)		
Patients who received assigned treatment in the fresh-embryo cycle — no.	327	325		
Patients who did not receive assigned treatment in the fresh-embryo cycle — no.¶	3	6		
Patients who did not receive assigned treatment in the frozen-and-thawed cycle — no.‖	60	—		
Pregnancies — no. (%)				
Fresh-embryo cycle	111 (33.6)	174 (52.6)	<0.001	11.4 to 26.5
Thawed-embryo cycle**	43 (24.3)	—		
Cumulative, fresh-embryo and thawed-embryo cycles††	158 (47.9)	174 (52.6)	0.24	-2.9 to 12.3
95% CI for the estimated cumulative rate — %	42.5 to 53.4	47.1 to 58.0		
Ectopic pregnancies — no.				
Fresh-embryo cycle	0	1		
Thawed-embryo cycle	1	—		

	Single-embryo-transfer	Double-embryo-transfer	95% CI of difference	P value
Spontaneous abortions at ≤12 weeks of gestation — no. (%)				
Fresh-embryo cycle	17 (15.3)	27 (15.5)		
Thawed-embryo cycle	13 (30.2)	—		
Spontaneous abortions at >12 weeks of gestation — no.				
Fresh-embryo cycle‡‡	2	3		
Thawed-embryo cycle	0	—		
Stillborn infants ≥28 weeks of gestation — no.				
Fresh-embryo cycle	1	1		
Thawed-embryo cycle	0	—		
Live births — no. (%)				
Fresh-embryo cycle	91 (27.6)	142 (42.9)	8.0 to 22.6	<0.001
Thawed-embryo cycle**	29 (16.4)	—		
Cumulative, fresh-embryo and thawed-embryo cycles§§	128 (38.8)	142 (42.9)	–03.4 to 11.6	0.30
95% CI for the estimated cumulative rate — %	33.5 to 44.3	37.5 to 48.4		
Multiple births — no. (%)¶¶	1 (0.8)	47 (33.1)		<0.001

* IVF denotes in vitro fertilization; ICSI, intracytoplasmic sperm injection; and CI, confidence interval. A *dash* denotes not applicable.

† Because of rounding, percentages may not total 100.

‡ *Mixed IVF and ICSI* denotes cycles in which 50% of the oocytes were fertilized by IVF and 50% by ICSI.

§ In the single-embryo-transfer group, 1 patient canceled the transfer owing to ovarian hyperstimulation syndrome. In the double-embryo-transfer group, 1 patient's embryos were lost during transfer.

¶ In the single-embryo-transfer group, 1 patient canceled the transfer because of ovarian hyperstimulation syndrome, and 2 patients requested a double-embryo transfer. In the double-embryo-transfer group, 1 patient's embryos were lost during transfer, 3 patients had only 1 embryo transferred because of ovarian hyperstimulation syndrome, and 2 patients requested a single-embryo transfer.

‖ Of the patients who did not receive treatment in the frozen-and-thawed cycle, 38 had no surviving embryos after freezing and thawing, 8 had a spontaneous pregnancy between the fresh and the frozen-and-thawed cycle, 5 had marital problems, 3 had severe illnesses, 1 patient's husband died, 1 changed clinics, 1 continued with a new fresh-embryo cycle after a fresh single-embryo transfer resulted in a stillborn child, and 3 received 2 or 3 embryos in the frozen-and-thawed cycle.

** The percentage was calculated on the basis of 177 thawed-embryo cycles.

†† In the single-embryo-transfer group, 4 patients had 2 pregnancies each, 1 from a cycle with a fresh embryo and 1 from a cycle with a frozen-and-thawed embryo. This group also includes 8 pregnancies that occurred after spontaneous conception between the cycle with the fresh embryo and the cycle with the frozen-and-thawed embryo.

‡‡ One patient in the single-embryo-transfer group underwent termination of pregnancy owing to fetal acrania and was included in the miscarriage group in the study.

§§ The single-embryo-transfer group includes 8 live births that occurred after spontaneous conception between the cycle with the fresh embryo and the cycle with the frozen-and-thawed embryo.

¶¶ The double-embryo-transfer group includes 1 multiple birth in which 1 fetus died in utero at 24 weeks of gestation.

Outcomes of Pregnancies Achieved by Donor Egg In Vitro Fertiization—A Comparison With Standard In Vitro Fertilization Pregnancies

Wiggins DA, Main E (California Pacific Med Ctr, San Francisco)

Am J Obstet Gynecol 192:2002-2008, 2005   20–6

Objective.—Prior studies on donor egg in vitro fertilization (DE-IVF) outcomes have been limited by the lack of an appropriate control group. Here, we review the obstetric and perinatal outcomes of pregnancies achieved by DE-IVF and compare these pregnancies with those of women who also needed similar assisted reproductive techniques, of similar socioeconomic status, and cared for by a small group of 8 physicians applying consistent diagnostic and treatment approaches.

Study Design.—A retrospective review of 50 consecutive pregnancies achieved by DE- IVF and 50 consecutive pregnancies achieved by standard IVF (STD-IVF) was performed. Comparisons were made for demographic and medical confounding factors and for outcome measures.

Results.—The 2 groups were nearly identical for gravidity, parity, and multiple gestations but did vary in maternal age. Average age of patients receiving DE-IVF was 41.9(±5.1), whereas the STD-IVF averaged 37.7(±3.6) years ($P < .001$). Key obstetric outcomes did not differ between the 2 groups with the exception of pregnancy-induced hypertension. In patients with DE-IVF, 26% had pregnancy-induced hypertension (PIH) develop, whereas this occurred in only 8% of the STD-IVF group ($P = .02$). Examining nulliparous patients only, 37.1% of DE-IVF had PIH develop, whereas only 8% of STD-IVF group achieved that diagnosis ($P < .003$). An analysis with a multiple logistic regression in nulliparous patients found odds ratios of 7.1 (95% CI, 1.4-36.7) in DE versus STD-IVF, odds ratio 4.9 (95% CI, 1.3-18.3) for multiple gestation versus singleton, and odds ratio 1.0 (95% CI, 0.9-1.1) for maternal age.

Conclusion.—Nulliparous pregnancies achieved by DE-IVF are associated with an increased risk of PIH; however, excellent outcomes can still be expected.

▶ The increasing use of assisted reproductive technologies has considerably expanded the choices available for infertile couples who seek to become pregnant. An important option for some women is the ability to utilize DE-IVF. Prior studies on DE-IVF outcomes have been limited by a lack of an appropriate control group. In this study by Wiggins and Main, obstetric and perinatal outcomes achieved by DE-IVF were compared with pregnancies of women who went through standard IVF procedures. The authors found a considerably increased risk for PIH. As more women seek to achieve pregnancy by assisted reproductive technologies, studies such as these provide important information for the counseling of women who will be choosing from an increasing array of reproductive options.

L. P. Shulman, MD

Dose-Finding Study of Daily GnRH Antagonist for the Prevention of Premature LH Surges in IVF/ICSI Patients: Optimal Changes in LH and Progesterone for Clinical Pregnancy

Huirne JAF, van Loenen ACD, Schats R, et al (Vrije Universiteit, Amsterdam)
Hum Reprod 20:359-367, 2005   20–7

Background.—An optimal range of LH concentrations for achieving pregnancy has not been established. The aim of this study was to investigate the effect of various LH levels induced by different GnRH antagonist doses on IVF outcome.

Methods.—This was a prospective, single centre study including 144 IVF patients, stimulated with recombinant FSH from cycle day 2, and co-treated with daily GnRH antagonist (antide/Iturelix) (2 mg/2 ml, 1 mg/ml, 0.5 mg/ml, 0.5 mg/0.5 ml or 0.25 mg/ml) from cycle day 7 onwards. Serum samples were taken three times daily.

Results.—Clinical pregnancies were only observed within a particular range of change in LH levels. The upper and lower thresholds for the mean LH area under the curve (AUC), adjusted for the baseline LH level before the antagonist was started (LH AUC^{-S6}; S6 = stimulation day 6) were -2.2 and 12.4 (IU/l) respectively (a negative value = below baseline levels). There were no clinical pregnancies outside these threshold values. Similar results were found for progesterone, the threshold levels of progesterone AUC^{-S6} were 3.98 and -1.21 ng/ml. Moreover, there were no pregnancies with progesterone levels >0.26 ng/ml/follicle on the day of hCG.

Conclusions.—Excessive or insufficient suppression of LH and progesterone levels during GnRH antagonist administration and high progesterone/follicle on hCG day seems to be associated with impaired clinical pregnancy rates.

▶ Investigators remain divided on the precise role of luteinizing hormone (LH) in oocyte maturation, and the necessity (or lack thereof) for LH supplementation in in vitro fertilization (IVF) gonadotropin stimulation regimens. The present study strives to establish a link between levels of endogenous LH after pituitary suppression and clinical pregnancy outcome. It makes teleological sense that there may be an optimal range of LH values to achieve the highest chance for IVF conception (as LH is clearly secreted throughout the follicular phase of the natural menstrual cycle) and that excessive or insufficient suppression of LH would correlate with negative outcomes. The present study may help to establish appropriate threshold levels for LH that may guide us to the optimal degree of LH supplementation to strive for in cycles of ovarian stimulation with follicle-stimulating hormone (FSH). It is likely that the preponderance of data will eventually show a need for modest concentrations of LH to demonstrate optimal clinical outcomes in IVF cycles. However, the debate continues in 2005, with both camps continuing to produce compelling data to demonstrate their points. Lisi et al[1] reported a significant increase in IVF implantation, and clinical pregnancy and delivery rates when recombinant LH was added to a standard FSH stimulation regimen after pituitary downregulation. In contrast, no such benefit was seen by Cedrin-Durnerin et al[2] in a similar study design, with the exception of gonadotropin-releasing hormone (GnRH) antagonist administration as opposed to pituitary downregulation.

M. R. Drews, MD

References

1. Lisi F, Rinaldi L, Fishel S, et al: Evaluation of two doses of recombinant luteinizing hormone supplementation in an unselected group of women undergoing follicular stimulation for in vitro fertilization. *Fertil Steril* 83:309-315, 2005.
2. Cedrin-Durnerin I, Grange-Dujardin D, Laffy A, et al: Recombinant human LH supplementation during GnRH antagonist administration in IVF/ICSI cycles: A prospective randomized study. *Hum Reprod* 19:1979-1984, 2004.

Abnormal Embryonic Development Diagnosed Embryoscopically in Early Intrauterine Deaths After In Vitro Fertilization: A Preliminary Report of 23 Cases
Philipp T, Feichtinger W, Van Allen MI, et al (Ludwig Boltzmann Inst of Clinical Gynecology and Obstetrics, Vienna)
Fertil Steril 82:1337-1342, 2004   20–8

Objective.—To provide data about the phenotypic appearance of the embryo of early failed pregnancies after IVF.
Design.—Clinical prospective descriptive study.
Setting.—Tertiary care center.
Patient(s).—Twenty-three women who had conceived by IVF and had a missed abortion before 12 weeks of gestation.
Intervention(s).—Embryoscopic examination of the embryo before curettage. Cytogenetic analysis of the chorionic villi by standard G-banding cytogenetic techniques or by comparative genomic hybridization in combination with flow cytometry analysis.
Main Outcome Measure(s).—Embryonic phenotype and karyotype were determined.
Result(s).—Twenty-one of 23 IVF embryos showed structural defects on embryoscopic examination. Seventeen of 23 specimens had a chromosomal abnormality. The majority were numerical aberrations such as monosomy X (2 cases). Trisomies for chromosomes 18 (one case), 16 (three cases), 15 (one case), 14 (two cases), 13 (one case), 12 (one case), 11 (one case), 10 (one case), 9 (one case), 8 (one case), and 3 (one case) were observed. A structural chromosome anomaly leading to a chromosomal trisomy was observed in one case. Aneuploidy explained the grossly abnormal embryonic development documented by embryoscopy in 15 of 21 cases.
Conclusion(s).—Aneuploidy is the major factor affecting normal embryonic development in missed abortions after IVF. Further investigation is needed to elucidate mechanisms that might prevent normal embryogenesis but evade detection by the cytogenetic techniques used in the present study.

▶ Despite advances in assisted reproductive technology, approximately 20% of clinical pregnancies conceived through IVF end in miscarriage. Limited data exist on the frequency of cytogenetic errors, and even less is known about morphologic abnormalities. In this prospective study of 23 women (mean age, 35.5 years) who had conceived by IVF and had a first-trimester miscarriage, embryoscopy was performed before dilatation and curettage. Twenty one embryos showed external abnormalities, of which 15 were found to be aneuploid. There were 2 normal-appearing embryos, 1 of which was trisomic. There were 15 trisomies, 6 of which would not have been tested for using the standard 9 chromosome probes (X, Y, 13-16, 18, 21, and 22) for preimplantation genetic diagnosis. Embryoscopy shows promise as a complementary technique, in addition to cytogenetic analysis, for the evaluation of miscarriage.

M. D. Stephenson, MD, MSc

Embryonic Soluble HLA-G as a Marker of Developmental Potential in Embryos

Noci I, Fuzzi B, Rizzo R, et al (Univ of Firenze, Italy; Careggi Hosp, Firenze, Italy; Univ of Ferrara, Italy)
Hum Reprod 20:138-146, 2004   20–9

Background.—In human reproduction, embryo implantation is complex and poorly understood. At present, no single markers are used in routine treatment to assay biochemical functions of the human embryo. Soluble human leukocyte antigen-G (sHLA-G) could be considered a possible marker of embryo developmental potential. It is localized primarily on the extravillous trophoblast, making this antigen a potential mediator of immune interaction at the maternal-fetal interface during gestation.

Methods.—Soluble-HLA-G levels were evaluated by an enzyme-linked immunosorbent assay (ELISA) employing monoclonal antibody MEM-G9. It was evaluated in 318 media of single embryo cultures. We correlated the presence of sHLA-G with embryo morphology and the pregnancy obtained in that treatment cycle.

Results.—No correlation was found between embryo morphology and sHLA-G levels. Pregnancy was observed only when the medium of at least one transferred embryo contained sHLA-G. In 26 out of 66 patients, none of the obtained embryos showed any detectable sHLA-G molecules and no pregnancy occurred.

Conclusions.—From our results, we propose sHLA-G as a potential marker of embryo development: the sHLA-G ELISA can be a useful biochemical assay in addition to embryo morphology in embryo selection for transfer in IVF treatment if there are other embryos with the same morphology.

▶ Since the advent of in vitro fertilization, noninvasive assessment of embryo implantation potential has largely been limited to evaluation of morphologic characteristics such as blastomere number, cleavage rate, and degree of fragmentation. Regardless of the sophistication of such assessment paradigms, they have all demonstrated limited ability to accurately select embryos with greatest chances of producing a conception, and thus have not proven helpful in our advancement toward the elusive goal of the highly successful single-embryo transfer. Assessment of HLA-G secretion from developing embryos has shown promise to provide embryologists with a more accurate means to noninvasively rate implantation potential for individual embryos, thus helping to limit the number of embryos transferred without sacrificing overall chances for pregnancy. Noci et al have overcome the experimental design problems of other similar investigations by culturing single oocytes and embryos in isolated wells as opposed to group culturing, so that each individual embryo may be assessed according to its specific secretion of HLA-G into its individual culture medium. A similar investigation by Yie et al[1] also concluded a striking correlation of embryonic secretion of HLA-G with conception of pregnancy, but was limited by this issue of grouping 2 or more embryos into each culture well, making individual embryo secretion assessment impossible. If HLA-G secretion is ever to realize its initial promise as a tool for embryo selection, all future investigations will need to follow the design of isolated single-embryo culture set forth in this investigation. Advances in the emerging science of microfluidics will also prove increasingly valuable in the assessment of miniscule changes in the concentrations of HLA-G and other molecules such as amino acids[2] in embryo culture media that may prove to be revealing markers of embryonic competency.

M. R. Drews, MD

References

1. Yie S, Balakier H, Motamedi G, et al: Secretion of human leukocyte antigen-G by human embryos is associated with a higher in vitro fertilization pregnancy rate. *Fertil Steril* 83:30-36, 2005.
2. Brison D, Houghton F, Falconer D, et al: Identification of viable embryos in IVF by non-invasive measurement of amino acid turnover. *Hum Reprod* 19:2319-2324, 2004.

21 Preimplantation Diagnosis

Preimplantation Genetic Diagnosis for Aneuploidy Screening in Patients With Unexplained Recurrent Miscarriages
Platteau P, Staessen C, Michiels A, et al (Vrije Universiteit Brussel, Belgium)
Fertil Steril 83:393-397, 2005   21–1

Objective.—To determine the aneuploidy rate in embryos of women with idiopathic recurrent miscarriages and to evaluate whether preimplantation genetic diagnosis for aneuploidy screening could be a feasible approach to improve the possibility of successful pregnancy in these couples.

Design.—Prospective cohort study.

Setting.—Tertiary university referral center.

Patient(s).—Women (n = 49) with recurrent idiopathic miscarriages (Table 1).

Intervention(s).—In vitro fertilization with preimplantation genetic diagnosis for aneuploidy screening.

TABLE 1.—Characteristics of the Patients, Stimulation, and FISH Results

	Patients <37 Years (35 Cycles)	Patients ≥37 Years (34 Cycles)
Mean age (y)	32.48 ± 2.72 yrs	40.15 ± 2.48 yrs
Mean no. of miscarriages	4.46 ± 2.10	4.93 ± 2.41
Mean no. of COC	13.84 ± 7.00	10.43 ± 5.92
Mean no. of MII	11.70 ± 5.83	8.88 ± 5.14
Mean no. of 2PN	8.69 ± 4.93	6.95 ± 3.89
No. embryos biopsied	240	173
Diagnosis		
% Normal	54.20% ± 21.74%	28.40% ± 28.69%
% Abnormal	43.85% ± 22.50%	66.95% ± 29.27%
% No diagnosis	1.94% ± 5.04%	4.63% ± 15.59%

Values are means ± SD.
Abreviations: FISH, Fluorescence in situ hybridization; *COC,* combined oocyte complexes; *MII,* metaphase II; *2PN,* 2 distinct pronuclei.
(Courtesy of Platteau P, Staessen C, Michiels A, et al: Preimplantation genetic diagnosis for aneuploidy screening in patients with unexplained recurrent miscarriages. *Fertil Steril* 83:393-397, 2005. Reprinted by permission from the American College of Surgeons.)

TABLE 3.—Pregnancy Outcome and Implantation Rates

	<37 Years	≥37 Years
Mean no. of embryos transferred	2.03 ± 0.79	2.05 ± 0.87
% No transfer	11.42% (4/35)	47.00% (16/34)
No. of clinical pregnancies	9	1
% Ongoing pregnancy/cycle	25.71%	2.94%
% Ongoing pregnancy/embryo transfer	29.03%	5.55%
Implantation rate	16.66% ± 30.32%	2.77% ± 11.78%

(Courtesy of Platteau P, Staessen C, Michiels A, et al: Preimplantation genetic diagnosis for aneuploidy screening in patients with unexplained recurrent miscarriages. *Fertil Steril* 83:393-397, 2005. Reprinted by permission from the American College of Surgeons.)

Main Outcome Measure(s).—Ongoing pregnancy rate (PR) and aneuploidy rate.

Result(s).—The aneuploidy rate was, respectively, 43.85% and 66.95% in the younger and older group. The ongoing PR per cycle was 25.71% in the younger and 2.94% in the older patients (Table 3).

Conclusion(s).—There is no therapeutic evidence to prescribe IVF with or without preimplantation genetic diagnosis for aneuploidy screening for this heterogeneous group of patients.

▶ The evaluation and management of recurrent miscarriage continue to be frustrating to the patient and clinician. Despite known genetic, endocrine, anatomic, and immunologic factors, approximately 40% of couples with recurrent miscarriage remain unexplained. Based on an observational report of 12 patients with recurrent miscarriage who had an ongoing pregnancy rate of 67% after in vitro fertilization (IVF), Balasch et al[1] suggested that replacement of multiple embryos may improve the maternal immune response to pregnancy as well as improve the chance of having a chromosomally normal embryo. Subsequently, Raziel et al[2] found no benefit of IVF in older women with recurrent miscarriage. Recent studies of preimplantation embryos have shown a high frequency of numeric chromosome errors, which has been linked to unexplained recurrent miscarriage.[3]

In this prospective study, 49 subjects with a history of unexplained recurrent miscarriage had IVF with intracytoplasmic sperm injection. Two blastomeres were removed from embryos of at least the 6-cell stage for preimplantation genetic diagnosis. Fluorescence in situ hybridization for chromosomes X, Y, 13, 16, 18, 21, and 22 was performed. Chromosomally normal blastocysts were transferred on day 5.

There were 25 subjects younger than 37 years and 24 subjects aged 37 or older. Patient characteristics are shown in Table 1. As expected, there were fewer normal embryos in the group of advanced maternal age: 130 of 240 (54%) versus 49 of 173 (28%). Despite such assisted reproductive technology, implantation and ongoing PRs were poor in the group aged 37 or older: 2.77% and 2.95%, respectively. In the group younger than 37, implantation and ongoing PRs were higher, but no better than if such technology had not been offered.

In summary, the results of this study can be used in counseling couples with unexplained recurrent miscarriage. IVF with preimplantation genetic diagnosis does not appear to improve subsequent pregnancy outcome in this cohort. Therefore, other evidence-based therapies should be explored.

M. D. Stephenson, MD, MSc

References

1. Balasch J, Creus M, Fabregues F, et al: In-vitro fertilization treatment for unexplained recurrent abortion: A pilot study. *Hum Reprod* 11:1579-1582, 1996.
2. Raziel A, Herman A, Strassburger D, et al: The outcome of in vitro fertilization in unexplained habitual aborters concurrent with secondary infertility. *Fertil Steril* 67:88-92, 1997.
3. Simon C, Rubio C, Vidal F, et al: Increased chromosome abnormalities in human preimplantation embryos after in-vitro fertilization in patients with recurrent miscarriage. *Reprod Fertil Dev* 10:87-92, 1998.

Comparison of Blastocyst Transfer With or Without Preimplantation Genetic Diagnosis for Aneuploidy Screening in Couples With Advanced Maternal Age: A Prospective Randomized Controlled Trial

Staessen C, Platteau P, Van Assche E, et al (Vrije Universiteit Brussel, Belgium)
Hum Reprod 19:2849-2858, 2004   21–2

Background.—It is generally accepted that the age-related increased aneuploidy rate is correlated with reduced implantation and a higher abortion rate. Therefore, advanced maternal age (AMA) couples are a good target group to assess the possible benefit of preimplantation genetic diagnosis for aneuploidy screening (PGD-AS) on the outcome after assisted reproductive technology (ART).

Methods.—A prospective randomized controlled clinical trial (RCT) was carried out comparing the outcome after blastocyst transfer combined with PGD-AS using fluorescence *in situ* hybridization (FISH) for the chromosomes X, Y, 13, 16, 18, 21 and 22 in AMA couples (aged ≥ 37 years) with a control group without PGD-AS. From the 400 (200 for PGD-AS and 200 controls) couples that were allocated to the trial, an oocyte pick-up was performed effectively in 289 cycles (148 PGD-AS cycles and 141 control cycles) (Fig 1).

Results.—Positive serum HCG rates per transfer and per cycle were the same for PGD-AS and controls: 35.8% (19.6%) [%/per embryo transfer (per cycle)] and 32.2% (27.7%), respectively (NS) (Table 2). Significantly fewer embryos were transferred in the PGD-AS group than in the control group ($P < 0.001$). The implantation rate (with fetal heart beat) was 17.1% in the PGD-AS group versus 11.5% in the control group (not significant; $P = 0.09$). We observed a normal diploid status in 36.8% of the embryos.

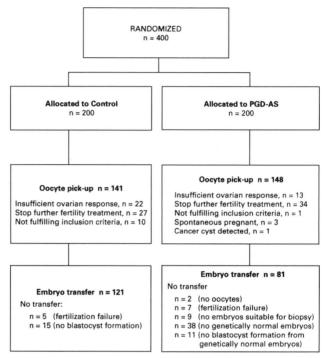

FIGURE 1.—Patient flow through the randomized controlled trial. (Courtesy of Staessen C, Platteau P, Van Assche E, et al: Comparison of blastocyst transfer with or without preimplantation genetic diagnosis for aneuploidy screening in couples with advanced maternal age: A prospective randomized controlled trial. *Hum Reprod* 19:2849-2858, 2004. Copyright European Society for Human Reproduction and Embryology, by permission of Oxford University Press/Human Reproduction.)

Conclusions.—This RCT provides no arguments in favour of PGD-AS for improving clinical outcome per initiated cycle in patients with AMA when there are no restrictions in the number of embryos to be transferred.

▶ With increasing pressures to reducing the risk of multiple pregnancy in ART, strategies have been developed to improve embryo selection. AMA is associated with an increased risk of trisomic pregnancies[1]; therefore, screening of embryos before transfer is an attractive hypothesis to improve implantation, reduce miscarriage rates, and avoid the birth of a child with a chromosome abnormality. Despite increasing use of PGD-AS for AMA, this report is the first published RCT to assess its effectiveness in ART.

Inclusion criteria consisted of (1) women aged 37 years or older, (2) need for in vitro fertilization with intracytoplasmic sperm injection, and (3) both partners with a normal cytogenetic analysis. Subjects were randomized before superovulation. A sample size calculation was performed, based on the primary outcome of an improved implantation rate of 15% per embryo in the PGD-AS group, with a result that at least 157 embryos had to be transferred in each group. Therefore, a total of 400 subjects were required: 200 in the

TABLE 2.—Clinical Results

	Control	PGD-AS	Statistics
Cycles (*n*)	141	148	
No. of cycles with			
Oocyte retrieval failure	0	2	
Fertilization failure	5	7	
All embryos arrested on day 3		9	
With biopsy	—	130	
With only genetically abnormal embryos	—	38	
With no morula or blastocyst formation from genetically normal embryos	—	11	
With no blastocyst formation	15	—	
No. of embryo transfers (ETs)	121	81	$P < 0.001^a$
Total number of embryos transferred	338	164	
Mean embryos transferred[b]	2.8 ± 1.2	2.0 ± 0.9	$P < 0.001^c$
No. of positive serum HCG	39	29	
% positive serum HCG per ET	32.2	35.8	
% positive serum HCG per cycle	27.7	19.6	
No. of implantations with fetal heartbeat (B)	39	28	
% of B per transferred embryo	11.5	17.1	$P = 0.09^a$
Outcome			
Preclinical abortions	9	7	
Clinical abortions and EUG	1	0	
Ongoing ≥12 weeks	29	22	
Singleton	23[d]	18	
Twin	6	3[e,f]	
Triplet		1	
No. of ongoing implantations (C)	35	27	
% of C per transferred embryo	10.4	16.5	$P = 0.06^a$

[a]χ^2 test.
[b]Expressed as mean $\pm$ SD per patient.
[c]*t*-test.
[d]Two triplet pregnancies (1 monozygotic twin and a singleton): reduced to a singleton pregnancy; 1 triplet reduced to a twin and spontaneously reduced further to a singleton pregnancy.
[e]One twin pregnancy resulting from a vanishing triplet pregnancy.
[f]One twin pregnancy lost at 21 weeks.
Abbreviations: PGD-AS, Preimplantation genetic diagnosis for aneuploidy screening; *HCG*, human chorionic gonadotropin; *EUG*, extrauterine gestation.
(Courtesy of Staessen C, Platteau P, Van Assche E, et al: Comparison of blastocyst transfer with or without reimplantation genetic diagnosis for aneuploidy screening in couples with advanced maternal age: A prospective randomized controlled trial. *Hum Reprod* 19:2849-2858, 2004. Copyright European Society for Human Reproduction and Embryology, by permission of Oxford University Press/ Human Reproduction.)

PGD-AS group and 200 in the control group. The randomization flow through chart is illustrated in Figure 1.

Characteristics of the subjects and treatment cycle embryology were similar in the 2 groups. As shown in Table 2, fewer embryos were transferred per cycle in the PGD-AS group: 2.0 versus 2.8 (*P* < .001). The implantation, miscarriage, and ongoing pregnancy rates were similar in the 2 groups.

Although this RCT was designed to assess the impact of PGD-AS on implantation rates rather than ongoing pregnancy rates, the outcomes suggest that PGD-AS is not advantageous in couples with AMA. Further trials are needed to confirm or dispute the results of this study.

M. D. Stephenson, MD, MSc

Reference

1. Hassold T, Chiu D: Maternal age-specific rates of numerical chromosome abnormalities with special reference to trisomy. *Hum Genet* 70:11-17, 1985.

Reliability of Comparative Genomic Hybridization to Detect Chromosome Abnormalities in First Polar Bodies and Metaphase II Oocytes
Gutiérrez-Mateo C, Wells D, Benet J, et al (Universitat Autònoma de Barcelona, Bellaterra, Spain; Inst for Reproductive Medicine and Science, West Orange, NJ; Institut Universitari Dexeus, Barcelona)
Hum Reprod 19:2118-2125, 2004   21–3

Background.—Preimplantation Genetic Diagnosis (PGD) using FISH to analyze up to nine chromosomes to discard chromosomally abnormal embryos has resulted in an increase of pregnancy rates in certain groups of patients. However, the number of chromosomes that can be analyzed is a clear limitation. We evaluate the reliability of using comparative genomic hybridization (CGH) to detect the whole set of chromosomes, as an alternative to PGD using FISH.

Method and Results.—We have analysed by CGH both, first polar bodies (1PBs) and metaphase II (MII) oocytes from 30 oocytes donated by 24 women. The aneuploidy rate was 48%. Considering two maternal age groups, a higher number of chromosome abnormalities were detected in the older group of oocytes (23% versus 75%, $P < 0.02$). About 33% of the 1PB-MII oocyte doublets diagnosed as aneuploid by CGH would have been misdiagnosed as normal if FISH with nine chromosome probes had been used.

Conclusion.—We demonstrate the reliability of 1PB analysis by CGH, to detect almost any chromosome abnormality in oocytes as well as unbalanced segregations of maternal translocations in a time frame compatible with regular *in vitro* fertilization (IVF). The selection of euploid oocytes could help to increase implantation and pregnancy rates of patients undergoing IVF treatment.

▶ CGH represents the next breakthrough in PGD, bringing with it far greater power to analyze early embryonic genetics than traditional fluorescent in situ hybridization (FISH). Up until now, the greatest limitation has been the time-consuming nature of amplifying any genetic material obtained from embryos for analysis. This has prevented CGH from becoming a clinically applicable PGD tool, as analysis could not be performed in a time frame consistent with clinical embryo culture and IVF-ET. Advancement of the technology to perform the task of amplification in a shorter time span now offers the promise to allow CGH to dramatically expand the accuracy and utility of PGD. Further work from this group and others as the technology is disseminated will be eagerly awaited, with hope for rapid application to the clinical setting.

M. R. Drews, MD

Detailed FISH Analysis of Day 5 Human Embryos Reveals the Mechanisms Leading to Mosaic Aneuploidy
Daphnis DD, Delhanty JDA, Jerkovic S, et al (Univ College London; London Fertility Centre)
Hum Reprod 20:129-137, 2004   21–4

Background.—Fluorescence *in situ* hybridization (FISH) analysis has shown that human embryos display a high level of chromosomal mosaicism at all preimplantation stages. The aim of this study was to investigate the mechanisms involved by the use of two probes for each of three autosomes at different loci and to determine the true level of aneuploid mosaicism by excluding FISH artefacts.

Methods.—Embryos were cultured in two different types of medium: group I were cultured in standard cleavage medium for up to day 5 and group II were cultured from day 3 to day 5 in blastocyst medium. Three rounds of FISH were performed. In round 1, the probes used were 1pTel, 11qTel and 18CEP; in round 2, the probes used were 1satII/III, 11CEP and 18qTel; in round 3, the probes used were 18CEP, XCEP and YCEP.

Results.—A total of 21 embryos were analysed in each group. The FISH results revealed one uniformly diploid and 20 mosaic embryos for group I, and two uniformly diploid and 19 mosaic embryos for group II. The predominant type of mosaicism was diploid/aneuploid. The use of two different probes per autosome was able to distinguish FISH artefacts affecting 5% of nuclei from true single cell anomalies.

Conclusions.—Post-zygotic chromosome loss was the most common mechanism leading to aneuploidy mosaicism for both groups, followed by chromosome gain, with fewer examples of mitotic non-disjunction.

Anaphase Lagging Mainly Explains Chromosomal Mosaicism in Human Preimplantation Embryos
Coonen E, Derhaag JG, Dumoulin JCM, et al (Maastricht Univ, The Netherlands)
Hum Reprod 19:316-324, 2004   21–5

Background.—Cleavage stage embryos as well as postimplantation embryos have been studied extensively over the years. However, our knowledge with respect to the chromosomal constitution of human embryos at the blastocyst stage is still rudimentary.

Methods.—In the present paper, a large series of human blastocysts was examined by means of fluorescent *in situ* hybridization (FISH).

Results.—It was found that only one in four blastocysts (25%) displayed a normal chromosomal pattern. We defined a group of blastocysts (26%) displaying a simple mosaic chromosome pattern (different cell lines resulting from one chromosomal error), an about equally large group of blastocysts (31%) displaying a complex mosaic chromosome pattern, and a smaller group of blastocysts (11%) showing a chaotic chromosome distribution pat-

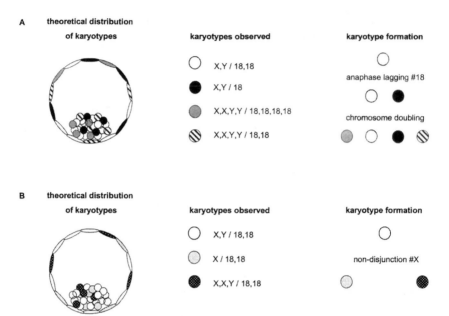

A theoretical distribution
of karyotypes

karyotypes observed

karyotype formation

X,Y / 18,18

X,Y / 18

anaphase lagging #18

X,X,Y,Y / 18,18,18,18

chromosome doubling

X,X,Y,Y / 18,18

B theoretical distribution
of karyotypes

karyotypes observed

karyotype formation

X,Y / 18,18

X / 18,18

non-disjunction #X

X,X,Y / 18,18

FIGURE 2.—Schematic representation of the etiology of chromosomal mosaicism observed in blastocysts. (Courtesy of Coonen E, Derhaag JG, Dumoulin JCM, et al: Anaphase lagging mainly explains chromosomal mosaicism in human preimplantation embryos. *Hum Reprod* 19:316-324, 2004. Copyright European Society for Human Reproduction and Embryology, by permission of Oxford University Press/Human Reproduction.)

tern (Fig 2). Six per cent of all blastocysts analysed could not be assigned one of the previously mentioned chromosomal patterns.

Conclusion.—Anaphase lagging appeared to be the major mechanism through which human embryos acquire a mosaic chromosome pattern during preimplantation development to the blastocyst stage.

▶ We have learned through preimplantation genetic diagnosis that a significant percentage of human embryos created through in vitro fertilization (IVF) possess aneuploidies at the cleavage stage. These initial findings helped to achieve a greater understanding of the genetic reasons for the observed inefficiency of IVF. The present studies (Abstracts 21–4 and 21–5) have taken this understanding to a higher level, demonstrating that significant mosaicism is seen within blastocysts, and that these issues may become amplified with postzygotic development. Unfortunately, we will likely never understand whether these genetic issues are unique to embryos created through ovarian stimulation and IVF, or if they represent part of the explanation for the relative inefficiency of human reproduction under natural in vivo conditions as well. Recent evidence from the murine model[1] and in hamsters[2] shows that both variations in gonadotropin superovulation regimens and in vitro culture conditions can dramatically alter spindle dynamics and microfilament formation in the oocyte. It is possible that many of the issues of aneuploidy and mosaicism that we observe in laboratory-derived embryos may be ironically occurring as a result of the processes necessary to obtain the multiple oocytes and embryos we require to overcome the inherent inefficiency of IVF.

M. R. Drews, MD

References

1. Sanfins A, Plancha C, Overstrom E, et al: Meiotic spindle morphogenesis in in vivo and in vitro matured mouse oocytes: Insights into the relationship between nuclear and cytoplasmic quality. *Hum Reprod* 19:2889-2899, 2004.
2. Lee S, Kim T, Cho M, et al: Development of a hamster superovulation program and adverse effects of gonadotropins on microfilament formation during oocyte development. *Fertil Steril* 83:1264S-1274S, 2005.

Telomere Length Predicts Embryo Fragmentation After In Vitro Fertilization in Women: Toward a Telomere Theory of Reproductive Aging in Women
Keefe DL, Franco S, Liu L, et al (Brown Med School, Providence, RI; MBL, Woods Hole, Mass; Tufts New England Med Ctr, Boston; et al)
Am J Obstet Gynecol 192:1256-1261, 2005   21–6

Objective.—Telomeres are DNA repeats which cap and protect chromosome ends, facilitate homologue pairing and chiasmata formation during early meiosis, and shorten with cell division and exposure to reactive oxygen to mediate aging. Early germ cells contain telomerase, a reverse transcriptase which adds telomeres to 3-prime DNA ends, but telomerase activity declines in oocytes, fixing telomere length earlier during development. Experimentally induced telomere shortening in mice disrupts meiosis, impairs chiasmata formation, halts embryonic cell cycles, and promotes apoptosis in embryos, a phenotype which mimics reproductive senescence in women. Ethical constraints limit study of human embryos to nondestructive assays, such as morphologic evaluation under transmission optics, but cytoplasmic fragmentation is a reliable marker of apoptosis.

Study Design.—Study design consisted of observational study of effect of telomere length in human eggs on cytoplasmic fragmentation, and on other morphologic features of preimplantation embryos. To test the hypothesis that telomere shortening triggers apoptosis in human embryos, we evaluated telomere length as a predictor of cytoplasmic fragmentation in embryos from women undergoing in vitro fertilization.

Results.—Telomere length negatively predicted fragmentation in day 3 preimplantation embryos, after controlling for patient age and basal follicle stimulating hormone level. Telomere length did not predict other features of preimplantation embryo morphology.

Conclusion.—The finding that telomere length in human eggs predicts cytoplasmic fragmentation in embryos provides evidence that telomere shortening induces apoptosis in human preimplantation embryos, consistent with a telomere theory of reproductive senescence in women.

▶ This study continues to expand our understanding of the genetic mechanisms of reproductive senescence in women. While not immediately applicable to the clinical setting, early work correlating telomere length in polar bodies with telomere length in oocytes may eventually lead us to yet another method of assessing oocyte and embryo implantation potential in the laboratory. Combined with other methods of noninvasive or minimally invasive embryo assessment, telomere length holds promise to contribute to the continued quest to maximize the efficiency of in vitro fertilization and the understanding of our age-dependent inefficiency in reproduction as a species.

M. R. Drews, MD

Noninvasive Imaging of Spindle Dynamics During Mammalia Oocyte Activation

Navarro PAAS, Liu L, Trimarchi JR, et al (Brown Univ, Providence, RI; Marine Biological Lab, Woods Hole, Mass; Univ of São Paulo, Brazil)
Fertil Steril 83:1197-1205, 2005   21–7

Objective.—To develop a method to evaluate spindle dynamics in living oocytes and in karyoplasts during the initial stages of activation and after pharmacological disruption of cytoskeleton.

Design.—Morphological study using a novel microscope.

Setting.—Translational research laboratory at marine biological laboratory.

Animal(s).—Six-week-old CD-1 or B6C3F1 mice superovulated with pregnant mare's serum gonadotropin and human chorionic gonadotropin (hCG).

Intervention(s).—Spindles of living oocytes and karyoplasts were imaged at 5-10 minute intervals using the Pol-Scope during the initial stages of oocyte activation and after pharmacological disruption of cytoskeleton.

Main Outcome Measure(s).—Assessment of spindle dynamics using Pol-Scope imaging.

Result(s).—During oocyte activation, spindle mid-region birefringence increased, followed by spindle rotation and second polar body extrusion in both intact oocytes and karyoplasts. Activation of protein kinase C (PKC) with phorbol 12-myristate 13-acetate failed to induce spindle activation in 60% of living oocytes and caused spindle disruption in some oocytes. Inhibition of PKC by a myristoylated PKC pseudosubstrate inhibited metaphase II release in most oocytes evaluated (86.7%). Cytochalasin D inhibited only spindle rotation and separation. Nocodazole disrupted spindles in less than 5 minutes after administration.

Conclusion(s).—Pol-Scope imaging allows investigation at near real time of spindle dynamics during activation of living oocytes. Spindles also showed evidence of activation even in karyoplasts. The procedure may be useful for detecting functional spindle aberrations in living oocytes. Further studies are needed to determine whether spindle dynamics predict clinical outcome.

▶ Noninvasive methods to assess reproductive competency of human oocytes and embryos will eventually provide the necessary tools to dramatically increase the efficacy of IVF-ET while simultaneously allowing for a reduction in the number of embryos transferred and, thus, a reduction in multiple pregnancy rates. The search for clinically applicable techniques is currently being conducted on 2 fronts: assessment of secretions or products of embryo metabolism in culture media, and observation of organelle dynamics with specific interest in the cytoskeleton and dynamics of the spindle. This investigation demonstrates possible clinical applications for Pol-Scope imaging to impact clinical care through potential noninvasive identification of spindle dysfunction. Through this technology, combined with examination of early embryonic secretions such as HLA-G, and traditional assessment of embryo morphology, a multifaceted paradigm is evolving for assessment and selection of those rare embryos with peak capacity to implant and produce viable conception.

M. R. Drews, MD

GYNECOLOGY

22 Pediatric and Adolescent Gynecology

Young Age at First Sexual Intercourse and Sexually Transmitted Infections in Adolescents and Young Adults

Kaestle CE, Halpern CT, Miller WC, et al (Univ of North Carolina at Chapel Hill)

Am J Epidemiol 161:774-780, 2005   22–1

Abstract.—The authors examined the relation between age at first vaginal intercourse and a positive nucleic acid amplification test for sexually transmitted infection (STI). A nationally representative sample of 9,844 respondents aged 18-26 years was tested for chlamydial infection, gonorrhea, and

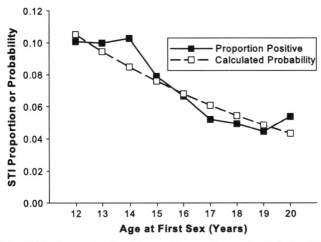

FIGURE 1.—Weighted proportion of participants with a sexually transmitted infection (STI) (*Chlamydia trachomatis, Neisseria gonorrhoeae*, or *Trichomonas vaginalis*) by age at first sexual intercourse, and corresponding probability of having an STI, as calculated from simple logistic regression before adjustment for demographic factors (*n* = 9,844), National Longitudinal Study of Adolescent Health, 2001–2002. (Courtesy of Kaestle CE, Halpern CT, Miller WC, et al: Young age at first sexual intercourse and sexually transmitted infections in adolescents and young adults. *Am J Epidemiol* 161:774-780, 2005, by permission of Oxford University Press.)

trichomoniasis in wave 3 (2001–2002) of the National Longitudinal Study of Adolescent Health. The authors used multiple logistic regression to assess the relation between age at first sexual intercourse and these STIs and to examine variation by current age, sex, race, and ethnicity. Younger ages at first intercourse were associated with higher odds of STI in comparison with older ages, but the effect diminished with increasing current age (Fig 1). For example, the odds of having an STI for an 18-year-old who first had intercourse at age 13 were more than twice those of an 18-year-old who first had intercourse at age 17 (prevalence odds ratio = 2.25, 95% confidence interval: 1.42, 3.59). In contrast, the odds of having an STI among 24-year-olds with first intercourse at age 13 versus those with first intercourse at age 17 were the same (prevalence odds ratio = 1.11, 95% confidence interval: 0.88, 1.39). Thus, earlier initiation of sexual intercourse is strongly associated with STIs for older adolescents but not for young adults over age 23 years.

▶ Adolescent behavior has long been associated with a variety of adverse outcomes. In this study from the University of North Carolina at Chapel Hill, Kaestle et al showed that there is a strong relationship between the age of first vaginal intercourse and a positive nucleic acid test for sexually transmitted diseases. Of further interest was that although the authors also found that early initiation of sexual intercourse was strongly associated with sexually transmitted infections for older adolescents, it was not associated with an increased risk of STIs for young adults older than 23 years. Studies such as these provide invaluable epidemiologic information concerning particular patient populations that may be at risk for adverse outcomes based on demographics or behavioral patterns or both. Such studies allow us to better identify those individuals and groups who may benefit from a different approach to disease prevention and thus improve overall outcomes in the near term and long term for these adolescents and young adults.

L. P. Shulman, MD

Promising to Wait: Virginity Pledges and Adolescent Sexual Behavior
Bersamin MM, Walker S, Waiters ED, et al (Pacific Inst for Research and Evaluation, Berkeley, Calif; Pacific Inst for Research and Evaluation, Calverton, Md)
J Adolesc Health 36:428-436, 2005   22–2

Purpose.—The current study examined the association between formal and non-formal virginity pledges and the initiation of genital play, oral sex, and vaginal intercourse among adolescents.

Methods.—Logistic regressions controlling for age, gender, race, expectancies, academic achievement, contraceptive education, perceived peer pledging behavior, and parental and peer attitudes were conducted to examine the relationship between pledging behavior and genital play, oral sex, and vaginal intercourse. A total of 870 adolescents aged 12-16 from 10 counties in northern and southern California participated in the current study.

Results.—The findings indicate that making a private pledge or promise to oneself to wait to have sexual intercourse until one is older reduces the likelihood that adolescents will engage in sexual intercourse and oral sex. The effect persists even when controlling for socio-demographic variables. Making a formal pledge did not appear to have an effect on sexual behavior.

Conclusions.—The findings raise questions about the effectiveness of formal virginity pledges in preventing adolescent sexual behavior. The findings suggest that sexual health programs may be more effective if they encourage young people to make a personal commitment to delay the onset of sex, foster social norms supportive of delaying sex, and raise awareness of how early sexual initiation may threaten future plans.

▶ The authors looked at the association between virginity pledges and the initiation of sexual behavior in adolescents, using longitudinal data. In the current climate of controversy regarding the effectiveness of abstinence-only programs, they looked at the virginity pledge specifically to see whether the effect extends to the delay of other sexual behaviors aside from sexual intercourse.

A total of 870 adolescents aged 12 to 16 years from California participated. Data were collected in 6-month intervals using in-home, computer-assisted, self-administered interviews and mail surveys. Logistic regression controlled for variables such as age, gender, race, academic achievement, contraceptive education, perceived peer pledging behavior, and parental and peer attitudes to examine the relationship between making virginity pledges and genital play, oral sex, and vaginal intercourse. Questions measured sexual activity, religiosity, virginity pledges, perceived peer pledging, expectancies (related to health and social consequences), parental and peer attitudes, sex education, academic achievement, and demographics. The authors did find that making a private pledge to oneself to wait to have sex did reduce the chances that an adolescent will engage in sexual behaviors; however, making a formal pledge did not make a difference. Making a private pledge did not extend to genital play. Private, nonformal pledges were associated with less likelihood of engaging in oral sex.

Understanding teen sexual behaviors is critical in education programs. Types of behaviors engaged in, such as oral sex, which is commonly preferred over vaginal intercourse, need to be understood and need to be included in the overall assessment of sexual behaviors.[1] These findings suggest that programs are more effective if they encourage teens to make a personal commitment rather than make a formal pledge. This is done by increasing awareness and educating teens about how initiation of sex affects their lives and future plans. To get a full understanding of these consequences, teens need to get all the information, including abstinence education and learning about making healthy choices.

E. A. Iglesias, MD

Reference

1. Halpern-Flesher BL, Cornell JL, Kropp RY, et al: Oral versus vaginal sex among adolescents: Perceptions, attitudes, and behavior. *Pediatrics* 115:845-851, 2005.

Oral Versus Vaginal Sex Among Adolescents: Perceptions, Attitudes, and Behavior

Halpern-Felsher BL, Cornell JL, Kropp RY, et al (Univ of California, San Francisco)
Pediatrics 115:845-851, 2005
22–3

Objective.—Despite studies indicating that a significant proportion of adolescents are having oral sex, the focus of most empirical studies and intervention efforts concerning adolescent sexuality have focused on vaginal intercourse. This narrow focus has created a void in our understanding of adolescents' perceptions of oral sex. This study is the first to investigate adolescents' perceptions of the health, social, and emotional consequences associated with having oral sex as compared with vaginal sex, as well as whether adolescents view oral sex as more acceptable and more prevalent than vaginal sex.

Methods.—Participants were 580 ethnically diverse ninth-grade adolescents (mean age: 14.54; 58% female) who participated in a longitudinal study on the relationship between risk and benefit perceptions and sexual activity. Participants completed a self-administered questionnaire that inquired about their sexual experiences and percent chance of experiencing outcomes from, attitudes toward, and perceived prevalence of oral versus vaginal sex among adolescents.

TABLE 2.—Adolescents' Chance Estimates of Experiencing Positive and Negative Outcomes for Vaginal Compared With Oral Sex

	Vaginal Sex, Mean % (SD)	Oral Sex, Mean % (SD)	F Value	P Value
Risks				
Get chlamydia	52.98 (25.40)	37.55 (28.86)	105.69	.000
Get HIV	49.92 (26.77)	37.64 (30.06)	77.01	.000
Become pregnant	67.63 (23.41)	16.71 (29.31)	824.86	.000
Relationship gets worse	42.13 (26.86)	35.61 (26.41)	37.47	.000
Bad reputation	41.46 (28.60)	37.58 (28.54)	10.54	.001
Get into trouble	71.71 (31.86)	63.16 (35.56)	64.77	.000
Feel bad about self	54.81 (34.11)	45.90 (34.91)	31.70	.000
Feel guilty	55.42 (33.85)	48.19 (35.43)	46.95	.000
Benefits				
Experience pleasure	72.03 (30.44)	59.19 (36.41)	43.93	.000
Feel good about self	40.01 (32.58)	40.26 (33.75)	.000	.999
Be more popular	27.13 (26.76)	26.85 (26.94)	.066	.797
Relationship gets better	41.29 (25.29)	39.71 (26.53)	.310	.578

Results.—More study participants reported having had oral sex (19.6%) than vaginal sex (13.5%), and more participants intended to have oral sex in the next 6 months (31.5%) than vaginal sex (26.3%). Adolescents evaluated oral sex as significantly less risky than vaginal sex on health, social, and emotional consequences (Table 2). Adolescents also believed that oral sex is more acceptable than vaginal sex for adolescents their own age in both dating and nondating situations, oral sex is less of a threat to their values and beliefs, and more of their peers will have oral sex than vaginal sex in the near future.

Conclusions.—Given that adolescents perceive oral sex as less risky, more prevalent, and more acceptable than vaginal sex, it stands to reason that adolescents are more likely to engage in oral sex. It is important that health care providers and others who work with youths recognize adolescents' views about oral sex and broaden their clinical preventive services to include screening, counseling, and education about oral sex.

▶ The authors' objective was to look at behaviors, perceptions, and attitudes relating to oral sex as opposed to vaginal intercourse, which has been extensively studied in the adolescent age group. Adolescents' opinions on oral sex, whether more prevalent and acceptable, and the emotional and perceived health consequences were evaluated. This longitudinal study was conducted using a self-administered questionnaire to obtain information about demographics, sexual experience, perceived risks of outcomes, attitudes towards oral sex, and perceived prevalence of oral sex versus vaginal sex in this age group.

A total of 580 ninth-grade students from 2 California public high schools participated and were surveyed every 6 months. Questions regarding engagement in and intentions to have oral and vaginal sex, estimates of the chances of experiencing risks and benefits of oral and vaginal sex, attitudes towards engaging in oral and vaginal sex, and perceived peer intention or engagement in oral and vaginal sex were asked. More study participants reported engaging in oral versus vaginal sex (19.6% vs 13.5%). More intended to have oral sex in the next 6 months (31.5%) than vaginal sex (26.3%). They evaluated oral sex as being less risky in regard to emotional and health consequences, such as getting chlamydia or HIV, than vaginal sex. They believed oral sex was more acceptable than vaginal sex and less of a threat to their morals and values, believing they are less likely to feel guilty or bad about themselves, compared with vaginal sex. They also perceived that more of their peers would have oral versus vaginal sex in the near future. Participants believed that oral sex was more acceptable for their age group than vaginal sex.

The percentage of high school students who have engaged in sexual intercourse has decreased from 1991 to 2003, from 54% to 47%.[1] Teen pregnancy rates have also decreased from 1990 to 2000.[2] A closer look at the types of sexual behaviors that teens are engaging in needs to be done in order to better direct pregnancy and sexually transmitted infection prevention programs. The results of this study lead to the conclusion that adolescents are more likely to engage in oral sex than vaginal sex. Risk prevention strategies should include addressing oral sex in education programs and having health care providers screen for these behaviors.

E. A. Iglesias, MD

References

1. Teen sexual activity in the United States. The national campaign to prevent teen pregnancy, 2005, http://www.teenpregnancy.org/resources/data/pdf/TeenSexActivityOnePager.pdf, accessed October 1, 2005.
2. Teen pregnancy rates in the United States, 1972-2000. The national campaign to prevent teen pregnancy, 2005, http://www.teenpregnancy.org/resources/data/pdf/TeenPregnancyRatesOnePager.pdf, accessed October 1, 2005.

Cervical Dysplasia in Adolescents
Wright JD, Davila RM, Pinto KR, et al (Washington Univ, St Louis; Baylor Univ, Dallas)
Obstet Gynecol 106:115-120, 2005   22–4

Background.—Although the incidence of cervical dysplasia in adolescents is increasing, a paucity of data exists regarding the outcomes of adolescents with Pap test abnormalities. We determined the natural history and outcome of adolescents with low-grade squamous intraepithelial lesions (LSIL) and high-grade squamous intraepithelial lesions (HSIL).

Methods.—A review of all women aged 18 years or younger with a cytologic diagnosis of LSIL or HSIL between 1997 and 2003 was performed. Follow-up cytologic and histologic samples were evaluated. The most significant abnormality was recorded for each patient. Rates of regression, persistence, and progression were calculated.

Results.—A total of 646 adolescents were identified. Follow-up was available for 477 teenagers with LSIL and for 55 with HSIL. Among adolescents with LSIL, 146 (35%) had negative follow-up. Low-grade abnormalities (atypical squamous cells of undetermined significance, LSIL, and cervical intraepithelial neoplasia grade 1) were seen in 199 (47%), whereas high-grade abnormalities were documented in 77 (18%). After 36 months, 62% had regressed, whereas 31% had progressive dysplasia. For the HSIL cohort, negative follow-up was documented in 12 (21.8%) adolescents, and 15 (27.3%) had low-grade abnormalities, whereas more than one half (50.9%) were found to have a high-grade abnormality. At 36 months, 31% of HSIL subjects had progressed to cervical intraepithelial neoplasia 3.

Conclusion.—Adolescents with LSIL and HSIL cytology are at significant risk for progression to high-grade cervical abnormalities. The rate of development of high-grade cervical abnormalities in adolescents is similar to adults. Adolescents with cytologic abnormalities mandate close follow-up.

▶ This study looked at the outcome of abnormal Pap smears in adolescents to help determine the natural progression in this age group. By studying this, the authors hope to contribute to the establishment of guidelines on how to manage LSIL and HSIL in the adolescent patient.

The study was a retrospective review using a database that identified 646 adolescents younger than 18 years (range, 12-18 years) who had LSIL or HSIL diagnosed between 1997 and 2003. Follow-up was available in 422 patients with LSIL and 55 with HSIL, yielding a total of 477 subjects. In general, patients had either repeat cytology or colposcopy with a histologic specimen available. The histologic and cytologic results for follow-up of LSIL were combined and evaluated. Histologic evaluation was available in 66.1% of LSIL. Of the subjects with LSIL, 35% had a negative follow-up, 47% had a low-grade abnormality such as atypical squamous cells of undetermined significance (ASCUS), LSIL, or cervical intraepithelial neoplasia (CIN) I, and 18% went on to have a high-grade abnormality (HSIL, CIN 2, CIN 3, and adenocarcinoma in situ). At 36 months, 61.7% of LSIL subjects regressed to normal, 31.3% progressed to moderate or severe lesions, and 6.9% had persistent low-grade abnormalities. In the group with the initial HSIL Pap, when histologic and cytologic follow-up was combined (histologic specimen was obtained in 91% of subjects), 21.8% had a negative follow-up, 27.3% had low-grade abnormalities, and 50.9% had high-grade abnormalities. One 18-year-old girl was found to have carcinoma in situ on biopsy. Thirty-one percent of subjects having HSIL progressed to CIN 3 in 36 months after the index Pap HSIL.

It has been noted that human papillomavirus (HPV) infections in this age group seem to be transient and rarely lead to invasive cervical disease.[1] New recommendations that allow for repeat cytology or HPV testing rather than direct referral to colposcopy appear to be safe in the adolescent age group.[2] The results of this study show that adolescents are at risk for the development of high-grade lesions, showing similar statistics to adult women. The timing of initial Pap smears and screening methods for adolescents are still topics of discussion. More prospective studies need to be done to help elucidate a more definitive protocol for this age group. These data support that adolescents need to be followed up closely, especially in light of the high risk of the population and problems with compliance and follow-up.

E. A. Iglesias, MD

References

1. Gray SH, Walzer TB: New strategies for cervical cancer screening in adolescents. *Curr Opin Pediatr* 16:344-349, 2004.
2. Moscicki AB: Cervical cytology testing in teens. *Curr Opin Obstet Gynecol* 17:471-475, 2005.

Fertility and Parental Consent for Minors to Receive Contraceptives
Zavodny M (Occidental College, Los Angeles)
Am J Public Health 94:1347-1351, 2004   22–5

Background.—Under Title X of the Public Health Service Act, family planning clinics that receive federal funds are required to provide their services without regard to age or marital status. A series of court decisions in the 1970s and 1980s found that clinics receiving Title X funding may not require parental consent or notification before providing birth control services to unmarried minors. However, in recent years, Congress and some state legislatures have considered requirements that publicly funded clinics notify parents before they provide contraceptives to minors. The effects of such a parental involvement requirement on births and abortions among minors were examined.

Methods.—Births and abortions among teens, relative to adults, in a suburban Illinois county that instituted a parental consent requirement in 1998 were compared with births and abortions in nearby counties from 1997 to 2000.

Results.—The relative proportion of births to women younger than 19 years in the study county increased significantly compared with nearby counties, while the relative proportion of abortions to women younger than 20 years decreased insignificantly, with a relative increase in the proportion of pregnancies (births and abortions) to young women in the county.

Conclusions.—It is thought that Title X has significantly reduced teen pregnancy rates by making available free or low-cost family planning services available to teens on a confidential basis. However, the mandate of a parental consent requirement for contraceptives but not abortions appeared to raise the frequency of pregnancies and births among young women. There is concern that a parental consent policy may also affect other aspects of the sexual health of teens, such a pregnancy testing and treatment for sexually transmitted disease.

Adolescents' Reports of Parental Knowledge of Adolescents' Use of Sexual Health Services and Their Reactions to Mandated Parental Notification for Prescription Contraception

Jones RK, Purcell A, Singh S, et al (Alan Guttmacher Inst, New York)
JAMA 293:340-348, 2005   22–6

Context.—Legislation has been proposed that would mandate parental notification for adolescents younger than 18 years (minors) obtaining prescription contraception from federally funded family planning clinics.

Objective.—To determine the extent to which parents are currently aware that their teenage daughters are accessing reproductive health services and how minors would react in the face of mandated parental involvement laws for prescription birth control.

Design, Setting, and Participants.—A total of 1526 female adolescents younger than 18 years seeking reproductive health services at a national sample of 79 family planning clinics were surveyed between May 2003 and February 2004.

Main Outcome Measures.—Proportions of minor females who reported that a parent or guardian was aware that they were at the family planning clinic and, under conditions of mandated parental involvement, proportions of minors who would access prescription contraceptives at family planning clinics or engage in unsafe sex.

Results.—Sixty percent of minors reported that a parent or guardian knew they were accessing sexual health services at the clinic. Fifty-nine percent of all adolescents would use the clinic for prescription contraception even if parental notification were mandated. This response was less common (29.5%) among adolescents whose parents were unaware of their clinic visits and more common (79%) among those whose parents were aware. Many adolescents gave more than 1 response to mandated parental involvement. Forty-six percent would use an over-the-counter method, and 18% would go to a private physician. Seven percent said that they would stop having sex as one response, but only 1% indicated this would be their only reaction. One in 5 adolescents would use no contraception or rely on withdrawal as one response to mandated notification.

Conclusions.—Most minor adolescent females seeking family planning services report that their parents are aware of their use of services. Most would continue to use clinic services if parental notification were mandated. However, mandated parental notification laws would likely increase risky or unsafe sexual behavior and, in turn, the incidence of adolescent pregnancy and sexually transmitted diseases.

▶ The issue of parental consent for family planning services has been controversial as long as these services have been available. Currently clinics that receive federal funding under Title X of the Public Health Services Act are required to provide services without regard to age or marital status.[1] This access is constantly being challenged and Congress, along with several state legislatures, are considering restrictions and regulations that would require parental consent for minors. These articles look at the consequences of such action in different ways.

Jones et al (Abstract 22–6) surveyed over 1500 adolescents younger than 18 years who were seeking reproductive health services to determine if their parents were aware they were utilizing these services and how their behavior would change if parental consent was mandated. In this sample, 60% reported that a parent or guardian knew they were accessing care at the family planning clinic and 59% stated they would continue to use the services even if parental consent was mandated. However, of the respondents whose parents were not aware, only 29.5% stated they would continue to use the clinic services and 6.4% of all respondents stated that if parental consent was required, they would continue to have sex, but not use contraception.

The above report was hypothetical, but Zavodny (Abstract 22–5) examined the actual effect of imposing mandatory parental consent. Zavodny compared the birth and abortion rates among adolescents in McHenry County, Ill., before and after parental consent requirements were enacted. She demonstrated an increase in the percentage of births to women younger than 19 years despite a decrease during the same time period in neighboring counties. She also documented a decrease in the relative proportion in abortions in women younger than 20 years during the same time period. She concluded that parental consent requirements for contraception increase the number of pregnancies and births among young women but do not significantly change the abortion rates.

The issue of parental consent requirements for access to family planning services is very controversial. These authors have shown that any action restricting care will have consequences in the form of either riskier sexual behaviors or increased unintended pregnancies. Providers and legislators should consider these consequences before mandating a "one size fits all" requirement on this extremely individual decision.

N. B. Zite, MD, MPH

Reference

1. Title X, Public Health Services Act, 42 USC. 300-300a-8.

Positive Experience of Teenage Motherhood: A Qualitative Study
Seamark CJ, Lings P (Honiton Group Practice, England; Peninsula Med School, Exeter, England)
Br J Gen Pract 54:813-818, 2004   22–7

Background.—Teenage pregnancy is seen as a cause for concern in the United Kingdom (UK). However, there has been little research from primary care looking at teenage motherhood and its implications.

Aim.—To investigate the experiences of teenage mothers in relation to their role as mothers and their expectations of their futures.

Design of Study: Qualitative study.

Setting.—East Devon, England.

Method.—Nine women who had conceived their first child while still a teenager agreed to participate. Semi-structured interviews were undertaken, audiotaped, transcribed, and analysed using interpretative phenomenological analysis.

Results.—The women expressed positive attitudes to being mothers and described how it had affected their lives. For some, motherhood had been the impetus to change direction and consider a career, because they had someone else for whom they were responsible. They recognised that they were still young enough to enter further education or other aspects of employment as their children grew up.

Conclusions.—For the women in this study, having been a teenage mother did not mean that their life and future were all over. Motherhood and bringing up children were valued in their own right. The women were realistic about their futures, often making plans to develop their careers.

▶ Authors in the UK looked at the implications of teenage motherhood. With teenage pregnancy being a concern in many countries, they looked at some of the well-deserved consequences and effects on teens. They investigated the attitudes of teen mothers and how pregnancy affected their lives in regard to future goals and expectations.

Seventeen subjects were approached and 9 subjects, who became mothers in their adolescent years, agreed to be interviewed. The interviews were audiotaped and interpreted. The authors found an overall positive attitude with immediate bonding felt by most of the mothers, and some describing actually being motivated to pursue careers because of the responsibility of having someone to care for. For these women, motherhood was valued in of itself, and they looked towards their futures with realistic goals and expectations.

Adolescent pregnancy rates and teen birth rates have decreased since the early 1990s.[1,2] This study brings some positive light to an otherwise negatively viewed outcome to teenage behaviors. These findings provide some food for thought, in a world where teenage pregnancy is so fought against and considered a problem.[3] This study illustrates the adaptability of teens and good outcomes, instead of only focusing on the negative.

E. A. Iglesias, MD

References

1. Teen birth rates in the United States 1940-2003. The national campaign to prevent teen pregnancy, 2005, http://www.teenpregnancy.org/resources/data/pdf/BirthRatesOnePager(05).pdf, accessed October 1, 2005.
2. Teen pregnancy rates in the United States, 1972-2000. National campaign to prevent teen pregnancy, 2005, http://www.teenpregnancy.org/resources/data/pdf/TeenPregnancyRatesOnePager .pdf, accessed October 1, 2005.
3. Teenager's sexual and reproductive health: Developed countries, facts in brief, 2002, http://www.agi-usa.org/pubs/fb_teens.html, accessed October 1, 2005.

Adolescents' Experience With the Combined Estrogen and Progestin Transdermal Contraceptive Method Ortho Evra

Harel Z, Riggs S, Vaz R, et al (Brown Univ, Providence, RI)
J Pediatr Adolesc Gynecol 18:85-90, 2005   22–8

Background.—The new combined estrogen & progestin contraceptive patch Ortho Evra was approved by the FDA in December 2001. To date, there is a paucity of data regarding its use in the adolescent age group. We examined adolescents' experience with this new contraceptive method.

Methods.—Using a questionnaire designed by the authors, care providers in a hospital based adolescent clinic interviewed and reviewed the charts of adolescent girls who had initiated Ortho Evra in 2002-2003.

Results.—Twenty-eight adolescent girls (age 18 ± 1 years, gyn age 6 ± 1 years, onset of sexual intercourse at 14 ± 1 years, body mass index (BMI) 27.6 ± 1.2, 57% Hispanic, 21% Caucasian, 11% African American, 7% biracial, 4% Indian American) who had used Ortho Evra for 7 ± 1 months were enrolled. Half (50%) were adolescent mothers, and 57% had a history of irregular menstrual periods. All (100%) girls reported regular menstrual periods while using Ortho Evra, with only 14% experiencing occasional breakthrough bleeding. Half reported a shorter duration and 36% reported a lighter flow of their periods. About a third (39%) reported a decrease and

11% reported an increase in dysmenorrhea symptoms. About a third (29%) of those with a history of recurrent headaches at initiation reported decrease in headaches, and about a third (33%) of those with acne at initiation reported decrease in facial acne while on Ortho Evra. There were no significant BMI changes during Ortho Evra use. Although condom use while on Ortho Evra was poor (only 15% reporting consistent condom use), there were no pregnancies reported. A majority (93%) reported that they remembered to apply the patches on time, and 40% stated that Ortho Evra was easier than previous contraceptive methods. Two thirds (68%) were very satisfied and 29% were somewhat satisfied with the method, and 93% stated that they would recommend the method to a friend/relative. The preferred application site was the buttock (40%) followed by the lower abdomen (32%). About a fifth (21%) experienced at least one episode of complete patch detachment and 32% reported partial peeling of the patch corners. About a third (32%) would prefer another patch color, and 25% would like a fourth week placebo patch. The most common side effects were mild temporary application site reactions (64%), some discomfort on patch removal (32%), nausea (18%), and breast tenderness (18%). Eleven girls (39%) discontinued Ortho Evra (three lost health insurance, three because of application site reactions, two found patch application schedule difficult to remember, two desired pregnancy, two because of nausea, one because of perceived weight gain).

Conclusions.—Ortho Evra provides excellent cycle control in adolescents. Most adolescents are satisfied with this method. Intensive efforts should be made to increase condom use by adolescents on Ortho Evra.

▶ The authors examined the experience of adolescents on the Ortho Evra contraceptive patch via a questionnaire used by health care providers to interview the subjects. Attitudes towards the patch as well as side effects experienced, including change in BMI, were evaluated.

There were 28 subjects aged 17 to 19 years. Some reported reasons to choose Ortho Evra were (1) difficulty in remembering the pill every day (46%), (2) side effects of other methods such as irregular bleeding, weight gain, or hair loss on Depo-Provera, (3) occurrence of vaginal infections with the vaginal ring, (4) wanting regular periods (36%), and (5) convenience (29%). Most subjects remembered to place the patch on time (93%), and 40% said it was an easier method than others. Sixty-eight percent were very satisfied, and 93% would recommend it to a friend or family member. All subjects had regular menses while on the patch, 14% reported spotting or breakthrough bleeding, 50% reported shorter periods, 36% reported lighter flow, and 4% reported a longer duration of menses. Subjects reported both a decrease and an increase in dysmenorrhea. Thirty-three percent reported an improvement in acne. No pregnancies were reported while on Ortho Evra. There was no significant change in BMI during use. Twenty-nine percent had a perceived weight loss, and 14% had a perceived weight gain while on the patch. The favored application site was the buttock (40%), followed by the lower abdomen (32%). The most common side effects were application site reactions that were mild (64%), removal discomfort (32%), nausea (18%), and breast tenderness

(18%). Twenty-one percent reported complete detachment of the patch. Fourteen percent reported fewer mood swings. As far as sexual activity, 78% reported unchanged libido, and 15% reported increased libido. There was a decrease in reported condom use while on Ortho Evra. Thirty-nine percent discontinued Ortho Evra secondary to a loss of health insurance, application site reactions, difficulty in remembering, wanting to get pregnant, nausea, and perceived weight gain.

The transdermal contraceptive patch first became available in 2002. Studies looking at the patch as well as patch versus oral contraceptive pills have found that efficacy and cycle control are similar. Compliance is good on the patch and better when compared with pills.[1,2] The side effect profile is similar to that of oral contraceptives.[3] Ortho Evra has gotten much negative publicity in recent months in regards to the risk of blood clots.[4] In spite of this, it remains a popular choice in the adolescent age group. It offers another good choice, especially in teens who commonly are noncompliant with other methods such as the pill.

E. A. Iglesias, MD

References

1. Audet MC, Moreau M, Koltun WD, et al: Evaluation of contraceptive efficacy and cycle control of a transdermal contraceptive patch vs an oral contraceptive: A randomized control trial. *JAMA* 285:2347-2354, 2001.
2. Smallwood GH, Meador ML, Lenihan JP, et al: Efficacy and safety of a transdermal contraceptive system. *Obstet Gynecol* 98:799-805, 2001.
3. Sibai BM, Odlind V, Meador ML, et al: A comparative and pooled analysis of the safety and tolerability of the contraceptive patch (Ortho Evra/Evra). *Fertil Steril* 77:S19-S26, 2002.
4. World Briefly, *Associated Press*, July 17, 2005.

Change in Bone Mineral Density Among Adolescent Women Using and Discontinuing Depot Medroxyprogesterone Acetate Contraception

Scholes D, LaCroix AZ, Ichikawa LE, et al (Group Health Cooperative, Seattle; Univ of Washington, Seattle; Fred Hutchinson Cancer Resarch Ctr, Seattle; et al)

Arch Pediatr Adolesc Med 159:139-144, 2005   22–9

Background.—Several studies report an association between depot medroxyprogesterone acetate (DMPA) injectable contraception and decreased bone mineral density. Adolescents, who are still gaining bone, may be particularly affected, but there has been little study of the association in adolescent users and none following discontinuation.

Objective.—To evaluate bone mineral density changes in adolescents using and discontinuing use of DMPA contraception.

Design.—A population-based prospective cohort study.

Participants.—One hundred seventy adolescent women, aged 14 to 18 years; 80 baseline DMPA users and 90 age-similar, unexposed comparison women. Sixty-one participants discontinued DMPA use during follow-up.

Main Outcome Measure.—Bone mineral density, measured every 6 months for 24 to 36 months at the hip, spine, and whole body, comparing mean bone mineral density changes in DMPA users and discontinuers with nonusers.

Results.—Among DMPA users, bone mineral density declined significantly relative to nonusers at the hip and spine but not the whole body. Annualized mean percentage changes, adjusted for covariates, were hip, −1.81% vs −0.19%, *P* < .001; spine, −0.97% vs 1.32%, *P* < .001; and whole body, 0.73% vs 0.88%, *P* = .78 for DMPA users vs nonusers, respectively. New users lost bone mineral density more rapidly than prevalent users. Discontinuers experienced significantly increased bone mineral density relative to nonusers at all anatomical sites; annualized mean percentage changes were hip, 1.34% vs −0.19%, *P* = .004; spine, 2.86% vs 1.32%, *P* = .004; and whole body, 3.56% vs 0.88%, *P* < .001.

Conclusions.—Use of DMPA contraception in adolescents was associated with significant continuous losses of bone mineral density at the hip and spine. However, significant gains postdiscontinuation provide evidence that the loss of bone mass is apparently reversed.

▶ This study looked at the effects of DMPA contraceptive injection on bone mineral density (BMD) in adolescents compared with nonusers, and the effects on BMD upon discontinuation of DMPA. One hundred seventy women participated in this 3-year prospective study; 80 subjects were in the baseline DMPA group and 90 in the nonuser group. Sixty-one subjects discontinued DMPA use.

The age range of the subjects was 14 to 18 years. BMD was measured at baseline and then every 6 months for 24 to 36 months. Ninety percent of the subjects completed up to 6 months, decreasing to 78% by 24 months. There were 77 participants left at 36 months. A decline in BMD was found in the spine and hip of DMPA users, but not the whole-body BMD. Results were reported as mean percent change over the year. The percent change in BMD from baseline differed in the hip and spine in DMPA users versus nonusers. Hip BMD was −1.81% in DMPA users and −0.19% in nonusers (*P* < .001), whereas spine BMD was −0.97% in users versus 1.32% in nonusers (*P* < .001). The changes were greater comparing the new users versus those who had been on DMPA for a while. Whole-body BMD was 0.73% in DMPA users versus 0.88% in nonusers (*P* = 0.78). Subjects who discontinued DMPA showed improvement in BMD as compared with nonusers on all sites that were measured: hip, 1.34% versus −0.19% (*P* = .004); spine, 2.86% versus 1.32% (*P* = .004); and whole body, 3.56% versus 0.88% (*P* < .001).

Many studies have shown the link between DMPA use and loss of BMD.[1,2] This is one of the first studies done that shows the reversibility of DMPA-related bone loss in the adolescent age group. This gives practitioners some reassurance, but still leaves open the question of prolonged use and whether BMD will ever reach its maximum potential had no exposure occurred at all. Continued use with caution is therefore warranted in this age group. Risks and benefits still need to be weighed in regard to pregnancy prevention as well as the other noncontraceptive benefits of DMPA use.

E. A. Iglesias, MD

References

1. Comer BA, Stager M, Bonny A, et al: Depot medroxyprogesterone acetate, oral contraceptives and bone mineral density in a cohort of adolescent girls. *J Adolesc Health* 35:434-441, 2004.
2. Lara-Torre E, Edwards CP, Perlman S, et al: Bone mineral density in adolescent females using depot medroxyprogesterone acetate. *J Pediatr Adolesc Gynecol* 17:17-21, 2004.

Depot Medroxyprogesterone Acetate, Oral Contraceptives and Bone Mineral Density in a Cohort of Adolescent Girls
Cromer BA, Stager M, Bonney A, et al (MetroHealth Med Ctr, Cleveland, Ohio; Rainbow Babies & Children's Hosp, Cleveland, Ohio; The Children's Hosp at the Cleveland Clinic, Ohio; et al)
J Adolesc Health 35:434-441, 2004   22–10

Purpose.—To conduct a longitudinal comparison of bone mineral density (BMD) in 370 adolescent girls, aged 12-18, who self-selected depot medroxyprogesterone acetate (DMPA) or an oral contraceptive (OC) containing 20 µg ethinyl estradiol/100 µg levonorgestrel with that in girls who received no hormonal treatment (control group).

Methods.—Lumbar spine and femoral neck BMD measurements were obtained by dual energy x-ray absorptiometry at baseline and 12 months. Data were analyzed with repeated measures analysis of covariance methods.

Results.—Over 12 months, lumbar spine BMD decreased in the DMPA group (n = 29), with a mean percent change of -1.4% (95% confidence interval [CI] -2.73, -0.10), and increased by a mean of 3.8% (95% CI 3.11, 4.57) in the control group [n = 107 ($p < .001$)]. The increase in mean percent change in lumbar spine BMD in the OC group (n = 79), 2.3% (95% CI 1.49, 3.18), was significantly smaller than in the control group ($p = .03$). Over 12 months, the mean percent change in femoral neck BMD was -2.2% (95% CI -3.95, -0.39) in the DMPA group, but increased 2.3% (95% CI 1.29, 3.27) in the control group ($p < .001$). The increase in mean percent change at the femoral neck in the OC group, 0.3% (95% CI -0.87, 1.41), was significantly lower than in the control group ($p = .03$).

Conclusions.—Our study contributes to an increasing body of knowledge indicating a negative impact of DMPA on bone health in young women. Additional findings suggest a potential adverse effect of an OC containing 20 µg ethinyl estradiol/100 µg levonorgestrel on bone health in adolescents.

▶ This study is a longitudinal study of 370 adolescent girls comparing the effects of DMPA injection, low-dose (20 µg ethinyl estradiol) OC pills (OCP), and no hormone on BMD. Femoral neck and lumbar spine BMD were measured by using dual energy x-ray absorptiometry at baseline, 6 months, and at 1-year follow-up. This study is designed to be a 2-year analysis. The 1-year interim findings are reported in this article.

The age of the subjects ranged from 12 to 18 years. Two hundred fifteen subjects completed up to the 12-month study visit. There were 29 subjects in the DMPA group, 79 in the OCP group, and 107 in the no-hormone group. BMD in the lumbar spine and the femoral neck decreased in the DMPA group versus the OCP group and the no-hormone group, which both had an increase in BMD. This was reported as mean percent change over the year. The mean percent change in the lumbar spine BMD was −1.4% in the DMPA group compared with an increase in the control group of 3.8% ($P < .001$). The increase in percent change in lumbar spine BMD in the OCP group was smaller than in the control group (2.3%, $P = .03$). As far as femoral neck BMD, the mean percent change was −2.2% in the DMPA group and 2.3% in the controls ($P < .001$). The mean percent change in femoral neck BMD in the OCP group was only 0.3%, lower than in controls ($P = .03$).

This study is adding to a growing body of knowledge pertaining to the effects of progestin-only methods of contraception on BMD.[1-3] This is especially important in the adolescent years when attaining optimal BMD is critical. Patients choosing progestin-only methods should be counseled on risks and advised on dietary changes and calcium supplementation. BMD studies should be conducted on long-term users and on patients having a significant family history of osteopenia/osteoporosis. Comparing OCP use in this study adds to the evidence of the detrimental effects of low-dose estrogen pills on attaining peak bone mineral acquisition during these critical adolescent years.[2] The reversibility of these detrimental effects are currently being evaluated. Determining this information may be critical to preventing the future morbidity of osteopenia and osteoporosis in these patients; however, these findings have *not* been associated with adverse events in users of DMPA.

E. A. Iglesias, MD

References

1. Scholes D, La Croix AZ, Ichikawa LE, et al: The association between depot medroxyprogesterone acetate contraception and bone mineral density in adolescent women. *Contraception* 69:99-104, 2004.
2. Rome E, Ziegler J, Secic M, et al: Bone biochemical markers in adolescent girls using either depot medroxyprogesterone acetate or an oral contraceptive. *J Pediatr Adolesc Gynecol* 17:373-377, 2004.
3. Lara-Torre E, Edwards CP, Perlman S, et al: Bone mineral density in adolescent females using depot medroxyprogesterone acetate. *J Pediatr Adolesc Gynecol* 17:17-21, 2004.

23 Sexuality

Sexual Functioning After Total Compared With Supracervical Hysterectomy: A Randomized Trial
Kuppermann M, for the Total or Supracervical Hysterectomy (TOSH) Research Group (Univ of California, San Francisco; et al)
Obstet Gynecol 105:1309-1318, 2005   23–1

Objective.—To compare sexual functioning and health-related quality-of-life outcomes of total abdominal hysterectomy (TAH) and supracervical hysterectomy (SCH) among women with symptomatic uterine leiomyomata or abnormal uterine bleeding refractory to hormonal management.

Methods.—We randomly assigned 135 women scheduled to undergo abdominal hysterectomy in 4 U.S. clinical centers to either a total or supracervical procedure. The primary outcome was sexual functioning at 2 years, as assessed by the Medical Outcomes Study Sexual Problems Scale. Secondary outcomes included specific aspects of sexual functioning and health-related quality-of-life at 6 months and 2 years.

Results.—Sexual problems improved dramatically in both randomized groups during the first 6 months and plateaued by 1 year. Health-related quality-of-life scores also improved in both groups. At 2 years, both groups reported few problems with sexual functioning (mean score on the Sexual Problems Scale for SCH group 82, TAH group 80, on a 0-to-100 scale with 100 indicating an absence of problems; difference = +2, 95% confidence interval −8 to +11), and there were no significant differences between groups.

Conclusion.—Supracervical and total abdominal hysterectomy result in similar sexual functioning and health-related quality of life during 2 years of follow-up. This information can help guide physicians as they discuss surgical options with their patients.

▶ Hysterectomy is the most common nonobstetric major surgical procedure performed in the United States.[1] Although most are TAH procedures, early anecdotal reports have suggested that SCH procedures retaining the cervix may preserve sexual function.[2,3]

The TOSH study was a multicenter, randomized trial comparing the effectiveness of TAH and SCH in women scheduled to undergo abdominal hysterectomy for symptomatic uterine leiomyomata or abnormal uterine bleeding.[4]

This report focused on sexual functioning and quality-of-life outcomes during 2 years of follow-up.

The authors found no significant differences between the SCH and TAH groups on any of the outcome measures 2 years after hysterectomy. However, the SCH group showed significantly more improvement on the Medical Outcomes Study sexual problems scale at 6 months and some differences at 1-year posthysterectomy. This finding is significant since the Medical Outcomes Study was the primary outcome variable and the only validated instrument used. The authors attributed this finding to either baseline differences between the 2 groups in sexual functioning or a more rapid recovery after SCH.

Neither patients nor physicians were blinded to the procedure. Patients were not blinded because of the need for continued cervical screening in the SCH group. However, it seems reasonable that a blinded physician, not performing the surgery, could have evaluated patient response.

The authors conclude that there is no difference in sexual functioning or quality of life after SCH compared with TAH. While this conclusion is valid at 2 years, it cannot be stated for earlier periods. These preliminary results are helpful, but more longitudinal data are necessary for physicians and patients to make educated decisions on the best type of hysterectomy to maintain sexual function.

C. S. Brown, PharmD

References

1. DeFrances DJ, Hall MJ: 2002 National Hospital Discharge Survey. *Adv Data* 1-29, 2004.
2. Kilkku P, Gronroos M, Hirvonen T, et al: Supravaginal uterine amputation vs. hysterectomy: Effects on libido and orgasm. *Acta Obstet Gynecol Scand* 62:147-152, 1983.
3. Zussman L, Zussman S, Sunley R, et al: Sexual response after hysterectomy-oophorectomy: Recent studies and reconsideration of psychogenesis. *Am J Obstet Gynecol* 140:725-729, 1981.
4. Learman LA, Summitt RJ, Varner RE, et al: A randomized comparison of total or supracervical hysterectomy: Surgical complications and clinical outcomes. *Obstet Gynecol* 102:453-462, 2003.

▶ With the availability of effective cervical screening and the anecdotal reports of improved sexual functioning with cervical preservation at hysterectomy, much interest has been generated in subtotal hysterectomy.[1] This study agrees with similar randomized studies from Great Britain and Denmark that showed no difference in sexual functioning at 12 months.[2,3] The reviewed study excluded postmenopausal women and followed patients past 24 months. Additionally, the reviewed study showed sexual functioning improved dramatically in both groups after hysterectomy, suggesting a degree of sexual dysfunction related to the original indication for the hysterectomy. The data presented should provide physicians and patients additional reassurance that sexual function does not have to suffer if hysterectomy is performed and may be improved regardless of whether the cervix is retained or not.

G. H. Lipscomb, MD

References

1. Kilkku P, Gronroos M, Hirvonen T, et al: Supravaginal uterine amputation vs. hysterectomy: Effects on libido and orgasm. *Acta Obstet Gynecol Scand* 62:147-152, 1983.
2. Thakar R, Ayers S, Clarkson P, et al: Outcomes after total versus subtotal abdominal hysterectomy. *N Engl J Med* 347:1318-1325, 2002.
3. Gimbel H, Zobbe V, Andersen BM, et al: Randomised controlled trial of total compared with subtotal hysterectomy with one-year follow up results. *Br J Obstet Gynaecol* 110:1088-1098, 2003.

The Relative Effects of Hormones and Relationship Factors on Sexual Function of Women Through the Natural Menopausal Transition

Dennerstein L, Lehert P, Burger H (Univ of Melbourne, Parkville, Australia; Univ of Mons, Belgium; Monash Med Ctr, Clayton, Australia)
Fertil Steril 84:174-180, 2005   23–2

Objective.—To investigate the relative effects of hormonal and relationship factors on female sexual function during the natural menopausal transition.

Design.—Prospective population-based questionnaire study.

Setting.—Interviews were conducted in the patients' homes.

Patient(s).—Four hundred thirty-eight Australian-born women aged 45–55 years who were still menstruating at baseline. Eight years of longitudinal data were available for 336 of these women, none of whom were hysterectomized.

Intervention(s).—Hormonal levels, age, menopausal status, partner status, and feelings for partner were measured and evaluated with longitudinal structural equation modeling.

Main Outcome Measure(s).—Short personal experiences questionnaire.

Result(s).—Sexual response was predicted by prior level of sexual function, change in partner status, feelings for partner, and E_2 level ($R^2 = .65$); dyspareunia was predicted by prior level of dyspareunia and E_2 level ($R^2 = .53$); and frequency of sexual activities was predicted by prior level of sexual function, change in partner status, feelings for partner, and level of sexual response ($R^2 = .52$). The minimum effective dose needed to increase sexual response by 10% (700 pmol/L E_2) is twice that needed to decrease dyspareunia.

Conclusion(s).—Prior function and relationship factors are more important than hormonal determinants of sexual function of women in midlife.

▶ Women's sexual function is thought to be more dependent on psychosocial and relationship factors than that of men. This study investigated the relative effects of hormonal and relationship factors on female sexual function during the natural menopausal transition.

The investigators found that prior functioning and relationship factors were more important than hormonal determinants of sexual function of women in midlife. The level of E_2 needed to produce a minimal clinically relevant difference on sexual response was twice that needed to improve dyspareunia. This suggests that the low doses of estrogen currently advocated in hormone therapy would not be effective in sustaining women's sexual function. Testosterone measures did not have a significant effect on sexual domains, possibly because of the insensitivity of testosterone assays to measure the lower end of the normal female range reliably.

Strengths of the study include use of a large community-based sample; use of reliable, validated measures; and the length of the study period. Limitations include only once-yearly measurements of hormones and the attrition rate. By the end of the 8 years of follow-up, only 49% of the eligible study participants at baseline continued in the study.

This study points out the need to obtain information on the nonmedical aspects of sexual function when interviewing women. In light of the current use of low-dose hormone therapy, it is important to understand that these doses will effectively treat dyspareunia from vaginal atrophy but probably will not increase sexual response.

C. S. Brown, MSN, PharmD

Correlates of Circulating Androgens in Mid-Life Women: The Study of Women's Health Across the Nation
Santoro N, Torrens J, Crawford S, et al (Albert Einstein College of Medicine, Bronx, New York; Massachusetts Gen Hosp, Boston; Rush Univ, Chicago; et al)
J Clin Endocrinol Metab 90:4836-4845, 2005   23–3

Context.—Androgens influence sexual differentiation and behavior, body composition, and physical functioning in men, but their role in women is less well understood. Because circulating androgens decline with age, the use of androgen supplementation for women to improve health and well-being has been increasing.

Objective.—The aim of this study was to assess the association between androgens and a variety of end points thought to be affected by androgens.

Design.—In a community-based baseline cohort of women aged 42–52 yr from the Study of Women's Health Across the Nation, we measured circulating testosterone (T), dehydroepiandrosterone sulfate, and SHBG, and calculated a free androgen index (FAI) in 2961 women.

Main Outcome Measures.—Correlations of androgen measures with each other and with body mass index, waist circumference, and waist-hip ratio were computed, and odds ratios (OR) were estimated for the categorical outcomes of functional limitations, functional status, self-reported health, scores indicative of depressed mood, quality of life, sexual desire and arousal, and the presence of the metabolic syndrome.

Results.—Androgens, and particularly SHBG, were associated most strongly with body mass index, waist circumference, and waist-hip ratio. SHBG was associated prominently inversely with the metabolic syndrome

TABLE 5.—Associations of Log-Transformed Hormones With Indicators of Well-Being, Libido, and Presence of the Metabolic Syndrome Computed Comparing 75th Percentile of Log-Transformed Hormone With 25th Percentile of Log-Transformed Hormone, Adjusted for Log Waist Circumference, Ethnicity, Site, Age, and Smoking

	T	DHEAS	SHBG	FAI	E2	n
	OR (95% CI)					
Higher physical functioning	1.11 (0.97, 1.28)	1.21 (1.06, 1.39)[a]	0.90 (0.78, 1.05)	1.17 (1.00, 1.38)	1.00 (0.87, 1.15)	2812
Higher quality of life	1.01 (0.93, 1.11)	1.02 (0.93, 1.11)	0.93 (0.84, 1.02)	1.07 (0.97, 1.18)	1.00 (0.92, 1.10)	2787
Better self-reported health	1.17 (1.08, 1.28)[b]	1.26 (1.15, 1.39)[c]	0.93 (0.85, 1.02)	1.19 (1.08, 1.30)[b]	0.95 (0.87, 1.04)	2881
CES-D depressive symptomatology	0.88 (0.79, 0.99)[d]	0.95 (0.85, 1.06)	1.11 (0.98, 1.25)	0.84 (0.74, 0.95)[a]	1.05 (0.94, 1.18)	2881
Higher desire	1.06 (0.98, 1.16)	1.04 (0.96, 1.14)	0.93 (0.85, 1.02)	1.11 (1.091, 1.22)[d]	1.04 (0.95, 1.13)	2846
Higher arousal[e]	1.04 (0.95, 1.14)	1.04 (0.95, 1.15)	0.89 (0.80, 0.98)[d]	1.12 (1.01, 1.25)[d]	0.92 (0.83, 1.02)	2255
Metabolic syndrome[g]	1.30 (1.15, 1.48)[c]	0.86 (0.76, 0.98)[d]	0.30 (0.24, 0.37)[c,f]	2.61 (2.17, 3.13)[c,f]	0.67 (0.58, 0.77)[c,f]	2828

[a] $P < 0.01$.
[b] $P < 0.001$.
[c] $P < 0.0001$.
[d] $P < 0.05$.
[e] Sexually active participants only.
[f] Model includes quadratic term in log hormone.
[g] Not adjusted for log BMI, since BMI is highly correlated with waist, which is part of the definition of metabolic syndrome.
(Courtesy of Santoro N, Torrens J, Crawford S, et al: Correlates of circulating androgens in mid-life women: The study of women's health across the nation. J Clin Endocrinol Metab 90:4836-4845, 2005, copyright The Endocrine Society.)

(OR = 0.32; 95% confidence interval = 0.26–0.39), which was present in 17% of women at baseline. Dehydroepiandrosterone sulfate was associated modestly with functional status and self-reported health. T was associated minimally with increased sexual desire (OR = 1.09; 95% confidence interval = 1.00–1.18). The association of FAI with self-reported health and depressive symptomatology based on the Center for Epidemiologic Studies Depression Scale score was explained more by T than by SHBG, whereas the association of FAI with sexual arousal and metabolic syndrome was due more to SHBG than to T.

Conclusions.—Circulating SHBG and androgens are most strongly associated with physical characteristics and the metabolic syndrome in women in this community-based cohort. Androgens are related weakly to physical functioning and other symptoms to which they commonly are attributed, such as sexual desire, sexual arousal, and well-being (Table 5).

▶ The impact of androgens on the quality of life of menopausal women continues to cause controversy in clinical and research circles. This multicenter trial measured several androgen-related analytes and indexes in correlation with a variety of epidemiologic and demographic characteristics of the studied cohort. The authors found that circulating androgens and SHBG were most strongly associated with physical characteristics and metabolic syndrome and were only weakly associated with physical functioning and classic androgen-related symptoms such as sexual desire and arousal. Although this is a study of surrogate markers and was not powered to assess clinical outcomes with androgen therapies directly, this study may serve to clarify the actual role of androgens in menopause management as current literature provides little strong scientific evidence concerning the role of androgens in menopausal therapies.

L. P. Shulman, MD

Circulating Androgen Levels and Self-reported Sexual Function in Women

Davis SR, Davison SL, Donath S, et al (Monash Med School, Victoria, Australia; Jean Hailes Found, Victoria, Australia; Monash Univ, Victoria, Australia; et al)
JAMA 294:91-96, 2005   23–4

Context.—It has been proposed that low sexual desire and sexual dysfunction are associated with low blood testosterone levels in women. However, evidence to support this is lacking.

Objective.—To determine whether women with low self-reported sexual desire and sexual satisfaction are more likely to have low serum androgen levels than women without self-reported low sexual desire and sexual satisfaction.

Design, Setting, and Participants.—A community-based, cross-sectional study of 1423 women aged 18 to 75 years, who were randomly recruited via the electoral roll in Victoria, Australia, from April 2002 to August 2003.

Women were excluded from the analysis if they took psychiatric medication, had abnormal thyroid function, documented polycystic ovarian syndrome, or were younger than 45 years and using oral contraception.

Main Outcome Measures.—Domain scores of the Profile of Female Sexual Function (PFSF) and serum levels of total and free testosterone, androstenedione, and dehydroepiandrosterone sulfate.

Results.—A total of 1021 individuals were included in the final analysis. No clinically significant relationships between having a low score for any PFSF domain and having a low serum total or free testosterone or androstenedione level was demonstrated. A low domain score for sexual responsiveness for women aged 45 years or older was associated with higher odds of having a serum dehydroepiandrosterone sulfate level below the 10th percentile for this age group (odds ratio [OR], 3.90; 95% confidence interval [CI], 1.54-9.81; P=.004). For women aged 18 to 44 years, having a low domain score for sexual desire (OR, 3.86; 95% CI, 1.27-11.67; P=.02), sexual arousal (OR, 6.39; 95% CI, 2.30-17.73; P<.001), and sexual responsiveness (OR, 6.59; 95% CI, 2.37-18.34; P<.001) was associated with having a dehydroepiandrosterone sulfate level below the 10th percentile.

Conclusions.—No single androgen level is predictive of low female sexual function, and the majority of women with low dehydroepiandrosterone sulfate levels did not have low sexual function.

► Sexual dysfunction occurs in 43% of women, and low sexual desire is the most prevalent sexual problem.[1] It has been associated with increasing age and oophorectomy. The Princeton Consensus group formulated the "female androgen insufficiency" syndrome characterized by a constellation of symptoms and a low free testosterone level.[2] Therapeutic trials with testosterone have demonstrated improved libido in women. The Davis et al study tried to determine whether women with low sexual desire were more likely to have low serum androgen levels than women without low sexual desire.

Strengths of this study included the use of a validated instrument that was designed for use in women with low sexual desire, use of sensitive radioimmunoassays for measuring androgens, and use of a community-based population of women.

Major weaknesses were observed in subject selection. Only 9.1% of women identified eventually participated, introducing possible selection bias. There was lack of clarity on how subjects were defined as "low sexual function" versus "not low sexual function," and women were not screened for quality of relationship with their sex partners. Since relationship factors have been shown to be more important than hormonal determinants of sexual function in women,[3] this is a significant confounding variable.

The authors concluded that androgen levels are not informative and should not be used for the purpose of diagnosing androgen insufficiency in women. The danger in this conclusion is that it may lead clinicians to not measure hormones when working up a sexual dysfunction patient. Consequently, treatment may be initiated when androgen levels are normal or high, increasing the risk of side effects as well as possible nonresponse.

C. S. Brown, MSN, PharmD

References

1. Laumann E, Paik A, Rosen RC: Sexual dysfunction in the United States: Prevalence and predictors. *JAMA* 281:537-544, 1999.
2. Bachmann G, Bancroft J, Braunstein G, et al: Female androgen insufficiency: The Princeton consensus statement on definition, classification, and assessment. *Fertil Steril* 77:660-665, 2002.
3. Dennerstein L, Lehert P, Burger H: The relative effects of hormones and relationship factors on sexual function in women through the natural menopausal transition. *Fertil Steril* 84:174-180, 2005.

Testosterone Patch for Low Sexual Desire in Surgically Menopausal Women: A Randomized Trial

Buster JE, Kingsberg SA, Aguirre O, et al (Baylor College of Medicine, Houston; Case Western Reserve Univ, Cleveland, Ohio; Colorado Gynecology & Continence Ctr, Denver; et al)
Obstet Gynecol 105:944-952, 2005   23–5

Objective.—To assess the efficacy and safety of a 300 µg/d testosterone patch for the treatment of hypoactive sexual desire disorder in surgically menopausal women on concomitant estrogen therapy.

Methods.—Five hundred thirty-three women with hypoactive sexual desire disorder who had undergone previous hysterectomy and bilateral oophorectomy were enrolled in a 24-week, multicenter, double-blind, placebo-controlled trial. Patients were randomly assigned to receive placebo or the testosterone patch twice weekly. The primary efficacy endpoint was change from baseline at week 24 in the frequency of total satisfying sexual activity, measured by the Sexual Activity Log. Secondary measures included sexual desire using the Profile of Female Sexual Function and personal distress as measured by the Personal Distress Scale. Hormone levels, adverse events, and clinical laboratory measures were reviewed.

Results.—Total satisfying sexual activity significantly improved in the testosterone patch group compared with placebo after 24 weeks (mean change from baseline, 1.56 compared with 0.73 episodes per 4 weeks, $P = .001$). Treatment with the testosterone patch also significantly improved sexual desire (mean change, 10.57 compared with 4.29, $P < .001$) and decreased personal distress ($P = .009$). Serum free, total, and bioavailable testosterone concentrations increased from baseline. Overall, adverse events were similar in both groups ($P > .05$). The incidence of androgenic adverse events was higher in the testosterone group; most androgenic adverse events were mild.

Conclusion.—In surgically menopausal women with hypoactive sexual desire disorder, a 300 µg/d testosterone patch significantly increased satisfying sexual activity and sexual desire, while decreasing personal distress, and was well tolerated through up to 24 weeks of use.

► Hypoactive sexual desire disorder (HSDD), or loss of libido associated with distress, is one of the 4 types of female sexual dysfunction recognized by the

Diagnostic and Statistical Manual of Mental Disorders, 4th edition.[1] The International Consensus Development Conference on Females Sexual Dysfunction defined hypoactive sexual desire disorder as the persistent deficiency (or absence) of sexual fantasies or thoughts or desire for or receptivity to sexual activity, which results in personal distress.[2]

Studies involving oral, intramuscular, and subcutaneous implants have demonstrated significant improvements in sexual desire in postmenopausal women. However, injections and implants produce variable and often supraphysiologic doses, and oral preparations can lead to decreased levels of high-density lipoprotein cholesterol from the first-pass effect through the liver. Testosterone patches are currently in development to reduce these types of side effects.

The current study was designed to determine the efficacy and safety of testosterone patches for the treatment of HSDD in surgically menopausal women receiving estrogen treatment. The authors found that testosterone patches were significantly more effective than placebo in increasing the frequency of satisfying sexual activity and desire and decreasing distress and was well tolerated.

Strengths of the multicenter study included a large sample size, inclusion of women who were in stable relationships and were distressed over their condition, and well-validated instruments designed to measure changes in libido and distress.

Nevertheless, it is unclear how to evaluate the findings. Although there was a statistically significant increase in the number of satisfying sexual experiences per 4 weeks in women receiving active drug versus placebo (1.5 vs 0.75), one wonders if this is clinically significant. However, there were also statistically significant differences in all other end points, including desire and distress associated with HSDD, strengthening the conclusions.

Because the study was limited to 24 weeks, it cannot address the safety of use beyond this duration. The Food and Drug Administration Reproductive Advisory Committee unanimously recommended against approval of the testosterone patch in 2004, mainly because of inadequate data on longer term safety.[3] The committee was clearly influenced by the results of the Women's Health Initiative and cautioned against the long-term use of hormonal agents without better data on safety risks, requiring long-term studies.

Use of the testosterone patch should be evaluated like any other medication that has potential benefits and risks, assessing the risk-benefit ratio in each patient. It is important to keep in mind that the authors evaluated a fairly narrow population of women, and that these results should not be applied to other groups such as premenopausal women, naturally menopausal women, or postmenopausal women not receiving estrogen.

C. S. Brown, MSN, PharmD

References

1. American Psychiatric Association: *Diagnostic and Statistical Manual of Mental Disorders*, ed 4. Washington, DC, 2000, American Psychiatric Association.

2. Basson R, Berman J, Burnett A, et al: Report of the international consensus development conference on female sexual dysfunction: Definitions and classifications. *J Urol* 163:888-893, 2000.
3. U.S. Food and Drug Administration: Transcript of Advisory Committee for Reproductive Health Drugs, December 2, 2004. Available at: http://www.fda.gov/ohrms/dockets/ac/cder04.html#ReproductiveHealthDrugs. Accessed February 25, 2005.

Sexual Activity and Function in Postmenopausal Women With Heart Disease

Addis IB, Ireland CC, Vittinghoff E, et al (Univ of Arizona, Tucson; Univ of California, San Francisco; Univ of California, San Diego)

Obstet Gynecol 106:121-127, 2005   23–6

Objective.—To examine the prevalence and correlates of sexual activity and function in postmenopausal women with heart disease.

Methods.—We included baseline self-reported measures of sexual activity and the sexual problem scale from the Medical Outcomes Study in the Heart and Estrogen/Progestin Replacement Study (HERS), a study of 2,763 postmenopausal women, average age 67 years, with coronary disease and intact uteri. We used multivariable linear and logistic regression to identify independent correlates of sexual activity and dysfunction.

Results.—Approximately 39% of the women in HERS were sexually active, and 65% of these reported at least 1 of 5 sexual problems (lack of interest, inability to relax, difficulty in arousal or in orgasm, and discomfort with sex). In multivariable analysis, factors independently associated with being sexually active included younger age, fewer years since menopause, being married, better self-reported health, higher parity, moderate alcohol use, not smoking, lack of chest discomfort, and not being depressed. Among the 1,091 women who were sexually active, lower sexual problem scores were associated with being unmarried, being better educated, having better self-reported health, and having higher body mass index.

Conclusion.—Many women with heart disease continue to engage in sexual activity into their 70s, and two thirds of these report discomfort and other sexual function problems. Physicians should be aware that postmenopausal patients are sexually active and address the problems these women experience.

▶ Menopausal status has been associated with diminished sexual activity. Two common problems are decreased sexual desire and dyspareunia. Prevalence of sexual dysfunction in postmenopausal women varies from 68% to 87% and is generally attributed to the decline in estrogen and testosterone levels.

The authors analyzed data from a cohort of postmenopausal women with coronary heart disease enrolled in HERS.[1] Women who were surgically menopausal, were receiving hormone therapy, or who had a myocardial infarction or a coronary revascularization procedure in the previous 6 months were excluded.

The authors found that in this cohort of postmenopausal women with heart disease, many continue to engage in sexual activity well into their 70s. Two thirds of those reporting sexual activity reported sexual problems, a rate that is similar to that reported by younger populations. Significant correlates for sexual dysfunction included body mass index greater than 30, poor health, depression, and being married.

Strengths of the study include use of a large community sample and a validated instrument to measure sexual dysfunction. Limitations include the inability to generalize the findings to the general population of postmenopausal women, as the cohort had an average age of 67 years, had diagnosed heart disease, and was 87% white. Nevertheless, these findings suggest that physicians should ask about sexual concerns of all postmenopausal women, including those with chronic health conditions.

C. S. Brown, MSN, PharmD

Reference

1. Grady D, Applegate W, Bush T, et al: Replacement study (HERS): Design, methods, and baseline characteristics. *Control Clin Trials* 19:314-335, 1998.

Evaluation of the Role of Pudendal Nerve Integrity in Female Sexual Function Using Noninvasive Techniques
Connell K, Guess MK, La Combe J, et al (Albert Einstein College of Medicine, Bronx, NY)
Am J Obstet Gynecol 192:1712-1717, 2005   23–7

Objective.—Using quantitative sensory testing and a validated questionnaire, we investigated the role of pudendal nerve integrity in sexual function among women.

Study Design.—Participants completed the Pelvic Organ Prolapse/Urinary Incontinence Sexual Questionnaire (PISQ). Vibratory and pressure thresholds were measured at the S2 dermatome reflecting pudendal nerve distribution.

Results.—A total of 56 women enrolled; 29 (51.8%) were asymptomatic and 27 (48.2%) had 1 or more forms of female sexual dysfunction (total sexual dysfunction) including: desire disorder 16.1%, arousal disorder 26.8%, orgasmic disorder 25%, and pain disorder 12.5%. Age, parity, menopausal status, and body mass index were similar between groups. PISQ scores were lower in symptomatic subjects compared with controls ($P <$ .001). Decreased tactile sensation was found at the clitoris for women with total sexual dysfunction, desire disorder, and arousal disorder. Women with arousal disorder also had decreased tactile sensation at the perineum.

Conclusion.—Pudendal nerve integrity may play a role in female sexual dysfunction.

▶ This study raises interesting questions and provides insight as to why most of our remedies for female sexual dysfunction have limited success. The obvious question raised is how did the pudendal nerve injury occur, and could it be related to previous birth trauma? Unfortunately there was no analysis in this report of parity or route of delivery. The results also have to be reviewed as very preliminary in that, interestingly, the deficit was in tactile sensation but not in vibratory sensation. But this may account for why some patients can achieve orgasm with vibrating devices but not through more nonmechanical means.

D. S. Miller, MD

Brain Activation During Vaginocervical Self-stimulation and Orgasm in Women With Complete Spinal Cord Injury: fMRI Evidence of Mediation by the Vagus Nerves
Komisaruk BR, Whipple B, Crawford A, et al (State Univ of New Jersey, Newark; Univ of Medicine and Dentistry of New Jersey, Newark)
Brain Res 1024:77-88, 2004   23–8

Abstract.—Women diagnosed with complete spinal cord injury (SCI) at T10 or above report vaginal-cervical perceptual awareness. To test whether the Vagus nerves, which bypass the spinal cord, provide the afferent pathway for this response, we hypothesized that the Nucleus Tractus Solitarii (NTS) region of the medulla oblongata, to which the Vagus nerves project, is activated by vaginal-cervical self-stimulation (CSS) in such women, as visualized by functional magnetic resonance imaging (fMRI). Regional blood oxygen level-dependent (BOLD) signal intensity was imaged during CSS and other motor and sensory procedures, using statistical parametric mapping (SPM) analysis with head motion artifact correction. Physiatric examination and MRI established the location and extent of spinal cord injury. In order to demarcate the NTS, a gustatory stimulus and hand movement were used to activate the superior region of the NTS and the Nucleus Cuneatus adjacent to the inferior region of the NTS, respectively. Each of four women with interruption, or "complete" injury, of the spinal cord (ASIA criteria), and one woman with significant, but "incomplete" SCI, all at or above T10, showed activation of the inferior region of the NTS during CSS. Each woman showed analgesia, measured at the fingers, during CSS, confirming previous findings. Three women experienced orgasm during the CSS. The brain regions that showed activation during the orgasms included hypothalamic paraventricular nucleus, medial amygdala, anterior cingulate, frontal, parietal, and insular cortices, and cerebellum. We conclude that the Vagus nerves provide a spinal cord-bypass pathway for vaginal-cervical sensibility in women with complete spinal cord injury above the level of entry into spinal cord of the known genitospinal nerves (Fig 8).

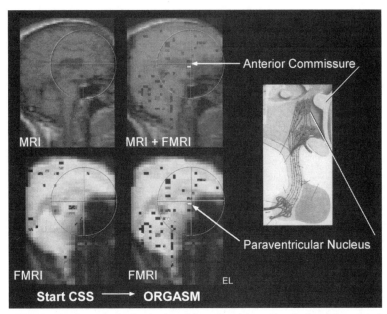

FIGURE 8.—Another example of activation of the region of the paraventricular nucleus of the hypothalamus at orgasm. This nucleus is localized in relation to the anterior commissure, as shown in the slightly modified schematic diagram of Netter [18]. The MRI (upper left) shows the midline sagittal anatomical view, the two lower images are "raw" fMRI images showing the activity during cervical self-stimulation (CSS) prior to orgasm (bottom left) and then at orgasm (bottom right). The fMRI activity at orgasm is superimposed on the anatomical MRI image (upper right). The crosshairs are situated at the anterior commissure. Note that the activated pixels (highlighted) are located slightly inferior and posterior to the anterior commissure. (Courtesy of Komisaruk BR, Whipple B, Crawford A, et al: Brain activation during vaginocervical self-stimulation and orgasm in women with complete spinal cord injury: fMRI evidence of mediation by the vagus nerves. *Brain Res* 1024:77-88. Copyright 2004 by Elsevier Science.)

▶ The sexual functioning of women with neurologic and spinal cord injuries is the subject of ongoing research. Unfortunately, little of this involves gynecologists. The authors showed that women with spinal interruption at T10 could perceive vaginal CSS that appeared to be mediated by the vagus nerve, and many experienced orgasm. While the mediation of gustatory satisfaction via the vagus nerve is well known to us in gynecology, its mediation of sexual satisfaction is less familiar to us. Nonetheless, this study serves as a reminder that the sexual challenges of patients with neurologic and spinal cord injury need to be addressed by gynecologists as they do in the intact patient.

D. S. Miller, MD

24 Contraception

Beyond the Pill: New Data and Options in Hormonal and Intrauterine Contraception
Kaunitz AM (Univ of Florida, Jacksonville)
Am J Obstet Gynecol 192:998-1004, 2005   24–1

Background.—The oral contraceptive was developed more than 40 years ago and is one of the best-studied medications. As of 2003, oral contraceptives are the reversible contraceptive most used by women in the United States. Although this form of contraception is highly effective for correct consistent users, inconsistent or incorrect use accounts for an annual failure rate of 8% in typical users. Thus, there is a need for hormonal and intrauterine contraceptives that do not require daily attention from the user. New approaches to hormonal and intrauterine contraception were outlined.

Overview.—New approaches to starting and taking oral contraceptives are being developed, as are new formulations to extend conventional oral contraceptive use from 3 weeks of hormonally active tablets followed by 1

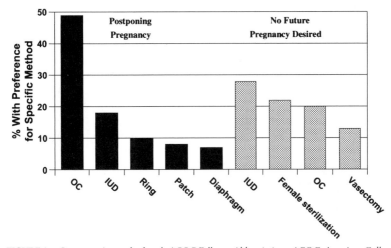

FIGURE 1.—Contraceptive use by female ACOG Fellows. *Abbreviations: ACOG,* American College of Obstetricians and Gynecologists; *OC,* oral contraceptive; *IUD,* intrauterine device. (From Kaunitz AM: Beyond the pill: New data and options in hormonal and intrauterine contraception. *Am J Obstet Gynecol* 192:998-1004. Copyright 2005 by Elsevier. Courtesy of American College of Obstetricians and Gynecologists: ACOG unveils survey of women ob-gyns at media briefing. *ACOG Today* 48:1,6, 2004. With permission.)

TABLE 5.—Indications for Methods Other Than Combined
(Estrogen-Progestin) Hormonal Contraception

In women with the following conditions, the use of progestin-only pills,
  DMPA, or a copper or levonorgestrel-releasing IUD may be safer
  then combination hormonal contraception:
Age >35 y and smoke cigarettes
Migraine headaches with vascular risk factors, vascular disease, or age
  >35 y
History of thromboembolic disease
Coronary artery disease
Cerebrovascular disease
Chronic liver disease
<2 weeks after delivery*
Hypertension with vascular disease or age >35 y
Diabetes mellitus with vascular disease or age >35 y
Systemic lupus erythematosus with vascular disease, nephritis, or
  antiphospholipid antibodies
Hypertriglyceridemia

*IUD insertion appropriate once uterine involution has occurred (approximately
6 weeks after delivery).
Abbreviations: DMPA, Depot medroxyprogesterone acetate; *IUD,* intrauterine
device.
(Courtesy of Kaunitz AM: Beyond the pill: New data and options in hormonal and
intrauterine contraception. *Am J Obstet Gynecol* 192:998-1004, 2005. Copyright
2005 by Elsevier. Reprinted by permission.)

placebo week to 12 weeks on followed by 1 week off. Injectable contraception (depot medroxyprogesterone acetate [DMPA]) was approved in 1992 and has been responsible for the declining rates of unintended pregnancies and abortions in the United States. However, there are concerns that the use of DMPA causes weight gain and an increased future risk of osteoporotic fractures, and these concerns continue to make some women reluctant to use this method of birth control despite its high effectiveness. Long-acting combination estrogen-progestin contraceptives have been approved in recent years, including a 1-week transdermal contraceptive patch and a contraceptive vaginal ring (Fig 1). Intrauterine devices (IUDs) can provide convenient, effective, reversible birth control. However, only 1% of the author's patients use IUDs. Much of the decline in IUD use is associated with concerns that they cause salpingitis and tubal infertility. Recent studies have shown that the risk of salpingitis associated with IUD use is small and is confined to the first month after insertion. The use of an IUD is not associated with a subsequent increased risk of tubal infertility. For most medical conditions, pregnancy is associated with more risks than the use of contraception (Table 5). Future contraceptives will include progestin-releasing contraceptive implants. It is hoped that an oral contraceptive–folic acid formulation will be available by 2010 to help reduce the incidence of neural tube defects, which are associated with inadequate intake of folic acid in pregnant women. Several approaches to effective, reversible hormonal contraception for men are under investigation.

Conclusions.—Birth control options have expanded well beyond the oral contraceptive pill. Clinicians who are knowledgeable about older contraceptive methods and new, longer-lasting contraceptives and emergency contraception can help their patients to minimize unintended pregnancy and induced abortion.

▶ In this clinical opinion, Dr Kaunitz provides an excellent overview of both new approaches to the pill and other nondaily options available to women today. As of 2003, the pill is the most common reversible method of contraception utilized by women,[1] but unfortunately discontinuations and typical use failure rates of up to 8%[2] contribute to unintended pregnancies. It is important for providers to have a good understanding of all the options available today, and to make sure they are offering all of these options to their patients—even women who have been using the pill for years.

Figure 1 graphically represents findings from a survey of American College of Obstetricians and Gynecologists (ACOG) fellows.[3] The difference between the 18% to 29% of these women and the 1% of the general public using intrauterine contraception[1] is staggering. Providers need to work to dispel myths and fears about these highly effective methods and emphasize the potential noncontraceptive benefits of these and all the hormonal methods currently available.

The article finishes by mentioning methods that will hopefully be available in the near future. Keeping current on contraceptive options and alerting patients of all options, including emergency contraception, is the only way that we are going to decrease the number of unintended pregnancies and abortions in the United States. Birth control is not a one-size-fits-all science, and providers need to allow women to determine what method fits best into their lifestyle to encourage successful contraception.

N. B. Zite, MD, MPH

References

1. Mosher W, Martinez GM, Chandra A, et al: Use of contraception and use of family planning services in the United States, 1982-2002. Advance data from *Vital and Health Statistics*, No 350. Hyattsville, Md, National Center for Health Statistics, 2004.
2. Tussel J: Contraceptive failure in the United States. *Contraception* 70:89-96, 2004.
3. ACOG unveils survey of women ob-gyns at media briefing. *ACOG Today* 48:1, 6, 2004.

Cost-Effectiveness and Contraceptive Effectiveness of the Transdermal Contraceptive Patch

Sonnenberg FA, Burkman RT, Speroff L, et al (Univ of Medicine and Dentistry of New Jersey, New Brunswick; Tufts Univ, Springfield, Mass; Oregon Health and Science Univ, Portland; et al)

Am J Obstet Gynecol 192:1-9, 2005   24–2

Objective.—The purpose of this study was to examine implications of increased perfect use on the cost-effectiveness of the contraceptive patch compared with combination oral contraceptives (COCs).

Study Design.—This study compared the patch with low-estrogen-dose COCs. It assumes that the risks of developing a medical condition during use are the same for both the patch and COCs. Differences in net cost and pregnancies avoided during use were modeled. With the use of a pharmacoeconomic model, both methods were compared with a hypothetical reference case of contraception nonuse. The base-case model considered women, ages

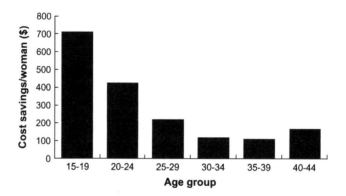

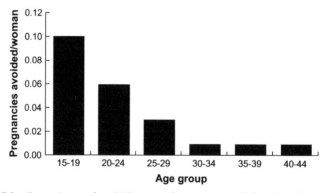

FIGURE 2.—Cost savings patch vs COCs (*top*) and pregnancies avoided patch vs COCs (*bottom*) per woman by age over 2 years. (Courtesy of Sonnenberg FA, Burkman RT, Speroff L, et al: Cost-effectiveness and contraceptive effectiveness of the transdermal contraceptive patch. *Am J Obstet Gynecol* 192:1-9. Copyright 2005 by Elsevier.)

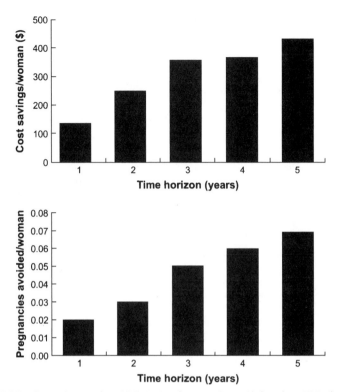

FIGURE 3.—Cost savings patch vs COCs (*top*) and pregnancies avoided patch vs COCs (*bottom*) per woman by time horizon. (Courtesy of Sonnenberg FA, Burkman RT, Speroff L, et al: Cost-effectiveness and contraceptive effectiveness of the transdermal contraceptive patch. *Am J Obstet Gynecol* 192:1-9. Copyright 2005 by Elsevier.)

15 to 50, in average health in a long-term, mutually monogamous, heterosexual relationship.

Results.—The base-case analysis showed that use of the patch resulted in a savings of 249 US dollars and 0.03 pregnancies per woman over 2 years compared with COCs (Figs 2 and 3).

Conclusion.—This analysis demonstrated that patch use would be cost saving compared with COC use, resulting in a net avoidance of pregnancy for this population. The cost savings are attributed to reduced costs of pregnancy.

▶ Unintended pregnancy is a major public health issue. In the United States alone there are 3 million unplanned pregnancies each year.[1] There are many costs associated with unintended pregnancy. In 2004, Sonnenberg et al[2] conducted a cost-utility analysis that demonstrated that compared with the use of no contraception, all types of contraception offer a cost savings in both health care dollars and quality-adjusted life years. In this analysis several of the same authors compare cost and efficacy between the transdermal contraceptive patch and oral contraceptives.

As with all cost-effectiveness analyses, several assumptions must be made from data from previous studies. The most concerning in this study is the assumption that women are not overweight. Given that 64% of adults in the United States are overweight or obese,[3] this assumption clearly weakens the study, especially when studies have demonstrated a decrease in efficacy among women weighing greater than 90 kg.[4] They also utilize data from Archer et al[5] that showed perfect use was increased in the transdermal system compared with oral contraceptives. Their conclusions were that transdermal contraception would have a net avoidance of pregnancy and therefore a cost savings compared with oral contraceptives.

This study was funded by an unrestricted educational grant from Ortho-McNeil Pharmaceuticals, the maker of the transdermal patch. Pharmaceutical company studies should not be discounted, but one must look at them critically. These study findings are not a surprise given that efficacy has been shown to be equal and compliance better, so at a public health level the patch may have benefits, but it is dangerous to extrapolate this to your patients and make global decisions. Contraception is still a very personal issue and for some individuals remembering something once a week may be more difficult than daily. Each patient, adolescent or older than 40 years, needs to be offered the chance to learn about all the safe and effective contraceptive options and determine which will best fit her lifestyle.

N. B. Zite, MD, MPH

References

1. Henshaw S: Unintended pregnancy in the United States. *Fam Plann Perspect* 30:24-9, 1998.
2. Sonnenberg FA, Burkman RT, Hagerty CG, et al: Cost and net health effects of contraception methods. *Contraception* 69:447-459, 2004.
3. National Health and Nutrition Examination Survey, 1999-2000.
4. Zieman M, Guillebaud J, Weisberg E, et al: Contraceptive efficacy and cycle control with the Ortho Evra/Evra transdermal system: The analysis of pooled data. *Fertil Steril* 77(suppl 2):s13-s18, 2002.
5. Archer DF, Cullins V, Creasy GW, et al: The impact of improved compliance with a weekly contraceptive transdermal system (Ortho Evra) on contraceptive efficacy. *Contraception* 69:189-195, 2004.

Levonorgestrel-Releasing Intrauterine System for Treating Menstrual Disorders: A Patient Satisfaction Questionnaire
Radesic B, Sharma A (Palmerston North Hosp, New Zealand)
Aust N Z J Obstet Gynaecol 44:247-251, 2004   24–3

Aims.—To establish the continuation and satisfaction rates and the reasons for removal of the levonorgestrel-releasing intrauterine system (LNG-IUS) in Palmerston North Hospital (PNH), New Zealand.

Sample and Setting.—All women (120) who had a LNG-IUS inserted at PNH between June 1998 and June 2002 were included in the study.

Methods.—A survey questionnaire regarding bleeding patterns, side-effects and satisfaction rates relating to the device as well as reasons for premature removal, current treatment for dysfunctional uterine bleeding (DUB) and contraception was sent to all 120 women. Seventy-eight of the 85 women who received the questionnaire (91%) responded to it. Thirty-five women were lost to follow-up and the overall response rate was 65%.

Results.—The LNG-IUS was prematurely removed from nine women and expulsion occurred in one case. The overall continuation rate was 87%. No women had LNG-IUS removed as a result of hormonal side-effects except for bleeding abnormalities. The overall satisfaction rate was 76%.

Conclusion.—Levonorgestrel-releasing intrauterine system is a well-accepted and efficacious therapy for heavy menstrual bleeding. These satisfaction and premature removal rates compare favourably with international figures. The response rate to the questionnaire was reasonably high given the highly mobile nature of the studied population.

▶ The use of the LNG-IUS for menorrhagia and menometrorrhagia has become commonplace in many parts of the world. The system is specifically approved for that indication in many countries including New Zealand, the country of origin of this article. Previous studies have shown a reduction in menstrual blood loss of 86% after 3 months and 97% after 12 months.[1]

This article looked at the satisfaction rate in patients treated with the device for menstrual dysfunction and showed a high continuation rate and good satisfaction. Unfortunately, the abstract alone leaves out many pertinent details of the study. Seventy percent of the patients had the device inserted for heavy menses and 29% for irregular menses, but as with many purely observational studies, no attempt was made to quantitate blood loss before or after treatment. In addition, there is little information on what workup for pathology was performed on these patients before treatment. The study implied that no anatomic pathology was present but did not elaborate further. This is not necessarily a problem, as this device has also been show to be quite effective in patients with bleeding from leiomyomata as well.

This article is worthwhile because it draws attention to what has become a standard treatment for uterine bleeding disorders in many countries. It would be worthwhile for the reader to obtain the entire article for further reading.

G. H. Lipscomb, MD

Reference

1. Andersson JK, Rybo G: Levonorgestrel-releasing intrauterine device in the treatment of menorrhagia. *Br J Obstet Gynaecol* 97:690-694, 1990.

The Use of Triphasic Oral Contraceptives in a Continuous Use Regimen

Shulman LP (Northwestern Univ, Chicago)

Contraception 72:105-110, 2005 24–4

Objective.—The objective of this study was to describe the characteristics of and outcomes and side effects in patients using triphasic oral contraceptives (OCs) in a continuous use regimen.

Methods.—A retrospective review of patient charts from four community-based physician practices was conducted. All patients had been using triphasic OCs in a continuous regimen (i.e., to prevent withdrawal bleeding) for a planned duration of at least three 28-day cycles. Data collected through retrospective chart abstraction included demographic and clinical indicators, duration of and reason for continuous triphasic OC use, prior OC history and side effect incidence and treatment.

Results.—Forty-three patients meeting the inclusion criteria had data of sufficient quality to be included in all analyses. These patients represented 603 total cycles. Nearly half of the patients (49%) indicated that their primary reason for continuous OC use was personal preference rather than medical reasons. More than half of the patients (56%) had previously used triphasic OCs in a noncontinuous regimen; 24% had no prior OC experience. The median duration of continuous use was 237 days (including right-censored patients; range, 55–994). Of the 39% of patients who terminated continuous use, the most common reason given was the desire to become pregnant (35%). Sixty-one percent of the patients reported no side effects from continuous use. The most common side effect occurring beyond Day 21 of continuous use was breakthrough bleeding (reported in four patients). Survival analysis indicated that time on continuous triphasic use was positively related to parity >0 ($p<.05$) and the absence of side effects ($p<.1$).

Conclusion.—The data suggest that successful continuous use is feasible with triphasic OCs, with few adverse side effects.

▶ Physicians have been prescribing OCs in a continuous regimen for decades to alleviate menstrual migraines, symptomatic endometriosis, and premenstrual symptoms.[1-3] More recently, it has become popular to initiate a continuous regimen for convenience.[4] Most of the studies looking at bleeding pattern and acceptability of extended regimens have utilized monophasic pills. Shulman challenges the notion that triphasic OCs would not be amenable to continuous use and would have high rates of unscheduled bleeding because of the hormonal fluctuations. In this retrospective survey he attempts to show that women were able to use triphasic OCs in an extended regimen without high rates of discontinuation for side effects.

Obviously, a randomized controlled trial is needed to provide irrefutable evidence that triphasic OCs do not have more side effects than monophasic pills when taken for longer than 21 days, but that would require a great deal of time and money. Of the 43 patients who were analyzed in this study, 61% reported no side effects. The most likely reason for a woman to discontinue her regimen was a desire for pregnancy (35%), and only 5% discontinued because of side effects. Breakthrough bleeding was the most common side effect reported beyond day 21, but it only occurred in 4 patients and only 2 of those terminated use for breakthrough bleeding.

This study has important clinical implications. Triphasic OCs are extremely popular and readily available pills. If a woman is already on a triphasic that she has no complaints with, she would not have to change pills to attempt a continuous regimen. The study also should help remind providers that side effects usually are self-limited, regardless of the regimen used, and if we counsel women thoroughly about expectations more women might continue their method.

N. B. Zite, MD, MPH

References

1. MacGregor A: Migraine associated with menstruation. *Funct Neurol* 77:143-153, 2000.
2. Vercellini P, De Giorgi O, Mosconi P, et al: Cyproterone acetate versus continuous monophasic oral contraceptive in the treatment of recurrent pelvic pain after conservative surgery for symptomatic endometriosis. *Fertil Steril* 77:52-61, 2002.
3. Loudon NB, Foxwell M, Potts DM, et al: Acceptability of an oral contraceptive that reduces the frequency of menstruation: The tri-cycle pill regimen. *Br Med J* 2:487-490, 1977.
4. Miller LK, Notter M: Menstrual reduction with extended use of combination oral contraceptive pills: A randomized controlled trial. *Obstet Gynecol* 98:771-778, 2001.

A Randomized Trial to Compare 24 h Versus 12 h Double Dose Regimen of Levonorgestrel for Emergency Contraception

Ngai SW, Fan S, Li S, et al (Univ of Hong Kong; Family Planning Assoc of Hong Kong; Inst of Shenzhen, China; et al)

Hum Reprod 20:307-311, 2004

24–5

Background.—Levonorgestrel (0.75 mg given for two doses 12 h apart) has been proven to be an effective regimen for emergency contraception when the first dose is given within 72 h of unprotected coitus. However, the

TABLE 3.—Pregnancy Rate and Prevented Fractions in Both Treatment Groups

Levonorgestrel Group	n	Pregnancies[a]	95% CI	Expected Pregnancies	Prevented Fraction (95% CI)
24 h	1038	20 (1.9)	1.2-2.9	71	72% (56.7-82.7)
12 h	1022	20 (2.0)	1.2-3.0	74	75% (59.0-83.7)

[a]Values in parentheses are percentages.
CI = confidence interval.
(Courtesy of Ngai SW, Fan S, Li S, et al: A Randomized trial to compare 24 h versus 12 h double dose regimen of levonorgestrel for emergency contraception. *Hum Reprod* 20:307-311, 2004. Copyright European Society for Human Reproduction and Embryology, by permission of Oxford University Press/Human Reproduction.)

TABLE 4.—The Effect of Further Acts of Intercourse on Pregnancy Rates in the 12 h and 24 h Group

Group	Pregnancy in Women With Further Acts of Intercourse n (%)	Pregnancy in Women With No Further Acts of Intercourse n (%)	P	Odds Ratio (95% CI)
24 h	4/225 (1.8)	16/792 (2.0)	0.82	0.88 (0.29-2.65)
12 h	10/221 (4.5)	10/774 (1.3)	0.003	3.62 (1.49-8.81)

CI = confidence interval.
(Courtesy of Ngai SW, Fan S, Li S, et al: A Randomized trial to compare 24 h versus 12 h double dose regimen of levonorgestrel for emergency contraception. *Hum Reprod* 20:307-311, 2004. Copyright European Society for Human Reproduction and Embryology, by permission of Oxford University Press/Human Reproduction.)

dosing interval is inconvenient for those taking the first dose in the afternoon. We conducted a randomized study to evaluate two levonorgestrel dosing regimens for emergency contraception. Two doses of levonorgestrel 0.75 mg were administered with the first dose given up to 120 h after unprotected intercourse. The second dose was given 12 h later in the first regimen and 24 h later in the second regimen.

Methods.—We conducted a double-blind, randomized trial between 1997 and 2003 at five centres in China. A total of 2071 women requesting emergency contraception within 120 h of unprotected intercourse were recruited. They were randomized to receive two doses of 0.75 mg of levonorgestrel, given either 24 h apart or 12 h apart.

Results.—Outcome was unknown for 53 women (24 in the 24 h group and 29 in the 12 h group). Among the remaining 2018 women, the crude pregnancy rate was 1.9% in the 24 h group [95% confidence interval (CI) 1.17–2.94] and 2.0% in the 12 h group (95% CI 1.19–2.99). The proportion of pregnancies prevented was estimated to be 72% in the 24 h group and 75% in the 12 h group (Table 3). Side-effects were mild in both groups. The efficacy of the 12 h regimen declined significantly when there were further acts of intercourse after treatment (5.0 versus 1.0%, $P < 0.01$) (Table 4). This was not observed in the 24 h group.

Conclusions.—Two doses of 0.75 mg levonorgestrel given either 24 or 12 h apart are effective for emergency contraception up to 120 h after unprotected intercourse. Further research to investigative more effective methods of emergency contraception is warranted.

▶ In 1974 Albert Yuzpe defined a regimen for emergency contraception (EC) that still bears his name.[1] This regimen was created by using an oral contraception that he had in his lab for another study (Ovral; Wyeth Laboratories, Philadelphia, Pa.) and used a 72-hour timeline for convenience. When he demonstrated a 2% failure rate he decided the regimen would include a repeat dose in 12 hours despite no evidence of improvement with this second dose.[2]

Since that time, numerous variations on the medications, doses, and timing of dosing have been studied. In 1998 a study was published that demonstrated improved response compared with Yuzpe's regimen with levonorgestrel (0.75

mg) alone with the same timing (2 doses, 12 hours apart, within 72 hours of unprotected coitus).[3] The World Health Organization studied levonorgestrel further and demonstrated that a single dose of 1.5 mg was as effective as the 12-hour-apart dosing interval.[4] The Ngai et al study also challenged the 12-hour interval between doses. More than 2000 Chinese women were randomized to doses either 12 or 24 hours apart, and the starting dose was also extended to be used within 120 hours of intercourse. There were only 40 pregnancies in the study, and several (n = 14) occurred in women who had further acts of intercourse between taking the levonorgestrel and their pregnancy.

EC has the potential to decrease the number of unintended pregnancies in the United States by half, and offering different dosing options may make it easier for some women to utilize.[5] This study reminds providers to recommend barrier methods or abstinence until menses occurs after EC use.

N. B. Zite, MD, MPH

References

1. Yuzpe A, Thurlow H, Ramzy I, et al: Post coital contraception: A pilot study. *J Reprod Med* 13:53-58, 1974.
2. Yuzpe A, Lancee W: Ethinylestradiol and dl-norgestrel as a postcoital contraceptive. *Fertil Steril* 28:932-936, 1977.
3. Task force on Postovulatory Methods of Fertility Regulation. Randomised Controlled trial of levonorgestrel versus the Yuzpe regimen of combined oral contraception. *Lancet* 352:428-433, 1998.
4. Von Hertzen H, Piaggio G, Ding J, et al: Low dose mifepristone and two regimens of levonorgestrel for emergency contraception: A WHO multicentre randomized trial. *Lancet* 360:1803-1810, 2002.
5. Trussel J, Stewart F, Guest F, et al: Emergency contraceptive pills: A simple proposal to reduce unintended pregnancies. *Fam Plann Perspect* 59:147-151, 1999.

Short-Term Oral Contraceptive Use and the Risk of Epithelial Ovarian Cancer

Greer JB, Modugno F, Allen GO, et al (Univ of Pittsburgh, Pa)
Am J Epidemiol 162:66-72, 2005

24–6

Abstract.—Oral contraceptive (OC) use has been consistently linked to a reduction in ovarian cancer in a dose-dependent fashion. Whether short-term OC use is protective remains controversial. In 1994–1998 in the Delaware Valley of Pennsylvania, the authors examined the association between short-term OC use and ovarian cancer in a population-based case-control study comparing 608 incident epithelial ovarian cancer cases with 926 community controls. Using unconditional logistic regression and adjusting for known confounders, they found a significant reduction in ovarian cancer risk for women who had used OCs for ≤ 6 months (odds ratio = 0.73, 95% confidence interval: 0.54, 0.99). This protective effect was observed in only that group who had used OCs for ≤ 6 months and stopped because of side effects (odds ratio = 0.59, 95% confidence interval: 0.40, 0.87 for side effects and odds ratio = 0.91, 95% confidence interval: 0.60, 1.37 for non-side-effects). Women who used OCs for >6 months were at a reduced risk independent of their reason for stopping. Results were similar when stratifying by parity and hormone therapy use. Thus, OC use for as little as 6 months provides significant protection against ovarian cancer risk, protection that appears limited to those women who stop using OCs because of side effects. Mediating factors may reflect endogenous hormone levels, OC metabolism, or OC bioactivity.

▶ The inability to consistently and accurately detect ovarian cancer in the early phases has lead to widespread study of a variety of US and serum markers that would allow such diagnosis. Unfortunately, no study has, as of yet, demonstrated the ability to consistently detect ovarian cancer in an earlier and more treatable stage of disease. However, various studies have demonstrated that the use of OCs can reduce the risk of developing ovarian cancer. These studies have demonstrated that long-term use of OCs has been effective in reducing the risk of developing epithelial ovarian cancer. In this study, Greer et al showed that short-term use of OCs is effective for providing significant protection against ovarian cancer. Indeed, the authors showed that as little as 6 months of use resulted in a considerable reduction in the frequency of ovarian cancer development. Women's health care providers need to be well versed in the risks and the noncontraceptive benefits of OCs and be ready to help patients make important decisions concerning not only the ability to prevent pregnancy but also the ability to choose amongst therapeutic options that will provide a wide spectrum of clinical benefit.

L. P. Shulman, MD

25 Abortion: Medical and Surgical

Attitudes of Obsetrics and Gynecology Residents Toward Abortion Participation: A Philadelphia Area Survey
Fischer RL, Schaeffer K, Hunter RL (Univ of Medicine and Dentistry of New Jersey–Robert Wood Johnson Med School at Camden)
Contraception 72:200-205, 2005   25–1

Objective.—The objective of this study was to evaluate the willingness of Philadelphia obstetrics and gynecology residents to participate in three abortion procedures for various fetal conditions.

Methods.—Anonymous questionnaires were distributed to 310 residents from 18 programs. The survey asked the residents whether they would participate in first trimester dilatation and evacuation (D&E), second trimester prostaglandin induction or second trimester D&E for the following conditions: lethal fetal anomaly, nonlethal anomaly with certain long-term functional consequences, possible long-term functional consequences, little or no long-term functional consequences and elective abortion of a normal fetus.

Results.—Of the 148 respondents, the percentage of residents who would participate in a second trimester D&E for each fetal condition was significantly lower than that for a first trimester D&E (p≤.001). Additionally, for each abortion procedure, the participation rates consistently fell for lesser degrees of fetal severity. Participation was significantly associated with preferences regarding abortion legislation and personal abortion stance.

Conclusion.—Resident attitudes regarding abortion participation were related to severity of the fetal condition, gestational age and procedure type.

▶ The continued availability of abortion services in this country is dependent on the willingness of obstetricians-gynecologists to do the procedure. Resident training has been positively linked to the practitioner's offering and performing abortions. The Accreditation Council on Graduate Medical Education recognized this fact and has stated that abortion training is a program requirement for obstetrics and gynecology resident training.

Nevertheless, concern still exists. This study attempts to define under what parameters would current obstetrics and gynecology residents perform abortions, and what other issues may influence their practice. In Philadelphia, 310 residents were surveyed by way of an anonymous questionnaire; about 48% responded. The survey defined degrees of severity of fetal anomalies (from lethal to long-term sequelae, to possible or few sequelae, to "elective" abortions). The residents were asked if they would perform or participate in abortions for these indications, and were also asked to define what procedure they would participate in; first-trimester D&E, second-trimester D&E, or second-trimester prostaglandin induction. Whereas almost 82% stated they would participate in a first-trimester procedure for a lethal fetal condition, only about 40% stated they would participate in procedures that were elective or indicated for conditions having few sequelae. For second-trimester procedures, the rates for participation were lower across the range of conditions, with those willing to do second-trimester D&E fewer than those willing to participate in prostaglandin inductions. As for purely elective procedures, the percentage of those willing to participate in second-trimester prostaglandin induction did not differ from the percentage willing to do a second-trimester D&E.

Residents' opinions may vary across programs and across regions of the country. The authors admit that attitudes in Philadelphia and in Philadelphia-based training programs may not be representative. Perhaps we might be encouraged that more than three fourths of residents would consider performing or participating in terminations for lethal conditions in the first and second trimesters, and that more than 40% would do so in elective cases. I would suppose that many more would state, if asked, that they would counsel about the option to terminate a pregnancy and would refer to a practitioner who would perform the procedure.

O. P. Phillips, MD

A Randomised Controlled Trial of 6 and 12 Hourly Administration of Vaginal Misoprostol for Second Trimester Pregnancy Termination

Herabutya Y, Chanrachakul B, Punyavachira P (Mahidol Univ, Bangkok, Thailand)

BJOG 112:1297-1301, 2005   25-2

Objective.—To compare the effectiveness of vaginal misoprostol administered 6 or 12 hourly for second trimester pregnancy termination.

Design.—A randomised controlled trial.

Setting.—University teaching hospital.

Sample.—Two hundred and seventy-nine pregnant women at gestations between 14 and 26 weeks undergoing pregnancy termination.

Methods.—Women were randomised to receive 600-µg misoprostol tablets vaginally either every 6 hours or every 12 hours until abortion occurred.

Main Outcome Measures.—Induction-abortion interval, success rate within 24 and 48 hours and adverse effects.

Results.—There was no significant difference in the median induction to abortion interval 6 hours (16 hours) and 12 hours (16 hours; $P = 0.80$). The total dose of misoprostol was higher in the 6-hour group (1800 vs 1200 µg). The cumulative abortion rates within 24 hours were 74% and 67% and within 48 hours 94% and 92%, in the 6- and 12-hour groups, respectively. Fever was more common in the 6-hour group (53%) versus the 12-hour group (31%; $P < 0.001$). The incidence of nausea, vomiting, diarrhoea, severe bleeding and abdominal pain were similar.

Conclusions.—Misoprostol (600 µg) administered at 12-hour intervals was associated with fewer adverse effects and was as effective as a 6-hour interval.

▶ Adverse effects of misoprostol include fever, nausea, vomiting, and abdominal pain and can add further to the distress of the patient undergoing a medically induced second-trimester abortion. In this study from Thailand, the authors tested the hypothesis that increasing the frequency of vaginally administrated misoprostol from every 12 hours to every 6 hours would increase the successful abortion rate within 24 hours and reduce the induction to abortion time interval. They expected the rate of adverse effects would not change, but that a reduction in the time to abortion would result in an improved side effect profile.

Women with pregnancies between 14 and 26 weeks were randomized to misoprostol 600-µg tablets vaginally every 6 hours (n = 140) or to every 12 hours (n = 139) until expulsion of the fetus. The average gestational age of 19 weeks was the same in each group as was the percentage that was nulliparous.

The cumulative success rate among women in pregnancies less than 18 weeks was no different in each group. In contrast, among women with pregnancies greater than 18 weeks, the success rate within 24 hours was significantly higher in the every 6-hour group (74%), compared with the every 12-hour group (61%). No other outcome differed between the groups, however. The induction to abortion interval, the rates of abortions within 24 hours and those within 48 hours, and the complete abortion rate did not differ between groups. The rates of side effects were similar between groups, with the exception of fever, which was more common in the every 6-hour group.

Reducing the dosing interval of misoprostol did not speed up the process of a second-trimester abortion or significantly reduce side effects. It is of interest to note that 29 women had had previous cesarean deliveries. No complications occurred.

O. P. Phillips, MD

Misoprostol Alone for Early Abortion: An Evaluation of Seven Potential Regimens

Blanchard K, Shochet T, Coyaji K, et al al (Ibis Reproductive Health, Cambridge; Univ of Michigan, Ann Arbor; KEM Hosp, Rasta Peth, Rao, India; et al)
Contraception 72:91-97, 2005   25–3

Introduction.—A growing body of literature has shown that misoprostol alone could be effective for early medical abortion. We evaluated seven potential regimens in women up to 56 days of gestation in order to potentially identify an optimal regimen.

Methods.—In phase I of the study, women requesting early abortion were randomized to one of three misoprostol regimens (4×400 µg po every 3 h, 2×800 µg po every 6 h, 1×600 pv µg); in phase II, women were randomized to one of two regimens (2×800 µg po every 3 h, 1×800 pv µg). In phase III, we consecutively tested two regimens (800 µg pv wetted with saline repeated after 24 h if intact gestational sac, 2×800 µg pv wetted with saline) to validate previously published results.

Results.—Although most women experienced some side effects, all regimens were tolerable and acceptable. Five of the seven regimens resulted in complete abortion rates of 60% or less. Only repeated doses of 800 µg pv misoprostol resulted in efficacy exceeding 60%.

Discussion.—Misoprostol-alone abortion regimens using oral misoprostol are too ineffective for clinical use or further investigation. Regimens with repeated dosing of misoprostol 800 µg pv warrant further study to find the optimal treatment protocol.

▶ The use of non-surgical approaches to pregnancy termination has considerably increased over the past decade. Initial and ongoing studies have shown that such approaches to abortion are safe and reliable in comparison to conventional surgical techniques. The decision to utilize a medical or surgical approach to pregnancy termination is usually determined by the gestational age of the pregnancy and personal desires by the woman requesting the abortion. However, this study by Blanchard and colleagues shows that the use of misoprostol alone for early pregnancy termination was not effective and resulted in considerable side effects and failed termination procedures. It is clear from the expanding literature on this topic that, although misoprostol plays an important role in the management of women who are seeking pregnancy termination or uterine evacuation for a non-viable gestation, its use as a stand alone agent for early first-trimester pregnancy terminations is considerably less efficacious than those regimens with mifepristone and other agents. Clinicians need to be aware of these issues when considering the use of medical interventions for pregnancy termination or uterine evacuation.

L. P. Shulman, MD

Fetal Pain: A Systematic Multidisciplinary Review of the Evidence
Lee SJ, Ralston HJP, Drey EA, et al (Univ of California, San Francisco)
JAMA 294:947-954, 2005   25–4

Context.—Proposed federal legislation would require physicians to inform women seeking abortions at 20 or more weeks after fertilization that the fetus feels pain and to offer anesthesia administered directly to the fetus. This article examines whether a fetus feels pain and if so, whether safe and effective techniques exist for providing direct fetal anesthesia or analgesia in the context of therapeutic procedures or abortion.

Evidence Acquisition.—Systematic search of PubMed for English-language articles focusing on human studies related to fetal pain, anesthesia, and analgesia. Included articles studied fetuses of less than 30 weeks' gestational age or specifically addressed fetal pain perception or nociception. Articles were reviewed for additional references. The search was performed without date limitations and was current as of June 6, 2005.

Evidence Synthesis.—Pain perception requires conscious recognition or awareness of a noxious stimulus. Neither withdrawal reflexes nor hormonal stress responses to invasive procedures prove the existence of fetal pain, because they can be elicited by nonpainful stimuli and occur without conscious cortical processing. Fetal awareness of noxious stimuli requires functional thalamocortical connections. Thalamocortical fibers begin appearing between 23 to 30 weeks' gestational age, while electroencephalography suggests the capacity for functional pain perception in preterm neonates probably does not exist before 29 or 30 weeks. For fetal surgery, women may receive general anesthesia and/or analgesics intended for placental transfer, and parenteral opioids may be administered to the fetus under direct or sonographic visualization. In these circumstances, administration of anesthesia and analgesia serves purposes unrelated to reduction of fetal pain, including inhibition of fetal movement, prevention of fetal hormonal stress responses, and induction of uterine atony.

Conclusions.—Evidence regarding the capacity for fetal pain is limited but indicates that fetal perception of pain is unlikely before the third trimester. Little or no evidence addresses the effectiveness of direct fetal anesthetic or analgesic techniques. Similarly, limited or no data exist on the safety of such techniques for pregnant women in the context of abortion. Anesthetic techniques currently used during fetal surgery are not directly applicable to abortion procedures.

▶ In the first paragraph, the authors begin with a political tone, referencing several states' attempts to place further barriers on abortion availability by requiring women to sign statements attesting to their understanding that an abortion causes the fetus "pain." The next 5 pages, however, are dedicated to a review of scientific articles that prove the fetus (at least a fetus <25 weeks' gestation) does not indeed feel pain.

First a definition of pain, which requires a high degree of cognitive, is not applicable to a first- or second-trimester fetus. Further, the authors provide research that finds the nerves that conduct pain stimuli (the thalamocortical circuits) are not developed until 24 to 26 weeks (from conception). Finally, the authors present ethical arguments against the assumption that the fetus may need anesthesia, where the risk to the mother would far outweigh the theoretic consideration of relieving fetal pain.

Considering we are dealing with another barrier created by some states to legalized abortion, we should suppose such an article stating common-sense axioms would be necessary. With almost 100 references, it seems to be a thorough review of the science. However, we shouldn't expect this article to alter anyone's opinions.

O. P. Phillips, MD

Safety of Mifepristone Abortions in Clinical Use
Henderson JT, Hwang AC, Harper CC, et al (Univ of California, San Francisco)
Contraception 72:175-178, 2005   25–5

Objectives.—Extensive data from clinical trials document mifepristone's safety and efficacy for induced abortion, but less information is available about its safety in routine clinical use.

Methods.—Data on mifepristone abortion use from the Planned Parenthood Federation of America, the largest provider of mifepristone abortion in the United States, from 2001 through the first quarter of 2004 were collected using a centralized reporting system. Over the study period, 95,163 mifepristone abortions were provided. Reportable events are complications requiring inpatient or outpatient hospital treatment.

Results.—Overall, 2.2 per 1000 women (95% CI 1.9-2.5) experienced a complication, most commonly, heavy bleeding. Mifepristone abortion mortality is estimated to be 1.1 per 100,000 based on one death (95% CI 0.3-5.9).

Conclusions.—The safety of mifepristone is high; few serious medical complications occur in routine clinical use.

▶ The authors take advantage of the huge database maintained through Planned Parenthood Federation of America and report on the complications from 95,163 mifepristone abortions performed over 3 years in 202 separate clinical sites. Their protocol was 200 mg of mifeprostine administered in the clinic, followed by patient self-administration of 800 μg of misoprostol within 24 to 72 hours if the patient's gestational age is less than 56 days from the last menstrual period, and within 24 to 48 hours if the patient's gestational age is 56 to 63 days. Overall, 79% of patients returned for a postabortion visit or were contacted by phone. However, failure to follow-up was not an exclusion criterion, and complication rates were calculated based on all procedures with the assumption that the clinics would be made aware of most complications.

The study found that the overall complication rate was 2.2 per 1000 procedures. This included heavy vaginal bleeding (1.3/1000), bleeding requiring transfusion (0.5/1000), endometritis (0.2/1000), and sepsis (2.1/100,000; 2

cases). There was one death and it was secondary to sepsis, for a death rate of 1.1 per 100,000. If only cases with follow-up were considered, the overall complication rate was 2.7 per 1000 procedures. Failed attempted abortions were reported separately, and the rate was 3.5 per 1000.

This represents the first large study of mifepristone in "routine clinical use in the United States." It clearly confirms the findings of smaller studies and clinical trials that first-trimester abortions induced with a mifepristone and misoprostol protocol are safe and efficacious. However, the authors did not make note of what number of patients (if any) required a surgical procedure for either bleeding or retained products.

O. P. Phillips, MD

Risk Factors for Complications of Induced Abortions in Nigeria
Mitsunaga TM, Larsen UM, Okonofua FE (MEASURE Evaluation/JSI, Arlington, Va; Univ of Maryland, College Park; Univ of Benin, Nigeria)
J Women's Health 14:515-528, 2005   25–6

Background.—The prevalence and risk factors for unsafe abortions and their complications are not well defined.

Methods.—A cross-sectional study of patient-reported reproductive history was conducted in three hospitals in southwest Nigeria from 1998 to 1999. Data on pregnancy outcomes and sociodemographic characteristics were collected for 1836 women ages 15-49 seeking family planning and antenatal services. Independent predictors for complications from induced abortion of first pregnancies were analyzed using logistic regression models.

Results.—Four hundred twenty-four women (29.7%) terminated their first pregnancy. As many as 43.1% of women unmarried at first pregnancy had an abortion, and being unmarried at pregnancy was the strongest predictor of abortion in the adjusted model. Almost 30% experienced complications at the time of abortion (heavy bleeding, high fever, and other), and 22.9% reported complications subsequent to and within 6 weeks of abortion. Heavy bleeding and 6-week complications were significantly associated with age at pregnancy, circumcision, and religion, and 87.6% of women with 6-week complications reported complications for 1 day. Type of provider was the sole significant predictor of fever, and doctor provider reduced the risk of fever. Induced abortion and related complications were common despite the widespread provision by doctors.

Conclusions.—Policies and programs should address improving abortion practices and postabortion care, increasing contraceptive use, and reducing the practice of female circumcision.

▶ This article attempts to define risk factors for complications for induced abortions in certain provinces of Nigeria. Although some pertinent information can be derived from the study, a great deal of insight is gained about abortions in such poor countries in reading the introduction and conclusions. In Nigeria, it is a crime to perform or obtain an abortion except to save the life of a mother;

however, one case law permits abortion for the indication of maternal mental health reasons. The World Health Organization estimates that 4.2 million unsafe abortions are performed in Africa each year. In Nigeria alone, the annual abortion rate is 25 per 1000 women. A significant proportion is illegal; and 20,000 women die from abortions annually in Nigeria.

For the study, women seeking family planning or antenatal services in 3 hospital sites were interviewed by nurse midwives trained in interviewing with a "value-free" technique. Abortion is illegal, and religious and cultural mores enforce a "no sex before marriage" code. Therefore, there may be underreporting. The women were asked about previous abortions and about the complications of bleeding and "fever" or infection 1 day after the procedure and up to 6 weeks after the procedure. Abortions made up more than 29% of all first pregnancies. These women were mostly likely to have been younger than 20 years at that time, students, and unmarried. They were likely to have been circumcised. A doctor performed the abortion in 51% of the cases. Almost 30% reported experiencing immediate complications, and about 23% reported complications up to 6 weeks. These self-reported complications were more common in younger women and with the more radical circumcisions. There were no differences if the procedure was performed by a doctor or nondoctor provider.

The authors describe the difficult choices women in Nigeria face. Pregnancy and childbirth before marriage are forbidden by tradition; however, a common belief held among countryman is that contraception may reduce future childbearing potential. And pregnancy is highly valued in marriage. It was unstated, but must be true, that women are unlikely to be truly consenting partners when they are students and unmarried teenagers. The final point to consider is our own country's future should legal, safe abortion ever be made unavailable.

O. P. Phillips, MD

26 Breast Health

Oral Contraceptive Use and Risk of Early-Onset Breast Cancer in Carriers and Noncarriers of *BRCA1* and *BRCA2* Mutations
Milne RL, for the Breast Cancer Family Registry (Univ of Melbourne; et al)
Cancer Epidemiol Biomarkers Prev 14:350-356, 2005   26–1

Background.—Recent oral contraceptive use has been associated with a small increase in breast cancer risk and a substantial decrease in ovarian cancer risk. The effects on risks for women with germ line mutations in *BRCA1* or *BRCA2* are unclear.

Methods.—Subjects were population-based samples of Caucasian women that comprised 1,156 incident cases of invasive breast cancer diagnosed before age 40 (including 47 *BRCA1* and 36 *BRCA2* mutation carriers) and 815 controls from the San Francisco Bay area, California, Ontario, Canada, and Melbourne and Sydney, Australia. Relative risks by carrier status were estimated using unconditional logistic regression, comparing oral contraceptive use in case groups defined by mutation status with that in controls.

Results.—After adjustment for potential confounders, oral contraceptive use for at least 12 months was associated with decreased breast cancer risk for *BRCA1* mutation carriers [odds ratio (OR), 0.22; 95% confidence interval (CI), 0.10-0.49; $P < 0.001$], but not for *BRCA2* mutation carriers (OR, 1.02; 95% CI, 0.34-3.09) or noncarriers (OR, 0.93; 95% CI, 0.69-1.24). First use during or before 1975 was associated with increased risk for noncarriers (OR, 1.52 per year of use before 1976; 95% CI, 1.22-1.91; $P < 0.001$).

Conclusions.—There was no evidence that use of current low-dose oral contraceptive formulations increases risk of early-onset breast cancer for mutation carriers, and there may be a reduced risk for *BRCA1* mutation carriers. Because current formulations of oral contraceptives may reduce, or at least not exacerbate, ovarian cancer risk for mutation carriers, they should not be contraindicated for a woman with a germ line mutation in *BRCA1* or *BRCA2*.

▶ Concerns regarding the use of hormonal therapies during the reproductive years and menopause continue to affect the use of such therapies by clinicians and patients alike. This concern continues to affect the use of hormonal therapies despite an increasing body of literature that shows that the use of such therapies does not increase the risk of adverse outcomes for most women and does provide noncontraceptive benefits. One well-recognized effect of oral contraceptive use is the reduction of the development of epithelial ovarian cancer in high-risk and low-risk women. However, many women who are at increased risk for developing ovarian cancer may also be at increased risk for developing breast cancer and thus may be concerned about the use of oral contraceptives during their reproductive years. This case-controlled study by Milne et al showed no increased risk for the development of early-onset breast cancer in high-risk women who were carriers or noncarriers of *BRCA1* and *BRCA2* gene mutations with the use of current low-dose oral contraceptives. As such formulations will likely reduce the risk of developing ovarian cancer, clinicians and women who are at increased risk for developing breast and ovarian cancer should feel confident that the use of conventional oral contraceptives will not increase the risk of breast cancer when used for reproductive or nonreproductive indications.

L. P. Shulman, MD

Secular Trends in the Incidence of Female Breast Cancer in the United States, 1973-1998

Nasseri K (Tri-Counties Public Health Inst, Santa Barbara, Calif)
Breast J 10:129-135, 2004
26–2

Abstract.—Statistical modeling suggests a causal association between the rapid increase in the incidence of female breast cancer (FBC) in the United States and the widespread use of screening mammography. Additional support for this suggestion is a shift in the stage at diagnosis that consists of an increase in early stage diagnosis followed by a decrease in late-stage diagnosis. This has not been reported in the United States. The objective of this study was to examine the secular trends in the incidence of FBC in search of empirical support for this shift. FBC cases in the Surveillance, Epidemiology, and End Results (SEER) database from 1973 through 1998 were dichotomized into early and late detection based. Early detection included all the in situ and invasive cases with local spread. Late detection included cases with regional spread and distant metastasis. Joinpoint segmented regression modeling was used for trend analysis. Early detection in white and black women followed a similar pattern of significant increase in the early 1980s that continued through 1998 with slight modification in 1987. The expected shift in stage was noticed only for white women when the incidence of late detection in them began to decline in 1987. The incidence of late detection in black women has remained stable. These results provide further support for the previously implied causal association between the use of screening mammography and the increased incidence of FBC in the United States. It also shows that the expected stage shift appeared in white women 50-69 years of age after an estimated detection lead time (DLT) of about 5 years. This is the first estimate of DLT in the United States that is based on actual data. The subsequent increase in late detection in white women since 1993 may be due to changes in case management and the increased use of sentinel lymph node biopsy (SLNB) rather than changes in the etiology or biology of FBC.

▶ The introduction of widespread mammography screening for women older than 50 years in 1982 resulted in a significant increase in the diagnosis of prevalent in situ and early-stage breast cancer. The subsequent age-adjusted rate of late disease appears to have been affected rather little in comparison. The authors conclude that an increase in the incidence of breast cancer diagnoses in the years since 1982 is likely due to a reduction in prevalent early and in situ tumors and not an actual increase in disease in the population. An equally dramatic reduction in late-stage disease and mortality has not been documented.

R. D. Arias, MD

The Association of Bloody Nipple Discharge With Breast Pathology
Sauter ER, Schlatter L, Lininger J, et al (Univ of Missouri-Columbia; Jefferson Cancer Network, Norristown, Pa)
Surgery 136:780-785, 2004   26–3

Background.—It is believed that bloody spontaneous nipple discharge (SND) portends a greater chance of malignancy than nonbloody discharge, and that cytologic evaluation of SND assists in treatment planning. Our aims were to assess (1) the pathology of women with/without SND who require diagnostic breast surgery, (2) whether bloody SND is associated with a different spectrum of pathologic findings than nonbloody, and (3) whether SND cytology is influenced by pathologic findings.

Methods.—One hundred seventy-five women who underwent breast operation were enrolled. Cytologic evaluation was performed on Papanicolaou-stained cytospin preparations of SND.

Results.—Papilloma and hyperplasia (both without atypia) were more frequent in breasts with than without SND; breast cancer was more common in breasts without SND ($P < .001$ for all) (Table 2). All cases of breast cancer with SND, but only 33% without, contained a papilloma or papillary features. Seventy-five percent of cancers presenting with SND were nonbloody. Papilloma was the most common diagnosis in breasts with bloody SND and was more common ($P = .017$) than in breasts without, whereas hyperplasia was the most common diagnosis in breasts with nonbloody SND and was more common ($P = .031$) than in breasts with bloody SND. SND cytology was not significantly influenced by pathology.

Conclusions.—Breast cancer can present as unilateral nonbloody SND, indicating the importance of surgical intervention. Papilloma was more common in women with SND than without and most often presented as bloody SND.

TABLE 2.—Pathologic Diagnosis in Breasts
With/Without SND

	SND (%)	
	Yes	No
Specimens	49*	141*
Diagnosis		
Normal	5 (10)	31 (22)
Hyperplasia		
Without atypia†	17 (35)	16 (11)
With atypia	0	7 (5)
Papilloma		
Without atypia†	19 (39)	2 (1)
With atypia	4 (8)	3 (2)
Lobular carcinoma in situ	0	5 (4)
Ductal carcinoma in situ†		
Papillary	1 (2)	5 (4)
Micropapillary	1 (2)	3 (2)
Cribiform	0	1 (1)
Solid	0	4 (3)
Comedo	0	4 (3)
Apocrine	0	1 (1)
Subtype not available	0	6 (4)
Invasive breast cancer†		
Ductal	2 (4)	49 (35)
Lobular	0	4 (3)

*One subject with bilateral SND and 14 subjects without SND had operation on both breasts. Thus, there are 49 SND specimens from 48 subjects and 141 non-SND specimens from 127 subjects.
†Difference between SND and non-SND groups, $P < .03$.
Abbreviation: SND, Spontaneous nipple discharge.
(Courtesy of Sauter ER, Schlatter L, Lininger J, et al: The association of bloody nipple discharge with breast pathology. *Surgery* 136:780-785. Copyright 2004 by Elsevier.)

▶ The management of reproducible, serous or bloody, unilateral single-duct discharge remains surgical excision. Mere cytologic evaluation of the effluent lacks both the sensitivity and specificity to make it useful in management. The fact that the large majority of these women do not have cancer and that no particular characteristic of the aspirate or the clinical setting improves the yield on this excision remains a source of frustration for both the surgeon and patient.

R. D. Arias, MD

Breast Cancer and Abortion

Lea RH, for the SOGC/GOC Joint Ad Hoc Committee on Breast Cancer (Halifax, NS, Canada; et al)
J Obstet Gynaecol 27:491, 2005

Background.—There has been confusion in recent years regarding the relationship between spontaneous and induced abortions and subsequent breast cancer. The nature of this relationship was clarified.

Overview.—A collaborative reanalysis was conducted of data from 53 epidemiologic studies including 83,000 women with breast cancer from 6 countries. In this analysis, it was found that the overall relative risk of breast cancer for women having one or more pregnancies that ended as a spontaneous abortion versus women with no such record was 0.98. The corresponding relative risk for induced abortion was 0.93. The risk of breast cancer was not significantly different among women with a prospectively documented spontaneous or induced abortion according to the number or timing for either type of abortion. Two later studies confirmed that neither form of abortion was associated with an increased risk of breast cancer. However, with an increased number of spontaneous abortions (≥ 3), the risk of breast cancer decreased in premenopausal women and increased in postmenopausal women.

Conclusions.—No association has been found between an induced or spontaneous abortion and an increased risk of breast cancer. Although some states have mandated a warning regarding such an association in any elective termination, patients who have had abortions can be reassured about their subsequent risk of breast cancer.

▶ Writing on behalf of the Society of Obstetricians and Gynaecologists of Canada and on behalf of the Society of Gynecologic Oncologists of Canada, the authors present a committee opinion on breast cancer risk and induced abortion based on 53 retrospective epidemiologic studies from 16 countries. This meta-analysis found a relative risk of 0.93 (95% confidence interval, 0.89-0.96; $P = .0002$). The analysis also found no difference in the risk for breast cancer in women who have had a spontaneous pregnancy loss.

This report of level II-2 evidence indicates there is no association between an induced abortion and an increased risk of breast cancer. Some states include this warning as a mandatory provision for an elective termination. However, patients who have had abortions may be reassured about their subsequent risk for breast cancer.

O. P. Phillips, MD

Breast Cancer Risk Associated With Being Treated for Infertility: Results From the French E3N Cohort Study
Gauthier E, for the E3N Group (INSERM, Villejuif Cedex, France; et al)
Hum Reprod 19:2216-2221, 2004   26–5

Background.—The use of fertility drugs (FDs) is steadily increasing in Western countries and concern has been raised as to the possible impact of fertility treatments on breast cancer risk.

Methods.—We analysed this association in the French E3N study. In this prospective cohort, data on treatment against infertility, duration and time of administration were collected at entry through self-administered questionnaires. Cox regression analysis was used to estimate adjusted relative risks (RRs).

TABLE 4.—Adjusted Relative Risks and 95% Confidence Intervals of Breast Cancer by Selected Indicators of Infertility Treatment: E3N Cohort Study, 1990-2000

		n	PY	Cases	RR[a]	95% CI
Specific drugs[b]						
Clomid®	Never received[c]	85 953	831 342	2388	1.00[d]	—
	Received	2390	23 089	66	0.96	0.75-1.23
GCE®	Never received	85 953	831 342	2388	1.00[d]	—
	Received	1888	18 203	56	0.97	0.74-1.27
Humegon®	Never received	85 953	831 342	2388	1.00[d]	—
	Received	789	7628	23	0.99	0.65-1.49
Overall duration of treatment (months)	Never treated	85 953	831 342	2388	1.00[d]	—
	≤6	1549	15 000	45	0.97	0.72-1.31
	>6	1516	14 653	43	0.92	0.68-1.24
Age at first use (years)	Never used	85 953	831 342	2388	1.00[d]	—
	<30	1638	15 862	46	0.98	0.73-1.32
	≥30	1292	12 479	38	0.90	0.65-1.25

[a]Relative risk adjusted for educational level, active smoking, body mass index (BMI), family history of breast cancer in first-degree relatives, personal history of benign breast disease, age at menarche, menopausal status, composite variable for parity and age at first full-term pregnancy.
[b]Women who had received other treatments exclusively are excluded.
[c]Never received infertility treatment.
[d]Reference category.
Abbreviations: PY, Person-years; *RR,* relative risk; *CI,* confidence interval.
(Courtesy of Gauthier E, for the E3N Group: Breast cancer risk associated with being treated for infertility: Results from the French E3N cohort study. *Hum Reprod* 19:2216-2221, 2004. Copyright European Society for Human Reproduction and Embryology, by permission of Oxford University Press/Human Reproduction.)

Results.—Among the 92,555 women from the study population, 6602 women were treated for infertility. During the 10 year follow-up period, 2571 cases of primary invasive breast cancer were diagnosed (183 in treated women). Our study showed no overall significant association between breast cancer risk and treatment for infertility (RR = 0.95, confidence interval 0.82-1.11), after surgery or FDs, and whatever the type, the duration of use and the age at first use of FDs (Table 4). However, infertility treatment was associated with an increased risk, of borderline significance, of breast cancer among women with a family history of breast cancer. This last result had limited statistical power.

Conclusions.—Our study provides evidence that treatment for infertility does not influence breast cancer risk overall. An interaction with a familial history of breast cancer is possible but should be investigated further.

▶ Because infertility and breast cancer are common disorders and because infertility treatments often increase ovarian estrogen production, albeit for relatively short periods, there is concern that infertility treatments may increase the risk of breast cancer. This prospective cohort study of more than 90,000 French women with over 2,500 cases of breast cancer after a mean follow-up of almost 10 years offers some assurance that FDs do not increase the risk of breast cancer. There was no overall significant association between breast cancer and treatment of infertility, with a relative risk of 0.95 and a confidence interval of 0.82 to 1.11. When evaluated individually, neither clomiphene nor human chorionic gonadotropin nor human menopausal gonadotropin treatment had any effect on breast cancer risk. This is probably the largest cohort study published investigating the risk of fertility treatment on breast cancer. It is in general agreement with previous studies which, for the most part, have not found an increased risk of breast cancer after fertility treatment.[1,2] However, there is an obvious need for continued surveillance, as larger studies and longer follow-up will be required for a definite answer.

R. Barnes, MD

References

1. Brinton LA, Moghissi KS, Scoccia B, et al: Ovulation induction and cancer risk. *Fertil Steril* 83:261-274, quiz 525-526, 2005.
2. Brinton LA, Scoccia B, Moghissi KS, et al: Breast cancer risk associated with ovulation-stimulating drugs. *Hum Reprod* 19:2005-2013, 2004.

Dietary Patterns and the Risk of Postmenopausal Breast Cancer
Fung TT, Hu FB, Holmes MD, et al (Simmons College, Boston; Harvard School of Public Health, Boston; Harvard Med School, Boston)
Int J Cancer 116:116-121, 2005   26–6

Abstract.—The association between individual foods and breast cancer has been inconsistent. Therefore, we examined the association between diet and risk of postmenopausal breast cancer by the alternative approach of dietary patterns. Dietary patterns were identified with factor analysis from food consumption data collected from a food frequency questionnaire in 1984. Relative risks were computed using proportional hazard models and adjusted for known risk factors for breast cancer. Between 1984 and 2000, we ascertained 3,026 incident cases of postmenopausal breast cancer. We identified 2 major dietary patterns. The prudent pattern is characterized by higher intake of fruits, vegetables, whole grains, low-fat dairy products, fish and poultry, while the Western pattern is characterized by higher intake of red and processed meats, refined grains, sweets and desserts and high-fat dairy products. Neither of the patterns was associated with overall risk of postmenopausal breast cancer. However, a positive association between the Western pattern score was observed among smokers at baseline (relative risk = 1.44, comparing top to bottom quintiles; 95% CI = 1.02–2.03; p for trend = 0.03). An inverse association was observed between the prudent pattern and estrogen receptor-negative cancer (relative risk = 0.62; 95% CI = 0.45–0.88; p for trend = 0.006). Among the major food groups, higher consumptions of fruits (relative risk for 1 serving/day increase = 0.88; 95% CI = 0.80–0.97; p = 0.009) and vegetables (relative risk = 0.94; 95% CI = 0.88–0.99; p = 0.03) were significantly associated with decreased risk for ER$^-$ breast cancer. In conclusion, we did not observe an overall association between the prudent or Western pattern and overall breast cancer risk. However, a Western-type diet may elevate risk of breast cancer among smokers, and a prudent diet may protect against estrogen receptive-negative tumors.

▶ Studies into the etiology and epidemiology of postmenopausal breast cancer serve to continue the ongoing struggle between environment and genomics. The study from the Harvard School of Public Health provides interesting information concerning the potential impact of food and the development of breast cancer. The association between individual foods and the development of breast cancer has thus far been inconsistent and not definitive. In this study, the authors compare 2 major dietary patterns, a prudent dietary pattern that was rich in vegetables, low-fat proteins, and high-fiber foods and another group characterized by a more "American" diet of foods with high levels of carbohydrates, high-fat meats, and small amounts of vegetables and fresh fruits. The authors did not observe an overall association between either food pattern and overall breast cancer risk. However, they did find in their subanalysis that the American-type diet was possibly associated with an increased risk of breast cancer among those who smoked and that the "prudent" diet may protect against estrogen receptor–negative tumors. These preliminary data serve to increase interest in the complex interactions between our environment and the development of breast cancer.

L. P. Shulman, MD

Alcohol Exposure and Breast Cancer: Results of the Women's Contraceptive and Reproductive Experiences Study
McDonald JA, Mandel MG, Marchbanks PA, et al (Ctrs for Disease Control and Prevention, Atlanta, Ga; Univ of Vermont, Burlington; Fred Hutchinson Cancer Research Ctr, Seattle; et al)
Cancer Epidemiol Biomarkers Prev 13:2106-2116, 2004   26–7

Objectives.—To explore associated biological outcomes and clarify the role of timing of exposure in the alcohol-breast cancer relationship.

Methods.—In a population-based study of 4,575 women ages 35 to 64 years diagnosed with invasive breast cancer between 1994 and 1998 and 4,682 controls, we collected details of lifetime alcohol use and factors that could confound or modify the alcohol-breast cancer relationship. We used conditional logistic regression to compute the odds of breast cancer among drinkers relative to nondrinkers at all ages and at ages 35 to 49 and 50 to 64 years separately.

Results.—Recent consumption (at reference age minus two) of ≥7 drinks per week was associated with increased risk [odds ratio (OR), 1.2; 95% CI, 1.01-1.3] and evidence of dose response was observed. Most of the excess was observed among women ages 50-64 years (OR 1.3; 95% CI, 1.1-1.6), although the test for age interaction was not statistically significant (Table 4). Exposure later in life seemed more important than early exposure. Excess breast cancer associated with recent consumption was restricted to localized disease. When outcome was examined according to tumor hormone recep-

TABLE 4.—Risk of Breast Cancer by Type of Alcoholic Beverage, Number of Drinks per Week 2 Years Before Reference Age, and Age Group (Women's CARE Study)

Type of Alcoholic Beverage	Overall			Ages 35-49 y			Ages 50-64 y		
	Case	Control	OR*	Case	Control	OR* (95% CI)	Case	Control	OR* (95% CI)
Beer†									
None	3,659	3,748	1.0	1,684	1,764	1.0	1,975	1,984	1.0
<7	754	779	0.9 (0.8-1.1)	446	494	0.9 (0.7-1.0)	308	285	1.0 (0.9-1.3)
≥7	114	112	1.0 (0.8-1.4)	76	73	1.1 (0.8-1.6)	38	39	1.0 (0.6-1.6)
Wine†									
None	3,065	3,210	1.0	1,414	1,538	1.0	1,651	1,672	1.0
<7	1,232	1,254	1.0 (0.9-1.1)	698	704	1.0 (0.9-1.2)	534	550	0.9 (0.7-1.0)
≥7	230	175	1.3 (1.1-1.6)	94	89	1.1 (0.8-1.6)	136	86	1.5 (1.1-2.0)
Liquor†									
None	3,413	3,543	1.0	1,642	1,733	1.0	1,771	1,810	1.0
<7	986	978	1.0 (0.9-1.2)	518	543	1.0 (0.8-1.1)	468	435	1.1 (0.9-1.3)
≥7	128	118	1.1 (0.8-1.4)	46	55	0.8 (0.5-1.3)	82	63	1.3 (0.9-1.9)

*ORs (versus none) were derived by conditional logistic regression (with study site, race, and 5-year age group as conditioning variables) and were adjusted for menopausal status, age at menarche, age at menopause, number of term pregnancies, age at first term pregnancy, body mass index, family history of breast cancer, use of hormone replacement therapy, and use of oral contraceptives. Women with missing values for any of the specified variables were excluded.

†Estimates are computed separately for beer, wine, and liquor, with all three factors in the model.

Abbreviations: CARE, Contraceptive and Reproductive Experiences; OR, odds ratio; CI, confidence interval.

(Courtesy of McDonald JA, Mandel MG, Marchbanks PA, et al: Alcohol exposure and breast cancer: Results of the Women's Contraceptive and Reproductive Experiences Study. *Cancer Epidemiol Biomarkers Prev* 13:2106-2116, 2004.)

tor status, highest risks were observed for estrogen receptor–positive/ progesterone receptor–negative tumors (OR 1.6; 95% CI, 1.2-2.3).

Conclusions.—The effect of timing of alcohol exposure on breast cancer risk is complicated and will require additional study focused on this one issue. Further work is needed to explain how alcohol exposure, sex hormones, and tumor receptor status interact.

▶ A small association between alcohol consumption and breast cancer diagnosis has been found by multiple investigators. This article stands out among them by examining the effect of timing of exposure on this admittedly small but reproducible risk. Here, early exposure had little effect on risk. It is interesting to note that excess risk was limited to localized disease.

R. D. Arias, MD

Consumption of Vegetables and Fruits and Risk of Breast Cancer
van Gils CH, Peeters PHM, Bueno-de-Mesquita HB, et al (Univ Med Ctr, Utrecht, The Netherlands; Natl Inst for Public Health and the Environment, Bilthoven, The Netherlands; German Inst of Human Nutrition Potsdam-Rehbrücke, Nuthetal, Germany; et al)
JAMA 293:183-193, 2005   26–8

Context.—The intake of vegetables and fruits has been thought to protect against breast cancer. Most of the evidence comes from case-control studies, but a recent pooled analysis of the relatively few published cohort studies suggests no significantly reduced breast cancer risk is associated with vegetable and fruit consumption.

Objective.—To examine the relation between total and specific vegetable and fruit intake and the incidence of breast cancer.

Design, Setting, and Participants.—Prospective study of 285,526 women between the ages of 25 and 70 years, participating in the European Prospective Investigation Into Cancer and Nutrition (EPIC) study, recruited from 8 of the 10 participating European countries. Participants completed a dietary questionnaire in 1992-1998 and were followed up for incidence of cancer until 2002.

Main Outcome Measures.—Relative risks for breast cancer by total and specific vegetable and fruit intake. Analyses were stratified by age at recruitment and study center. Relative risks were adjusted for established breast cancer risk factors.

Results.—During 1,486,402 person-years (median duration of follow-up, 5.4 years), 3659 invasive incident breast cancer cases were reported. No significant associations between vegetable or fruit intake and breast cancer risk were observed. Relative risks for the highest vs the lowest quintile were 0.98 (95% confidence interval [CI], 0.84-1.14) for total vegetables, 1.09 (95% CI, 0.94-1.25) for total fruit, and 1.05 (95% CI, 0.92-1.20) for fruit and vegetable juices. For 6 specific vegetable subgroups no associations with breast cancer risk were observed either.

Conclusion.—Although the period of follow-up is limited for now, the results suggest that total or specific vegetable and fruit intake is not associated with risk for breast cancer.

▶ Belief in a protective effect of fruit and vegetable consumption has been supported by a number of breast cancer case-control studies. This association, when found, has been quite modest, and the specific mechanism by which protection is exerted remains elusive. This analysis is derived from the large prospective data from the EPIC study. Sadly, the authors found no association between fruit and vegetable consumption and breast cancer risk, thus decreasing the evidence for this potentially modifiable risk factor.

R. D. Arias, MD

European Randomized, Multicenter Study of Goserelin (Zoladex) in the Management of Mastalgia
Mansel RE, Goyal A, Preece P, et al (Cardiff Univ, Wales; Ninewells Hosp, Dundee, Scotland; Univ of East Anglia, Norwich, England; et al)
Am J Obstet Gynecol 191:1942-1949, 2004   26–9

Background.—Breast pain is a common symptom in patients attending breast clinics. The purpose of this study was to evaluate the efficacy of goserelin (Zoladex) as compared with sham injection in patients with mastalgia.

Study Design.—One hundred forty-seven premenopausal women were randomized to treatment with either goserelin injection (3.6 mg/month) or sham injection for a total of 6 injections. Patients' daily self-assessment of breast pain using Cardiff breast pain chart was recorded during the 6-month treatment period and for 6 months in the posttreatment period.

Results.—A significant treatment difference between the 2 groups in favor of goserelin was noted during the treatment period. Mean breast pain score improved by 67% in the goserelin group and 35% in the sham group during the treatment period. The mean pain scores increased in both groups in the posttreatment period. No significant posttreatment difference was found between the two groups. Side effects were more common with goserelin than sham injection. Patients receiving goserelin experienced vaginal dryness, hot flushes, decreased libido, oily skin or hair, and a decrease in breast size more frequently than sham patients.

Conclusion.—Goserelin is an effective short-term treatment for mastalgia. However, side effects are common, and thus, goserelin should be kept in reserve for patients who are refractory to other forms of treatment. Potentially, goserelin could be used to induce a rapid relief of symptoms that could be maintained with alternative therapies.

▶ The search for a pharmacologic intervention for women with mastalgia continues. Currently, the only Food and Drug Administration–approved drug with an indication for the treatment of mastalgia is danazol. Its use is substantially limited by its side effect profile. This evaluation of goserelin revealed similar limitations. It should be noted that the use of this potent gonadotropin-releasing hormone analogue did reduce the concomitant use of analgesics compared with a sham injection. When a safe, effective, alternative therapy becomes available, there may be a place for a short course of goserelin to initiate rapid relief of symptoms.

R. D. Arias, MD

Fertility Pattern Does Not Explain Social Gradient in Breast Cancer in Denmark

Danø H, Hansen KD, Jensen P, et al (Univ of Copenhagen; Univ of Aarhus, Denmark)
Int J Cancer 111:451-456, 2004   26–10

Abstract.—The present study was undertaken to assess the impact of reproductive behavior on the social class gradient in breast cancer occurrence in Denmark. Objectives were to study whether the gradient across socioeconomic groups could be explained by fertility differences, whether the gradient across educational groups could be explained by fertility differences and whether the effect of socioeconomic group on breast cancer incidence and mortality could be explained by education and vice versa. We studied 674,084 women aged 20-39 at the census on 9 November 1970 for whom we had complete data on fertility history. The cohort was followed up for breast cancer incidence and mortality until 8 November 1998. Fertility history varied considerably across socioeconomic group, where 38% of the academics were childless at the age of 30, in contrast to only 8% of women in agriculture. The academics had the highest risk of breast cancer and women in agriculture had the lowest risk. For incidence, the gradient in the relative risks was 1.74, which changed to 1.49 when fertility history was incorporated and to 1.29 when school education was also taken into account. For school education, women with ≥ 12 years of schooling had the highest risk and women with ≤ 7 years of schooling had the lowest risk. For incidence, the gradient in the relative risk was 1.38, which changed to 1.26 when fertility history was incorporated and to 1.22 when socioeconomic group was also taken into account.

▶ The small but well-established association between higher education and breast cancer risk is evaluated for confounding effect in this Danish cohort study. In this population, fertility history accounted for one third of the excess risk associated with socioeconomic standing. The remaining excess risk must be accounted for in other ways that distinguish the more privileged woman. The observation that breast cancer mortality was highest in academics and lowest in agricultural workers is surprising. These authors expect the dramatic increase in well-educated Danish women will herald an increase in breast cancer incidence.

R. D. Arias, MD

27 Ectopic Pregnancy

The Role of Sonographic Endometrial Patterns and Endometrial Thickness in the Differential Diagnosis of Ectopic Pregnancy
Hammoud AO, Hammoud I, Bujold E, et al (Wayne State Univ, Detroit; Henry Ford Hosp, Detroit)
Am J Obstet Gynecol 192:1370-1375, 2005   27–1

Objective.—The purpose of this study was to examine the usefulness of the endometrial trilaminar pattern and thickness in the diagnosis of ectopic pregnancy.

Study Design.—We reviewed patient records for clinical and ultrasonographic data for patients with the suspicion of ectopic pregnancy. The trilaminar pattern (Fig 1) and endometrial thickness were tested as predictors for the diagnosis of ectopic pregnancy.

Results.—The trilaminar pattern had a specificity of 94% and sensitivity of 38% (n = 403 women). The mean endometrial thickness was thinner in patients with ectopic, compared with normal pregnancy (9.5 ± 5.7 mm vs 12.4 ± 5.9 mm; $P = .035$). Patients with normal pregnancy or first-trimester losses had comparable thicknesses (12.4 ± 5.9 mm vs 12.5 ± 8.0 mm). The receiver operator curve showed that there was no thickness value useful for the diagnosis of ectopic pregnancy.

Conclusion.—The trilaminar pattern is specific for the diagnosis of ectopic pregnancy, but it is associated with low sensitivity. The endometrial thickness tends to be thinner in patients with an ectopic pregnancy. Comment:

▶ US remains an important element in the diagnosis, but is rarely diagnostic by itself. Diagnosis with US has primarily relied on the presence or absence of an intrauterine pregnancy or, more rarely, an identified extrauterine pregnancy. However, there are other US findings that may be useful in the diagnosis of an ectopic pregnancy, such as nonspecific but suspicious adnexal masses. The appearance of the endometrial stripe can also be suggestive of an ectopic pregnancy. It has been known for some time that a thin endometrial stripe is more likely to be associated with an ectopic pregnancy than a thick stripe, but the wide range of normal values has limited its usedfulness.[1,2] The trilaminar pattern has also been suggested as predictive of ectopic pregnancy.[3] This study is by far the largest to investigate this pattern (403 patients). The study's findings are consistent with those of previous smaller studies that found a

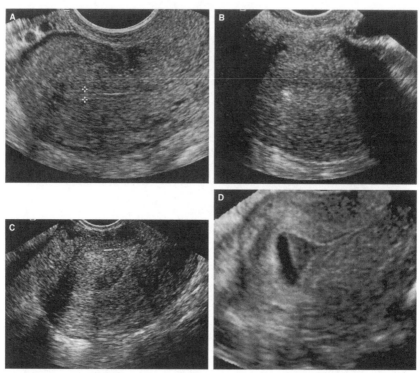

FIGURE 1.—Classification of endometrial patterns on transvaginal ultrasound. **A,** Sagittal view of the uterus with an endometrial trilaminar pattern. **B,** Transverse view of a homogenous hyperechoic endometrial pattern. **C,** Sagittal view of a heterogeneous endometrial pattern. **D,** Sagittal view of a pseudogestational sac that contains fluid and debris. (Courtesy of Hammoud AO, Hammoud I, Bujold E, et al: The role of sonographic endometrial patterns and endometrial thickness in the differential diagnosis of ectopic pregnancy. *Am J Obstet Gynecol* 192:1370-1375, 2005. Copyright 2005 by Elsevier. Reprinted by permission.)

poor sensitivity but an excellent specificity when a trilaminar pattern was found.[3] This study would suggest that the endometrial trilaminar pattern, if present, should be highly suggestive of ectopic pregnancy.

G. H. Lipscomb, MD

References

1. Spandorfer SD, Barnhart KT: Endometrial stripe thickness as a predictor of ectopic pregnancy. *Fertil Steril* 66:474-477, 1996.
2. Mol BW, Hajenius PJ, Engelsbel S, et al: Are gestational age and endometrial thickness alternatives for serum human chorionic gonadotropin as criteria for the diagnosis of ectopic pregnancy? *Fertil Steril* 72:643-645, 1999.
3. Lavie O, Boldes R, Neuman M, et al: Ultrasonographic "endometrial three-layer" pattern: A unique finding in ectopic pregnancy. *J Clin Ultrasound* 24:179-183, 1996.

Symptomatic Patients With an Early Viable Intrauterine Pregnancy: hCG Curves Redefined

Barnhart KT, Sammel MD, Rinaudo PF, et al (Univ of Pennsylvania, Philadelphia)

Obstet Gynecol 104:50-55, 2004   27–2

Objective.—To analyze the change in serial human chorionic gonadotropin (hCG) levels in women symptomatic with pain or bleeding who presented with nondiagnostic ultrasonography but were ultimately confirmed to have a viable intrauterine pregnancy.

Methods.—The rise in serial hCG measures were modeled over time, with the start point defined in 2 ways: by last menstrual period and by date of presentation for care. Both semiparametric (spline) curves and linear random-effects models were explored. The slope and projected increase of hCG were calculated to define 99% of viable intrauterine pregnancies.

Results.—A total of 287 subjects met inclusion criteria and contributed 861 measurements of hCG. On average, these subjects contributed 3.00 observations and were followed up for 5.25 days. A linear increase in log hCG best described the pattern of rise. Curves derived from last menstrual period and day of presentation do not differ substantially. The median slope for a rise of hCG after 1 day was 1.50, (or a 50% increase); 2.24 after 2 days (or a 124% rise), and 5.00 after 4 days. The fastest rise was 1.81 at 1 day, 3.28 at 2 days, and 10.76 at 4 days. The slowest or minimal rise for a normal viable intrauterine pregnancy was 24% at 1 day and 53% at 2 days.

Conclusion.—These data define the slowest rise in serial hCG values for a potentially viable gestation and will aid in distinguishing a viable early pregnancy from a miscarriage or ectopic pregnancy. The minimal rise in serial hCG values for women with a viable intrauterine pregnancy is "slower" than previously reported, suggesting that intervention to diagnosis and treat an abnormal gestation should be more conservative.

▶ The use of serial hCG titers is crucial for the modern nonsurgical algorithms to diagnose early ectopic pregnancies. Although there is consensus that the rise in hCG titers is distinctly different between most ectopic pregnancies and normal intrauterine pregnancies, there is less agreement on the appropriate rise in normal viable pregnancies. Previous studies were frequently performed with relatively small numbers of patients and performed on populations that might not be generalized to women at risk for ectopic pregnancy or miscarriage. For example, the frequently quoted 66% rise over 2 days was arrived after the study of only 20 patients.[1] This study is important in that women symptomatic for pain or bleeding and with a nondiagnositic US but who were ultimately found to have a viable intrauterine pregnancy were included. Since this population is precisely the group that would be screened for potential ectopic pregnancy, delineation of the cutoff points for hCG rise for viable pregnancies is of utmost importance. Although this study did reveal a much slower rise in hCG titers for viable pregnancies in this at-risk group, it did confirm the frequently used cutoff for nonviable pregnancies of less than a 50% rise in 48 hours. All viable pregnancies had a minimum of a 53% hCG rise over 48 hours.

G. H. Lipscomb, MD

Reference

1. Kadar N, Caldwell BV, Romero R: A method of screening for ectopic pregnancy and its indications. *Obstet Gynecol* 58:162-166, 1981.

Presence of a Yolk Sac on Transvaginal Sonography Is the Most Reliable Predictor of Single-Dose Methotrexate Treatment Failure in Ectopic Pregnancy

Bixby S, Tello R, Kuligowska E (Boston Univ)
J Ultrasound Med 24:591-598, 2005   27–3

Objective.—The purpose of this study was to determine which imaging characteristics can be used as prognostic indicators in conjunction with β-human chorionic gonadotropin (β-hCG) levels in the treatment of ectopic pregnancy (EP) with single-dose methotrexate (MTX).

Methods.—A retrospective study was performed on 62 patients (age range, 16-47 years; mean, 29 years) treated with MTX for EP from November 2000 to August 2003. The transvaginal sonographic findings in each case were analyzed for the presence and size of an extraovarian mass or a pseudogestational sac, amount of free fluid, presence of a yolk sac, and fetal heart motion. Patient age and β-hCG level were also noted. Success of treat-

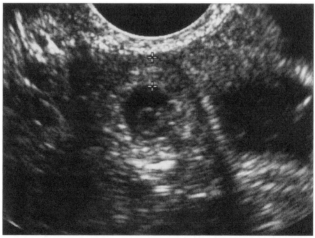

FIGURE 4.—Extraovarian mass containing a yolk sac in a patient who had single-dose methotrexate treatment failure. (Courtesy of Bixby S, Tello R, Kuligowska E: Presence of a yolk sac on transvaginal sonography is the most reliable predictor of single-dose methotrexate treatment failure in ectopic pregnancy. *J Ultrasound Med* 24:591-598, 2005. Publisher AIUM)

ment was defined as a single dose of MTX that resulted in appropriate lowering of β-hCG levels.

Results.—Of 62 patients, 17 (27%) had single-dose MTX treatment failure. A yolk sac was identified in 15 (88%) of the 17 treatment failures and in none of the cases in which treatment was successful (positive predictive value, 100%) (Fig 4). The average β-hCG level in the cohort of patients who had single-dose treatment failure was 3282 mIU/mL compared with 1544 mIU/mL in the treatment success cohort. The presence of fetal heart motion was seen in only 1 patient, and this patient had treatment failure. The age of the patient, size of the extraovarian mass, presence of a pseudogestational sac, and amount of free fluid did not correlate with outcome.

Conclusions.—The presence of a yolk sac was always associated with treatment failure in single-dose MTX treatment of EP and was the most reliable predictor of failure among all features analyzed. The β-hCG level was a useful adjunct. A prediction rule was created correlating the probability of treatment success with the β-hCG level.

▶ Traditional risk factors for failure of MTX treatment of EP include ectopic size, serum hCG levels, serum progesterone levels, and the presence or absence of ectopic fetal cardiac activity or free peritoneal blood. Recently, a history of previous EP and the presence of a yolk sac have also been suggested as risk factors.[1,2] The reviewed study presents further data on the effect of a yolk sac on MTX treatment failure.

This article was a retrospective analysis of pharmacy records of any patients receiving MTX for EP at the authors' institution over a 3-year period. Patients were apparently diagnosed and treated by multiple physicians, raising some concerns about the uniformity of diagnostic and treatment protocols. As with many similar studies on risk factors for failure, the treatment group was small and totaled only 63 patients. Of the 84 patients initially identified as having MTX ordered, 9 subsequently had a spontaneous abortion of an intrauterine pregnancy. This raises doubts about the accuracy of the diagnosis for the group. However, of the 62 patients actually included in the review, 60 did undergo dilatation and curettage (D&C) before treatment. Success in this study was defined as either an increase in hCG of 50% between days 4 and 7 or a need for a second course of MTX. This is different than generally used in this type of study. The biggest limitation was the failure to perform a multiple regression analysis to confirm that the presence of a yolk sac was an independent risk factor for failure rather than a co-indicator of elevated hCG as has been shown for many other markers.[3] The level of hCG was noted to be higher in failures than success. However, statistical analysis was not provided, nor were data presented in the article to allow for the calculation of the influence of hCG on failure rates. While this study provides further data to suggest that the presence of a yolk sac may be a risk factor for failure of medical therapy for EP, the data presented are not of sufficient quality to currently recommend using this factor to decide on candidates for medical therapy.

G. H. Lipscomb, MD

References

1. Lipscomb GH, Givens VA, Meyer ML, et al: Previous ectopic pregnancy as a risk factor for failure of systemic methotrexate therapy. *Fertil Steril* 81:1221-1224, 2004.
2. Potter MB, Lepine LA, Jamieson DJ: Predictors of success with methotrexate treatment of tubal ectopic pregnancy at Grady Memorial Hospital. *Am J Obstet Gynecol* 188:1192-1194, 2003.
3. Lipscomb GH, McCord ML, Huff G, et al: Predictors of success of methotrexate treatment in women with tubal ectopic pregnancies. *N Engl J Med* 341:1874-1878, 1999.

Frozen Section Examination of Endometrial Curettings in the Diagnosis of Ectopic Pregnancy
Barak S, Oettinger M, Perri A, et al (Israel Inst of Technology, Haifa)
Acta Obstet Gynecol Scand 84:43-47, 2005   27–4

Background.—The aim of our study was to determine the accuracy and validity of frozen section analysis of endometrial curettings in differentiating between abnormal intrauterine and ectopic pregnancies.

Methods.—A retrospective analysis of the database of the Department of Obstetrics and Gynecology in our institute was performed from January 1998 to September 1999. In 70 women with a suspected ectopic pregnancy a diagnostic curettage was sent for frozen section examination because products of conception could not be identified macroscopically in the curettings. Routine paraffin fixation specimens were also prepared from the endometrial curettings. A frozen section diagnosis was considered correct if it concurred with the final pathologic diagnosis, and incorrect if it differed. The sensitivity, specificity, positive predictive value and negative predictive value of a frozen section in identification of conception products were calculated.

Results.—Of the 70 frozen section studies the diagnosis was correct in 63 (90%), and incorrect in 7 (10%) cases. Of 50 specimens interpreted as negative on frozen sections (no products of conception noted), 6 (12%) were found to contain conception products on final pathologic review. One of the 20 (5%) specimens interpreted as positive by a frozen section failed to demonstrate products of conception on a final pathologic section. The sensitivity of frozen sections in the diagnosis of ectopic pregnancy was 76%, specificity 97.8%; positive predictive value 95%; negative predictive value 88% and accuracy 90%.

Conclusions.—Frozen section examination is a rapid and accurate method for identifying products of conception in endometrial curettings, and may reduce delay in the diagnosis of an ectopic pregnancy and in the institution of therapy.

▶ In patients undergoing dilatation and curettage (D&C) for presumed ectopic pregnancy, the diagnosis is frequently delayed while waiting for repeat human chorionic gonadotropin (hCG) levels or final pathology. This article examines the use of frozen section for rapid diagnosis in patients in whom villi could not be identified macroscopically with saline floatation. Overall, frozen section was most accurate when villi were obtained. Even then, 1 (5%) of 20 villi-positive specimens was a false positive. Likewise, 12% of negative specimens were ultimately found to have villi on final pathology. Several factors should be considered when interpreting this study. The number of patients studied (70) makes drawing conclusions risky. However, this study does agree with other generally small studies that indicated frozen section is most accurate if villi are found.[1-3] However, most studies have found that even when final pathology found no villi, that a large proportion of such patients will ultimately be diagnosed as a completed abortion or a resolving pregnancy of undetermined site. The majority of patients will still require serial hCG levels to arrive at an accurate diagnosis. As such, the use of frozen section examination of curettings in patients undergoing D&C for presumed ectopic pregnancy has limited clinical utility.

G. H. Lipscomb, MD

References

1. Spandorfer SD, Menzin AW, Barnhart KT, et al: Efficacy of frozen-section evaluation of uterine curettings in the diagnosis of ectopic pregnancy. *Am J Obstet Gynecol* 175:603-605, 1996.
2. Lindahl B, Ahlgren M: Identification of choronic villi in abortion specimens. *Obstet Gynecol* 67:79-81, 1986.
3. Kristiansen JD, Clausen I, Nielsen MN, et al: Steriomicroscopic demonstration of chorionic villi: Differentiation between miscarriage and ectopic pregnancy. *Br J Obstet Gynaecol* 100:839-841, 1993.

Do We Need to Follow Up Complete Miscarriages With Serum Human Chorionic Gonadotrophin Levels?
Condous G, Okaro E, Khalid A, et al (St George's Hosp, London)
BJOG 112:827-829, 2005   27–5

Abstract.—Despite a history of heavy vaginal bleeding with clots, a proportion of women diagnosed with complete miscarriage, using transvaginal sonography (TVS), have an underlying ectopic pregnancy (EP). We evaluated the need for hormonal follow up in women with history and scan findings suggestive of complete miscarriage. One hundred and fifty-two consecutive women with findings suggesting complete miscarriage at presentation based on their history and TVS were presented to the Early Pregnancy Unit. Serum human chorionic gonadotrophin (hCG) levels were taken at presentation and 48 hours. All women were followed up until hCG was <5 u/L or a pregnancy was visualised on TVS either inside or outside the uterus. Overall, 9 (5.9%) of 152 women with an apparent complete miscarriage had an underlying EP. A diagnosis of complete miscarriage based on history and scan findings alone is unreliable. These women should be managed as 'pregnancies of unknown location' with serum hCG follow up.

▶ Although this study was only a "short communication," it is important because it illustrates the need for vigilance in patients with an apparent complete miscarriage. In this series, 5.9% were diagnosed as an EP. The study group was a subset of the larger group of patients who present with a provable miscarriage. All patients presented with a positive pregnancy test and heavy bleeding with passage of clots but without tissue available for pathology or prior documentation of an intrauterine pregnancy. Unfortunately, the diagnosis of EP may be questioned in some of these patients. Patients with rising hCG levels did not undergo dilatation and curettage, and the use of the presence of an adnexal mass on US as a confirmatory test is suspect unless a gestational pole, yolk sac, or cardiac activity is seen. Unfortunately, this was not elaborated in the brief article. Nevertheless, 6 of the 9 EPs diagnosed with US were confirmed with laparoscopy. In addition, there is the possibility that at least some of the patients ultimately diagnosed as a miscarriage had resolving EPs. This would be of academic interest only and would not be clinically significant, since they resolved without incidence. While this study could be improved, it does suggest that the use of serial hCG titers in patients with presumed but unproved miscarriages would be prudent.

G. H. Lipscomb, MD

Comparison of Multidose and Single-Dose Methotrexate Protocols for the Treatment of Ectopic Pregnancy
Lipscomb GH, Givens VM, Meyer NL, et al (Univ of Tennessee, Memphis)
Am J Obstet Gynecol 192:1844-1848, 2005   27–6

Background.—Intramuscular methotrexate therapy has become the most common medical treatment for ectopic pregnancy. However, the most appropriate treatment protocol has remained controversial. The 2 most commonly used treatment protocols in the United States involve either a multidose or a single-dose protocol. There has been no direct comparison of these 2 protocols, but a recent meta-analysis found that the single-dose protocol was associated with a significantly increased failure rate. Success rates for treatment of ectopic pregnancy with either the multidose or single-dose methotrexate regimen were compared in 643 patients from the same database.

Methods.—The comparison included demographics, gestational age, serum human chorionic gonadotropin levels, progesterone levels, ectopic sac size and volume, overall ectopic mass size and volume, ectopic cardiac activity, history of ectopic pregnancy, number of treatment days, methotrexate doses, and outcome in consecutive patients with ectopic pregnancy who were treated with methotrexate.

Results.—Success rates were comparable between patients with multidose and single-dose therapy (95% vs 90%, respectively). The 2 treatment protocols were also comparable in terms of human chorionic gonadotropin and progesterone levels, gestational age, ectopic size, ectopic volume, and ectopic mass volume. Patients who received single-dose methotrexate therapy were significantly heavier (146 lb vs 159 lb), had greater ectopic cardiac activity (3.1% vs. 10.3%), and received fewer doses of methotrexate.

Conclusions.—Single-dose methotrexate therapy appears to be as effective as multidose therapy for the treatment of ectopic pregnancy.

▶ The ideal treatment protocol for medical treatment of ectopic pregnancy with methotrexate remains undetermined. In the United States, most medical protocols use variants of either the "multidose" or "single-dose" protocol. Because of its simplicity and low complication rate, the single-dose protocol is most commonly used. However, there has been a long-standing debate on which protocol is the most appropriate and most effective. Unfortunately, a direct comparison between the 2 protocols has never been performed. An excellent meta-analysis of 260 multidose patients and 1067 single-dose patients showed that multidose was superior to single-dose methotrexate.[1] One disadvantage of meta-analysis is that patients cannot be directly compared; instead, compiled data from the included studies rather than individual raw data must be compared. Likewise, 100 of the 260 multidose patients and 350 of the 1067 single-dose patients in the meta-analysis were from the reviewed study's database, thus heavily weighting the study with those patients. The advantages of the reviewed study were that the authors were able to directly compare individual patient data, and that both patient groups were treated by essentially the same physician at the same institution, albeit during different time periods. A total of 677 patients from the same institution were compared. This is the largest series of such patients yet reported. Although this study suggests that single-dose methotrexate is as effective as multidose methotrexate, a definitive study has not yet been performed.

G. H. Lipscomb, MD

Reference

1. Barnhart KT, Gosman G, Ashby R, et al: The medical management of ectopic pregnancy: A meta-analysis comparing "single dose" and "multidose" regimens. *Obstet Gynecol* 101:778-784, 2003.

Medical Treatment of Ruptured With Hemodynamically Stable and Unruptured Ectopic Pregnancy Patients
Kumtepe Y, Kadanali S (Ataturk Univ, Erzurum, Turkey)
Eur J Obstet Gynecol Reprod Biol 116:221-225, 2004   27–7

Objective.—To determine the success rate of methotrexate treatment of ruptured ectopic pregnancy with hemodynamically stable and unruptured ectopic pregnancy patients.

Study Design.—This prospective clinical study was carried out on 161 patients with suspected tubal ectopic pregnancy. Forty-six patients have been accepted as ruptured ectopic pregnancy with hemodynamically stable and 115 patients have been accepted as unruptured ectopic pregnancy. All patients diagnosed with ectopic pregnancy were treated by single dose (50 mg/m²) methotrexate if they have stable hemodynamia and fulfill the criteria of methotrexate treatment. Weekly β-hCG level was measured and if this level was under 10 IU/L, the treatment has been accepted as successful. Mann-Whitney and Fisher's exact tests were used (SPSS, 10.0) for statistical analysis.

Results.—The success rates of methotrexate treatments in ruptured ectopic pregnancy patients with hemodynamically stable and in patients with unruptured ectopic pregnancy were observed as 62% and 81%, respectively (*P* < 0.001). The treatment was successfully completed in all expectant management patients.

Conclusion.—Although methotrexate treatment of ruptured ectopic pregnancy with hemodynamically stable patients is not as successful as in unruptured ectopic pregnancy group, 62% success rate in this group may promise a treatment choice before surgery application.

▶ Most physicians would be appalled at the idea of medically treating a ruptured ectopic pregnancy. However, the authors correctly point out that many "ruptured" ectopic pregnancies have intra-abdominal bleeding from tubal bleeding or tubal abortion without rupture, and that some true ruptures do not continue to have active bleeding. The title is thus somewhat misleading in that most of these patients were not true tubal ruptures. The diagnosis of "rupture" was made based on US findings of 380 mL of pelvic fluid. The fact that many patients with ectopic pregnancies and at least some hematoperitoneum have an intact tube is well documented in the literature but not necessarily well known by many physicians. Using culdocentesis to document hematoperitoneum, Vermesh et al[1] noted that more than 50% of ectopic pregnacies with a positive culdocentesis had an unruptured fallopian tube.

In this study, surgery was performed on "ruptured" medically treated ectopic patients for a falling hematocrit or the development of rebound tenderness. Although patients with hemodynamically "ruptured" ectopic pregnancies had a higher failure rate (38%) than patients with "unruptured" ectopic pregnancies (19%), the study does demonstrate that a considerable number of patients with free fluid in the pelvis will be successful with medical therapy. This confirms the experience at the University of Tennessee where free fluid, presumably blood, confined to the pelvis is not considered a contraindication in hemodynamically stable patients with ectopic pregnancies. In fact, blood confined to the pelvis was not a risk factor for failure of methotrexate therapy in a review of 360 consecutively treated patients.[2] However, it is not clear how many of these patients would have more than 380 mL as required in this study.

G. H. Lipscomb, MD

References

1. Vermesh M, Graczykowski JW, Sauer MV: Reevaluation of the role of culdocentesis in the management of ectopic pregnancy. *Am J Obstet Gynecol* 162:411-413, 1990.
2. Lipscomb GH, Mccord ML, Stovall TG, et al: Predictors of success of methotrexate treatment in women with tubal ectopic pregnancies. *N Engl J Med* 341:1974-1978, 1999.

Cost-effectiveness of Presumptively Medically Treating Women at Risk for Ectopic Pregnancy Compared With First Performing a Dilatation and Curettage
Ailawadi M, Lorch SA, Barnhart KT (Univ of Pennsylvania, Philadelphia; Children's Hosp of Philadelphia)
Fertil Steril 83:376-382, 2005
27–8

Objective.—To compare the cost and complication rate of two alternative strategies for the diagnosis and medical management of ectopic pregnancy when ultrasound is nondiagnostic.

Design.—A decision tree was constructed to compare [1] dilatation and curettage (D&C) followed by treatment of all ectopic pregnancies with methotrexate versus [2] empiric treatment of all patients with possible ectopic pregnancies with methotrexate without D&C.

Setting.—University setting.

Patient(s).—Ten thousand hypothetical women with nonviable pregnancies and a known incidence of ectopic pregnancy were entered into a computer model.

Main Outcome Measure(s).—The two approaches were compared with respect to the number of missed ectopic pregnancies, complications, procedures performed, admissions to the hospital, and cost.

Result(s).—The D&C group had 1% more failed managements of ectopic pregnancies and 13.4% fewer patients with a miscarriage undergo a second treatment for resolution. The D&C group had 13.7% fewer complications including 6.3% fewer hospitalizations. D&C costs $173 to $223 more than empiric use of methotrexate per patient.

Conclusion(s).—Empirically treating women at risk for ectopic pregnancy with methotrexate does not reduce complications or save money. In the absence of such savings, the desire to make an accurate and definitive diagnosis, allowing objective prognosis on future fertility and risk of repeat ectopic pregnancy, supports the need to distinguish a miscarriage from ectopic pregnancy before treatment with methotrexate.

▶ Patients with suspected ectopic pregnancy based on inappropriately rising human chorionic gonadotropin levels below the discriminatory zone of transvaginal US typically undergo D&C to eliminate the possibility of a failed intrauterine pregnancy. Some authorities have suggested treating all such patients with methotrexate to avoid the cost and morbidity of D&C. Since there are no randomized trials to evaluate these treatment strategies, the authors have performed a decision analysis to theoretically compare the two. The final analysis failed to show any substantial differences in overall cost or complications. This analysis would seem to argue that without any proven advantage to eliminating D&C, the value of having a proven diagnosis on which to base treatment and counseling for future pregnancies favors retaining D&C in these situations. In any decision analysis, the final result is totally dependent on the accuracy of the data imputed. Many of these imputed values must be an estimate based on the best evidence available, and if inaccurate, would invalidate the analysis. Since the incidence of ectopic pregnancy, the accuracy of diagnosis, and the severity of complications may vary widely between patient populations, hospitals, and physicians, there may be situations where these factors could make one treatment method far superior.

G. H. Lipscomb, MD

28 Infectious Disease

Vulvovaginal Symptoms in Women With Bacterial Vaginosis
Klebanoff MA, Schwebke JR, Zhang J, et al (NIH, Bethesda, Md; Univ of Alabama at Birmingham)
Obstet Gynecol 104:267-272, 2004   28–1

Objective.—A substantial, but highly variable, percentage of women with bacterial vaginosis are said to be asymptomatic. The purpose of this study was to estimate the prevalence of symptoms among women with bacterial vaginosis compared with women without bacterial vaginosis by direct, explicit, and detailed questioning of these women.

Methods.—Women presenting for a routine health care visit at 12 health department clinics in Birmingham, Alabama, were recruited to participate in a longitudinal study of vaginal flora. At the first visit, they underwent a pelvic examination, lower genital tract microbiological evaluation, and an interview that included detailed questions regarding lower genital tract symptoms. The prevalence of symptoms among women with and without bacterial vaginosis (Gram stain score 7 or higher) was compared.

Results.—Among 2,888 women without gonorrhea, *Chlamydia*, or trichomonas, 75% of women with and 82% of women without bacterial vaginosis never noted any vaginal odor in the past 6 months ($P < .001$). The corresponding values were 63% and 65% for never noting vaginal "wetness" ($P = .02$); 58% and 57% for vaginal discharge ($P = .65$); 91% and 86% for irritation ($P = .004$); 88% and 85% for itching ($P = .64$); and 96% and 94% for dysuria ($P = .002$), respectively. Cumulatively, 58% of women with bacterial vaginosis noted odor, discharge, and/or wetness in the past 6 months compared with 57% of women without bacterial vaginosis ($P = .70$).

Conclusion.—The 2 classic symptoms of bacterial vaginosis discharge and odor are each reported by a minority of women with bacterial vaginosis and are only slightly more prevalent than among women without bacterial vaginosis.

▶ Some women with bacterial vaginosis are thought to be asymptomatic. These authors investigated the prevalance of common symptoms usually associated with bacterial vaginosis compared with a cohort of women without bacterial vaginosis. They found that the 2 classic symptoms of bacterial vaginosis, discharge and odor, were each reported by a minority of women with bacterial vaginosis and were only slightly more common than in women without bacterial vaginosis. The vast majority of women did not report any vaginal discharge, wetness, or odor, even upon explicit questioning. The authors conclude that further research should determine factors among women with bacterial vaginosis that would result in the reporting of symptoms.

G. D. Wendel, Jr, MD

Maintenance Fluconazole Therapy for Recurrent Vulvovaginal Candidiasis

Sobel JD, Wiesenfeld HC, Martens M, et al (Wayne State Univ, Detroit; Univ of Pittsburgh, Pa; Hennepin County Med Ctr, Minneapolis; et al)
N Engl J Med 351:876-883, 2004   28–2

Background.—No safe and convenient regimen has proved to be effective for the management of recurrent vulvovaginal candidiasis.

Methods.—After inducing clinical remission with open-label fluconazole given in three 150-mg doses at 72-hour intervals, we randomly assigned 387 women with recurrent vulvovaginal candidiasis to receive treatment with fluconazole (150 mg) or placebo weekly for six months, followed by six months of observation without therapy. The primary outcome measure was the proportion of women in clinical remission at the end of the first six-month period. Secondary efficacy measures were the clinical outcome at 12 months, vaginal mycologic status, and time to recurrence on the basis of Kaplan-Meier analysis.

Results.—Weekly treatment with fluconazole was effective in preventing symptomatic vulvovaginal candidiasis. The proportions of women who remained disease-free at 6, 9, and 12 months in the fluconazole group were 90.8 percent, 73.2 percent, and 42.9 percent, as compared with 35.9 percent, 27.8 percent, and 21.9 percent, respectively, in the placebo group (P<0.001). The median time to clinical recurrence in the fluconazole group was 10.2 months, as compared with 4.0 months in the placebo group (P<0.001). There was no evidence of fluconazole resistance in isolates of *Candida albicans* or of superinfection with *C. glabrata*. Fluconazole was discontinued in one patient because of headache.

Conclusions.—Long-term weekly treatment with fluconazole can reduce the rate of recurrence of symptomatic vulvovaginal candidiasis. However, a long-term cure remains difficult to achieve.

▶ These investigators addressed an important clinical dilemma—how to prevent recurrent vulvovaginal candidiasis. They performed a randomized, prospective clinical trial assigning women with recurrent vulvovaginal candidiasis to treatment with fluconazole (150 mg) or placebo weekly for 6 months. They found that the weekly fluconazole maintenance therapy was associated with a significant reduction in symptomatic vulvovaginal candidiasis. Further, the median time to clinical recurrence was 10 months compared with 4 months in the placebo group. There was no evidence of fluconazole resistance or superinfection with resistant yeast. They conclude that long-term weekly therapy with fluconazole can reduce the rate of recurrence of symptomatic vulvovaginal candidiasis over 6 months of treatment and subsequent follow-up for 6 more months. Unfortunately, data on the long-term effects for cure remain uncertain.

G. D. Wendel, Jr, MD

Bacterial Vaginosis and Risk of Pelvic Inflammatory Disease
Ness RB, Hillier SL, Kip KE, et al (Univ of Pittsburgh, Pa; Boston Med Ctr; Med Univ of South Carolina, Charleston; et al)
Obstet Gynecol 104:761-769, 2004   28–3

Background.—Bacterial vaginosis commonly is found in women with pelvic inflammatory disease (PID), but it is unclear whether bacterial vaginosis leads to incident PID.

Methods.—Women (n = 1,179) from 5 U.S. centers were evaluated for a median of 3 years. Every 6-12 months, vaginal swabs were obtained for gram stain and culture of microflora. A vaginal microflora gram stain score of 7-10 was categorized as bacterial vaginosis. Pelvic inflammatory disease was diagnosed by presence of either histologic endometritis or pelvic pain and tenderness plus one of the following: oral temperature greater than 38.3°C; sedimentation rate greater than 15 mm/hour; white blood count greater than 10,000; or lower genital tract detection of leukorrhea, mucopus, or *Neisseria gonorrhoeae* or *Chlamydia trachomatis.*

Results.—After adjustment for relevant demographic and lifestyle factors, baseline bacterial vaginosis was not associated with the development of PID (adjusted hazard ratio 0.89, 95% confidence interval 0.55-1.45). Carriage of bacterial vaginosis in the previous 6 months before a diagnosis (adjusted risk ratio 1.31, 95% confidence interval 0.71-2.42) also was not significantly associated with PID. Similarly, neither absence of hydrogen peroxide–producing *Lactobacillus* nor high levels of *Gardnerella vaginalis* significantly increased the risk of PID. Dense growth of pigmented, anaerobic gram-negative rods in the 6 months before diagnosis did significantly increase a woman's risk of PID ($P = .04$). One subgroup of women, women with 2 or more recent sexual partners, demonstrated associations among bacterial vaginosis, *Gardnerella vaginalis*, anaerobic gram-negative rods, and PID.

Conclusion.—In this cohort of high-risk women, after adjustment for confounding factors, we found no overall increased risk of developing incident PID among women with bacterial vaginosis.

▶ Bacterial vaginosis (BV) commonly is found in women with acute PID, and it is presumed that untreated BV may lead to upper genital tract infection. This study describes a cohort of women from 5 centers followed up longitudinally over 3 years with vaginal swabs obtained every 6 to 12 months for assessment of BV. After adjustment for relevant factors, BV was not associated with the development of acute PID, even in the 6 months before a diagnosis of PID. In addition, there was no association between absence of hydrogen peroxide–producing *Lactobacillus* or high levels of *G vaginalis* (a common organism with BV) and the risk of PID. The authors conclude that in this high-risk cohort, there was no overall increased risk of developing PID among women with BV. This study provides evidence that questions the need to screen nonpregnant women for BV to prevent the development of PID. However, the authors did note that women with multiple sex partners may be at increased risk for PID from BV and pigmented, anaerobic gram-negative rods.

G. D. Wendel, Jr, MD

Successful Treatment of Bacterial Vaginosis With a Policarbophil-Carbopol Acidic Vaginal Gel: Results From a Randomised Double-blind, Placebo-controlled Trial
Fiorilli A, Molteni B, Milani M ("Ospedale Civile di Vimercate, Presidio di Carate," Milan, Italy; R&D Mipharm, Milan, Italy)
Eur J Obstet Gynecol Reprod Biol 120:202-205, 2005   28–4

Objective.—We evaluated the efficacy of a mucoadhesive vaginal gel (MVG, Miphil©) with acidic-buffering properties in bacterial vaginosis (BV).

Study Design.—Double-blind, placebo-controlled, 12-week trial.

Subjects.—A total of 45 non-pregnant women with BV were enrolled in the trial. Patients were treated with MVG 2.5 g or the corresponding placebo (P) daily for the first week and then every 3 days for the following 5 weeks (treatment phase) in a 2:1 ratio. All patients were followed for an additional 6 weeks without treatments (follow-up phase). Clinical cure was defined as absence of vaginal discharge, vaginal pH <4.5, a negative fish odour test and a Nugent score <7.

Vaginal pH

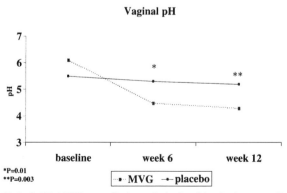

*P=0.01
**P=0.003

⋯■⋯ MVG   ─■─ placebo

FIGURE 2.—Vaginal pH in MVG (mucoadhesive vaginal gel) and the placebo group. (Courtesy of Fiorilli A, Molteni B, Milani M: Successful treatment of bacterial vaginosis with a policarbophil-carbopol acidic vaginal gel: Results from a randomised double-blind, placebo-controlled trial. *Eur J Obstet Gynecol Reprod Biol* 120:202-205. Copyright 2005 with permission from the American Society for Reproductive Medicine.)

Results.—At week 6, 28 out of 30 women (93%) in the MVG group were clinically cured in comparison with only 1 out of 15 (6%) in the P group (P=0.0001). At week 12, 86% of MVG treated women remained cured in comparison with 8% in P group ($P = 0.0001$). At baseline, the vaginal pH was 6.1 ± 0.7 in the MVG and 5.5 ± 0.7 in the P group (Fig 2). Vaginal pH significantly ($P = 0.003$) decreased to 4.3 ± 0.3 in the MVG group. In P group non-significant modifications of vaginal pH were observed (5.1 ± 0.5).

Conclusion.—Our results demonstrated that this MVG is an effective treatment of BV. Comment:

▶ BV remains one the most common causes of vaginal discharge in women throughout the reproductive years. BV is also considered an important risk factor for obstetric complications such as preterm birth and postpartum endometritis. Antibiotics such as metronidazole and clindamycin are well recognized as effective therapies for BV; however, the use of both antibiotic regimens is associated with a high risk of recurrence. A common finding among women with recurrent BV is a persistently elevated vaginal pH. Accordingly, the authors from Milan, Italy, sought to evaluate an intravaginal therapy that reduced vaginal pH and maintained that reduction for a period of time. This double-blind, placebo-controlled, 12-week trial demonstrated that this MVG was significantly more effective in treating women with BV than was placebo. The authors found that vaginal pH was significantly decreased in the MVG group and maintained at a reduced level compared with women using the placebo regimen. The use of a nonantibiotic, nonhormonal intravaginal therapy is an interesting new option for the treatment of BV and deserves serious consideration as an important option for gynecologic and obstetric patients who are afflicted with this common vaginal infection.

L. P. Shulman, MD

Vaginal–Perianal Compared With Vaginal–Rectal Cultures for Identification of Group B Streptococci

Jamie WE, Edwards RK, Duff P (Univ of Florida, Gainesville)
Obstet Gynecol 104:1058-1061, 2004   28–5

Objective.—To estimate whether the rates of recovery of group B streptococci from combined vaginal and perianal cultures and combined vaginal and rectal cultures are equivalent.

Methods.—We performed a prospective cohort study of vaginal-perianal versus vaginal-rectal culture for group B streptococci. Two hundred pregnant women in the third trimester were enrolled. Three specimens were collected from each patient in the following order: lower third of the vagina, perianal skin, and rectum. Each specimen was cultured serially in selective broth media, then on sheep's blood agar. Suspicious colonies were confirmed by latex agglutination. Culture positivity rates from the combined sites of vagina and perianal skin were compared with vagina and rectum. Laboratory personnel were blinded to the collection site of each individual swab.

Results.—Of the 200 subjects, 71 (36%) had a positive culture from at least 1 site. Vaginal culture was positive in 55 patients (28%), compared with 48 patients (24%) with positive perianal cultures and 50 patients (25%) with positive rectal cultures. Results of combined vaginal and perianal cultures were positive in 68 patients (34%); results of combined vaginal and rectal cultures were positive in 67 patients (34%) ($P = 1.0$).

Conclusion.—The group B streptococci detection rate from vaginal-perianal specimens is not significantly different from the detection rate from vaginal-rectal specimens. Therefore, pregnant women do not need to be subjected to the discomfort of collection of a rectal specimen.

▶ The current Centers for Disease Control and Prevention recommendations call for screening all pregnant women for group B streptococcal colonization at 35 to 37 weeks' gestation to identify candidates for intrapartum antibiotic prophylaxis. The method of specimen collection involves swabbing both the lower third of the vagina and rectum based on older studies that indicated rectal cultures were positive more often than vaginal cultures (17.9% vs 10.2%). These investigators performed a prospective, cohort study of vaginal-perianal versus vaginal-rectal cultures for group B streptococci. Each patient collected a specimen from the lower third of the vagina, the perianal skin, and the rectum, in order. Thirty-six percent of the patients had a positive culture from at least one site, most commonly the vagina, followed by the perineum and rectum in about 25% of patients in each group. There was no difference in the rate of combined vaginal and perianal cultures that were positive (34%) compared with combined vaginal and rectal cultures (34%). The authors conclude that pregnant women do not need to be subjected to rectal specimen collection, which is sometimes inconvenient and uncomfortable to collect.

G. D. Wendel, Jr, MD

29 Ultrasound

Integrated FDG PET/CT in Patients With Persistent Ovarian Cancer: Correlation With Histologic Findings
Sironi S, Messa C, Mangili G, et al (Univ of Milano-Bicocca, Italy; Natl Research Council of Italy, Milan; Univ Vita-Salute, Milan, Italy)
Radiology 233:433-440, 2004   29–1

Purpose.—To prospectively evaluate the accuracy of integrated positron emission tomography (PET) and computed tomography (CT) for depiction of persistent ovarian carcinoma after first-line treatment, with use of histologic findings as the reference standard.

Materials and Methods.—Thirty-one women (mean age, 55.9 years) with ovarian carcinoma treated with primary cytoreductive surgery and followed up with platinum regimen chemotherapy were included. All 31 patients were scheduled for surgical second-look. Before surgical second-look, all patients underwent fluorodeoxyglucose (FDG) PET/CT. At PET/CT, three main categories of persistent disease were considered for data analysis: lymph nodal lesion, peritoneal lesion, and pelvic lesion. In all patients, imaging findings were compared with results of histologic examination after surgical second-look to determine the diagnostic accuracy of PET/CT in the evaluation of disease status. The κ statistic (Cohen κ) was used for statistical analysis.

Results.—Seventeen (55%) of 31 patients had persistent tumor at histologic analysis after surgical second-look, and fourteen (45%) had no histologically proved tumor. The total number of lesions that was positive for tumor cells at histologic analysis was 41 (lymph nodes, $n = 16$; peritoneal lesions, $n = 21$; pelvic lesions, $n = 4$); maximum diameter of these lesions was 0.3–3.2 cm (mean, 1.7 cm). A correlation was found between PET/CT and histologic analysis ($κ = 0.48$). The overall lesion-based sensitivity, specificity, accuracy, positive predictive value, and negative predictive value of PET/CT were 78%, 75%, 77%, 89% and 57%, respectively. In the detection of a tumor, a size threshold could be set at 0.5 cm, as this was the largest diameter of a lesion missed at PET/CT.

Conclusion.—Integrated PET/CT depicts persistent ovarian carcinoma with a high positive predictive value.

Preoperative Sonographic Features of Borderline Ovarian Tumors

Exacoustos C, Romanini ME, Rinaldo D, et al (Università degli Studi di Roma 'Tor Vergata,' Rome)

Ultrasound Obstet Gynecol 25:50-59, 2005   29–2

Objective.—To determine the sonographic findings that distinguish borderline ovarian tumors (BOT) from both benign and invasive malignant tumors, thus allowing conservative treatment and laparoscopic management of these tumors.

Methods.—We reviewed retrospectively transvaginal sonograms of 33 women who, when evaluated further by surgery and histology, were found to have BOT. Twenty-three were premenopausal and 10 were postmenopausal (mean age ± SD, 45.8 ± 15.7 years). For each mass, size and morphological features and power Doppler characteristics were evaluated. We compared these findings with those of 337 patients with benign ovarian tumors and those of 82 patients with invasive malignant ovarian tumors. Patients with dermoid cysts were not included in the study.

Results.—Of the 33 BOT, 15 were mucinous and 18 were serous cystadenomas. The presence of papillae, defined as a small number of solid tissue projections, 1–15 mm in height and 1–10 mm in width (base) and length (base), into the cyst cavity from the cyst wall, was significantly more frequent in BOT (48%) than it was in benign (4%) and invasive (4%) malignant tumors. Intracystic solid tissue (> 15 mm in height or > 10 mm in width or length) was observed in 48% of invasive malignant masses but in only 18% of BOT and in 7% of benign tumors ($P < 0.001$). No sonographically unilocular, hypoechoic, smooth-walled adnexal cysts were invasively malignant but three unilocular cysts with a diameter of > 6 cm were serous BOT. Although close attention was paid to the cyst wall at ultrasound examination we did not observe in these three cysts the very small papillae which were found at histological analysis.

Conclusions.—The most frequent diagnostic feature on imaging BOT is the presence of papillae within the cyst. However, neither papillae nor other sonographic features constituted highly sensitive sonographic markers of BOT.

Sonographic Assessment of Non-malignant Ovarian Cysts: Does Sonohistology Exist?

de Kroon CD, van der Sandt HAGM, van Houwelingen JC, et al (Leiden Univ, The Netherlands)

Hum Reprod 19:2138-2143, 2004   29–3

Background.—Transvaginal ultrasound (TVU) is feasible and accurate in the differentiation between non-malignant and malignant ovarian abnormalities. However, despite the clinical relevance, the accuracy of TVU in the differentiation between the many different non-malignant cysts is unknown.

Methods.—Between 1992 and 2002, all women who had surgery at our centre because of a non-malignant ovarian cyst were included prospectively in this study. The sonographic characteristics as well as the expected histological diagnosis (the 'sonohistological diagnosis') were evaluated preoperatively. This diagnosis was compared with the histopathological diagnosis, and diagnostic parameters [with 95% confidence interval (CI)] of the sonohistological diagnosis were calculated. Logistic models, with the sonographic characteristics as variables, were constructed for each histopathological diagnosis.

Results.—A total of 406 women were included consecutively. The overall diagnostic accuracy of the sonohistological diagnosis was 60% (95% CI 0.56–0.65). Only in cases of simple ovarian cysts did the diagnostic accuracy of the respective logistic model exceed that of the sonohistological diagnosis (0.88 versus 0.81, $P < 0.01$). The diagnostic accuracy of the sonohistological diagnosis for endometriotic and dermoid ovarian cysts was significantly better compared with the respective logistic model (0.84 versus 0.71, $P < 0.01$ and 0.87 versus 0.82, $P = 0.03$, respectively).

Conclusion.—In approximately half of the non-malignant ovarian cysts, TVU is capable of distinguishing between the different histopathological diagnoses of non-malignant ovarian masses. Only in the diagnosis of simple ovarian cysts might use of the logistic models be helpful.

▶ The use of imaging technology to predict a wide variety of outcomes with ovarian pathology continues to gain popularity. These 3 studies assess the role of radiologic imaging to predict clinical outcomes in a spectrum of patients with ovarian pathology. The first study by Sironi et al used PET/CT to evaluate patients who had undergone initial therapy for ovarian carcinoma. The authors found that integrated PET/CT was able to depict persistent ovarian carcinoma with a high positive predictive value. Such technology may provide a highly sensitive, noninvasive approach to determining persistence or recurrence of ovarian cancer for patients who have undergone optimal first-line therapy. The study by Exacoustos et al sought to describe the preoperative sonographic features of borderline ovarian tumors. This class of ovarian tumors represents a particularly challenging clinical situation for gynecologists and oncologists, as decisions regarding therapy and follow-up of these borderline tumors continues to spark heated debate among researchers and clinicians. This group found that the most frequent diagnostic feature of borderline ovarian tumors was the presence of papillae within the cyst. However, in contrast to the findings of the first report, this particular ultrasonographic finding was not a sensitive or specific marker for borderline ovarian tumors. The third study evaluates a topic of considerable interest to clinicians who care for women. Specifically, can TVU differentiate between nonmalignant and malignant ovarian abnormalities? Although TVU has been shown to be highly accurate in the evaluation of ovarian cysts, its ability to differentiate between malignant and nonmalignant cysts is decidedly less robust. Unfortunately, the results of this study demonstrated clinical outcomes comparable to earlier studies. Specifically, TVU was neither sensitive nor specific in its ability to differentiate between malignant and nonmalignant ovarian cysts. We are thus left with core radiographic and serum markers for the detection of earlier and thus more successfully treatable stages of ovarian cancer. Further work will undoubtedly be performed and will hopefully be able to demonstrate effective protocols to enable us to detect ovarian cancer at a more successfully treatable stage.

L. P. Shulman, MD

Transvaginal Ultrasound-Guided Aspiration for Treatment of Tubo-Ovarian Abscess: A Study of 302 Cases
Gjelland K, Ekerhovd E, Granberg S (Haukeland Univ, Bergen, Norway; Sahlgrenska Univ, Göteborg, Sweden; Karolinska Univ, Stockholm)
Am J Obstet Gynecol 193:1323-1330, 2005   29–4

Objective.—Our purpose was to evaluate the effectiveness and safety of transvaginal ultrasound-guided aspiration together with antibiotic therapy for treatment of tubo-ovarian abscess.

Study Design.—A review of women treated with transvaginal ultrasound-guided aspiration for tubo-ovarian abscess at Haukeland University Hospital, Bergen, Norway, between June 1986 and July 2003 was performed. Immediate clinical response and longer-term follow-up results were assessed.

Results.—A total of 449 transvaginal aspirations were performed on 302 women. A total of 282 women (93.4%) were successfully treated for transvaginal aspiration of purulent fluid, together with antibiotic therapy. In the other 20 women (6.6%), surgery was performed. The main indications for surgery were diagnostic or therapeutic uncertainty, such as suspected residual tubo-ovarian abscess or pain. No procedure-related complications were diagnosed.

Conclusion.—Transvaginal ultrasound-guided aspiration combined with antibiotics is an effective and safe treatment regimen for tubo-ovarian abscess. The high success rate indicates that it should be a first-line procedure.

▶ This study describes a longitudinal cohort observed over 17 years that included more than 300 consecutive women admitted for the treatment of acute salpingitis with tubo-ovarian abscess in Norway. The authors performed a single aspiration in almost two thirds of the patients, whereas an additional one third required up to 4 aspirations of purulent material. Women were concomitantly treated with broad-spectrum antibiotics, and only 6.6% required surgical intervention. While this is not a prospective comparative trial, the success rate is impressive, especially given that the investigators aspirated 80 to 90 mL on average from each patient. Transvaginal US-guided aspiration under antibiotic treatment seems a reasonable intervention in cases of tubo-ovarian abscess or pyosalpinx. This treatment regimen has several advantages compared with surgical or laparoscopic intervention. The procedure takes 15 to 30 minutes, is well tolerated, inexpensive, and minimally invasive. Lacking from this study are data regarding the ultimate course in these women regarding the effects of this treatment regimen on future fertility and chronic pelvic pain.

G. D. Wendel, Jr, MD

Preoperative Ultrasound to Predict Infraumbilical Adhesions: A Study of Diagnostic Accuracy

Tu FF, Lamvu GM, Hartmann KE, et al (Univ of North Carolina, Chapel Hill)
Am J Obstet Gynecol 192:74-79, 2005   29–5

Objective.—The purpose of this study was to determine the test characteristics of preoperative abdominal ultrasound in predicting infraumbilical adhesions in women.

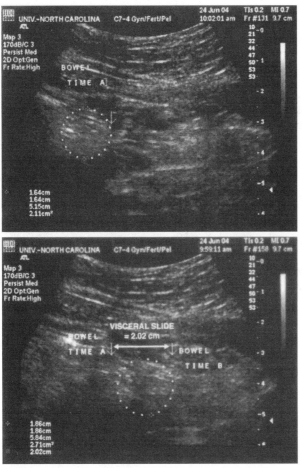

FIGURE 2.—Ultrasound visualization of movement of abdominal viscera (visceral slide) during inspiration in an adhesion-free volunteer. The ultrasound transducer is positioned longitudinally over the umbilicus, and the woman is asked to take deep breaths in and out. *Time A* is at expiration, *time B* is after inspiration. The bowel (discernable by the presence of a round echogenic focus with peristaltic activity inside) moves inferiorly with inspiration away from the diaphragm (**left-hand side of each ultrasound**) toward the pelvis (**right-hand side of each ultrasound**). Distance traversed by the bowel (*dotted circles*) longitudinally is measured as visceral slide (here, 2.02 cm). (Courtesy of Tu FF, Lamvu GM, Hartmann KE, et al: Preoperative ultrasound to predict infraumbilical adhesions: A study of diagnostic accuracy. *Am J Obstet Gynecol* 192:74-79, 2005. Copyright 2005 by Elsevier. Reprinted by permission.)

Study Design.—This was a diagnostic test study of 60 women at risk for intra-abdominal adhesions undergoing laparoscopy or vertical laparotomy. Participants underwent periumbilical sonographic measurement of visceral slide (longitudinal movement of the viscera during a cycle of respiration; Fig 2).

Results.—Prevalence of infraumbilical bowel adhesions was 12%. A visceral slide threshold <1 cm to predict adhesions had sensitivity = 86%, specificity = 91%, positive predictive value = 55%, and negative predictive value = 98%. On stratifying visceral slide (<0.8 cm, ≥0.8 and <1 cm, and ≥1 cm), the likelihood ratios for detecting adhesions were 15.1, 5.0, and 0.2, respectively.

Conclusion.—Measuring visceral slide improves preoperative prediction of both presence and absence of bowel adhesions in patients with previous abdominal operations or infection; this technique may assist in avoiding iatrogenic bowel injury.

▶ Bowel injury, recognized or unrecognized, remains an area of great concern for laparoscopists. As noted by the authors of this article, there is no valid method of predicting intra-abdominal adhesions. This study evaluated the use of US to predict infraumbilical adhesions by measuring the longitudinal distance the intestines and omentum traveled during an exaggerated inspiration-expiration cycle. Confirmation of adhesions was made surgically. Overall, the value of this test appears to be in its negative predictive value of 98%. When the test was positive, only 6 of 11 patients had adhesions (positive predictive value, 55%). Although this test seems to have some utility, it is unlikely to have widespread use, as most gynecologists will not find it very practical and will simply approach patients who would be considered at risk with an alternative entry site of open laparoscopy.

V. A. M. Givens, MD

30 Surgery

Ignorance of Electrosurgery Among Obstetricians and Gynaecologists
Mayooran Z, Pearce S, Tsaltas J, et al (Monash Univ, Clayton, Victoria, Australia; Oxford Univ, England)
BJOG 111:1413-1418, 2004   30–1

Objective.—The purpose of this study was to assess the level of skill of laparoscopic surgeons in electrosurgery.

Design.—Subjects were asked to complete a practical diathermy station and a written test of electrosurgical knowledge.

Setting.—Tests were held in teaching and non-teaching hospitals.

Sample.—Twenty specialists in obstetrics and gynaecology were randomly selected and tested on the Monash University gynaecological laparoscopic pelvi-trainer. Twelve candidates were consultants with 9-28 years of practice in operative laparoscopy, and 8 were registrars with up to six years of practice in operative laparoscopy. Seven consultants and one registrar were from rural Australia, and three consultants were from New Zealand.

Methods.—Candidates were marked with checklist criteria resulting in a pass/fail score, as well as a weighted scoring system. We retested 11 candidates one year later with the same stations.

Main Outcome Measures.—No improvement in electrosurgery skill in one year of obstetric and gynaecological practice.

Results.—No candidate successfully completed the written electrosurgery station in the initial test. A slight improvement in the pass rate to 18% was observed in the second test. The pass rate of the diathermy station dropped from 50% to 36% in the second test.

Conclusion.—The study found ignorance of electrosurgery/diathermy among gynaecological surgeons. One year later, skills were no better.

▶ Electrosurgical instruments are present in virtually all operative suites and are used on a regular basis by surgeons for specialties. Unfortunately, most surgeons are probably unaware of even basic electrosurgical principles. Although better design and safety features have reduced electrosurgical injuries, dangers still exist. This study used a written questionnaire based on a freely available booklet by a well-known electrosurgical manufacturer along with a practical test. For those familiar with electrosurgery, the questions asked seem basic. This study has confirmed in a small subgroup of physicians what many of us who lecture on the subject believe applies to a much broader group of physicians—that basic knowledge of electrosurgical principles and safety is inadequate.

V. A. M. Givens, MD

A Double-Blind Randomised Controlled Trial of Laparoscopic Uterine Nerve Ablation for Women With Chronic Pelvic Pain

Johnson NP, Farquhar CM, Crossley S, et al (Univ of Auckland, New Zealand)
BJOG 111:950-959, 2004   30–2

Objective.—To determine the effectiveness of laparoscopic uterine nerve ablation (LUNA) for chronic pelvic pain in women with endometriosis and women with no laparoscopic evidence of endometriosis.

Design.—A prospective double-blind randomised controlled trial (RCT).

Setting.—Single-centre, secondary-level gynaecology outpatient service and tertiary-level pelvic pain and endometriosis outpatient service in Auckland, New Zealand.

Population.—One hundred and twenty-three women undergoing laparoscopy for investigation and management of chronic pelvic pain, 56 with no laparoscopic evidence of endometriosis and 67 with endometriosis.

Methods.—Women were randomised from the two populations, firstly those with no evidence of endometriosis and secondly those undergoing laparoscopic surgical treatment for endometriosis, to receive LUNA or no LUNA. Participant and assessor blinding was employed. Follow up for pain outcomes was undertaken at 24 hours, 3 months and 12 months.

Main Outcome Measures.—Changes in non-menstrual pelvic pain, dysmenorrhoea, deep dyspareunia and dyschezia were assessed primarily by whether there was a decrease in visual analogue score for these types of pain of 50% or more from baseline and additionally whether there was a significantly different change in median visual analogue score. The numbers requiring further surgery or starting a new medical treatment for pelvic pain and complications were also measured.

Results.—There was a significant reduction in dysmenorrhoea at 12 month follow up in women with chronic pelvic pain in the absence of endometriosis who underwent LUNA (median change in visual analogue scale (VAS) from baseline -4.8 *versus* -0.8 ($P = 0.039$), 42.1% *versus* 14.3% experiencing a successful treatment defined as a 50% or greater reduction in visual analogue pain scale for dysmenorrhoea ($P = 0.045$). There was no significant difference in non-menstrual pelvic pain, deep dyspareunia or dyschezia in women with no endometriosis undergoing LUNA versus no LUNA. The addition of LUNA to laparoscopic surgical treatment of endometriosis was not associated with a significant difference in any pain outcomes.

Conclusions.—LUNA is effective for dysmenorrhoea in the absence of endometriosis, although there is no evidence of effectiveness of LUNA for non-dysmenorrhoeic chronic pelvic pain or for any type of chronic pelvic pain related to endometriosis.

▶ The use of LUNA for chronic pain conditions remains controversial. In this study, patients underwent interoperative randomization to LUNA or no LUNA after laparoscopy had been performed for chronic pain. Patients were subdivided into those with laparoscopic evidence of endometriosis or those with no evidence of endometriosis. Patients and the data collector were blinded from the assignment. Six patients subsequently had additional surgery and were excluded from data collection, but 10 other patients had additional medical treatment, such as oral contraceptives, gonadotropin-releasing hormone, and other treatments. Data collection was continued in these patients, and it is difficult to determine what if any effect these treatments had on the final results. The conclusion supports the findings of a recent meta-analysis[1] which showed that LUNA was effective for dysmenorrhoea in the absence of endometriosis but not for dysmenorrhoea in the presence of endometriosis, or for dyspareunia.

V. A. M. Givens, MD

Reference

1. Johnson N, Wilson M, Farquhar C: Surgical pelvic neuroablation for chronic pelvic pain. *Gynaecol Endosc* 9:351-361, 2000.

Tying a Loop-to-Strand Suture: Is It Safe?
Hurt J, Unger JB, Ivy JJ, et al (Louisiana State Univ, Shreveport)
Am J Obstet Gynecol 192:1094-1097, 2005   30–3

Objective.—This study was undertaken to evaluate the integrity of the loop-to-strand knot when tied with square and nonidentical sliding knots.

Study Design.—The synthetic absorbable monofilament suture poliglecaprone 25 in 0 and 2-0 suture gauges was used in this experiment. For each suture gauge, 3 groups of knots were tested: (1) single strand-to-single strand, flat square knot, (2) loop-to-single strand, flat square knot, and (3) loop-to-single strand, nonidentical sliding knot. All knots were tied with 6 throws. The proportion of knots becoming untied was compared among the 3 groups for each suture gauge. Ultimate load required to untie or break knots within each group was also evaluated.

Results.—The loop-to-strand knot performed well in both suture gauges tested as long as it was tied with a flat square knot. The loop-to-strand knot tied with a nonidentical sliding knot had an unacceptably high failure rate.

Conclusion.—The loop-to-strand termination of a continuous suture may be acceptable when tied with a 6-throw flat square knot but not acceptable if tied with sliding knots.

▶ When terminating a single running suture, many surgeons will use a "loop-to-strand" knot. However, this may be an unwise choice when using a monofilament suture and had been advised against by Ethicon in 1994. This is the first study to actually test the reliability of a loop-to-strand knot compared with a "strand-to-strand" knot, which in practice requires running 2 sutures to the midline and tying the 2 strands to each other. Further complicating the issue is that many surgeons actually tie nonidentical sliding knots instead of flat knots (often unwary of the fact).[1] In this study, none of the square strand-to-strand knots failed by unraveling, while a high percentage of the loop-to-strand knots failed by unraveling. With the use of size 0 sutures, 86% of nonidentical knots and 15% of flat knots unraveled before breaking. Although use of square knots reduced the rate of failure, it would seem prudent to avoid the loop-to-strand knot when using monofilament suture in critical applications that may be subject to tension.

V. A. M. Givens, MD

Reference

1. Trimbos JB: Security of various knots commonly used in surgical practice. *Obstet Gynecol* 64:274-280, 1984.

Ovarian Conservation at the Time of Hysterectomy for Benign Disease
Parker WH, Broder MS, Liu Z, et al (Univ of California, Los Angeles; Cerner Health Insights, Beverly Hills, Calif; Univ of Southern California, Los Angeles; et al)
Obstet Gynecol 106:219-226, 2005   30–4

Objective.—Prophylactic oophorectomy is often recommended concurrent with hysterectomy for benign disease. The optimal age for this recommendation in women at average risk for ovarian cancer has not been determined.

Methods.—Using published age-specific data for absolute and relative risk, both with and without oophorectomy, for ovarian cancer, coronary heart disease, hip fracture, breast cancer, and stroke, a Markov decision analysis model was used to estimate the optimal strategy for maximizing survival for women at average risk of ovarian cancer. For each 5-year age group from 40 to 80 years, 4 strategies were compared: ovarian conservation or oophorectomy, and use of estrogen therapy or nonuse. Outcomes, as proportion of women alive at age 80 years, were measured. Sensitivity analyses were performed, varying both relative and absolute risk estimates across the range of reported values.

Results.—Ovarian conservation until age 65 benefits long-term survival for women undergoing hysterectomy for benign disease. Women with oophorectomy before age 55 have 8.58% excess mortality by age 80, and those with oophorectomy before age 59 have 3.92% excess mortality. There is sustained, but decreasing, benefit until the age of 75, when excess mortality for oophorectomy is less than 1%. These results were unchanged following multiple sensitivity analyses and were most sensitive to the risk of coronary heart disease.

Conclusion.—Ovarian conservation until at least age 65 benefits long-term survival for women at average risk of ovarian cancer when undergoing hysterectomy for benign disease.

▶ This article purports to confront dogma with evidence. However, careful reading shows that it might not be all it is made to appear. For many years, gynecologists have been telling their patients that they should have their normal ovaries removed at the time of hysterectomy after a certain age, which varies from institution to institution. This report uses Markov modeling to show that prophylactic oophorectomy at the time of hysterectomy in women not at high risk of developing ovarian cancer is associated with increased mortality rate. The problem with studies using Markov modeling is that the results depend on the assumptions used in the model. Some of those used in this study are questionable, such as assuming that postmenopausal estrogen therapy decreases cardiac mortality rate. Thus, this study should be considered with the skepticism mentioned but not applied in the accompanying editorial.[1] However, there is clearly a grain of truth here and an important issue is raised that must be confronted by data. This study adds to the body of literature that has yet to show a survival advantage for prophylactic oophorectomy in patients not at high risk for ovarian cancer. If we cannot show any benefits for our interventions, then we, at least, should be sure that we are doing no harm.

D. S. Miller, MD

Reference

1. Olive DL: Dogma, skepsis, and the analytic method. The role of prophylactic oophorectomy at the time of hysterectomy. *Obstet Gynecol* 106:214-215, 2005.

A Randomized Trial That Compared Povidone Iodine and Chlorhexidine as Antiseptics for Vaginal Hysterectomy
Culligan PJ, Kubik K, Murphy M, et al (Univ of Louisville, Ky)
Am J Obstet Gynecol 192:422-425, 2005   30–5

Objective.—The purpose of this study was to compare the efficacy of chlorhexidine and povidone iodine for cleansing the operative field for vaginal surgery.

Study Design.—This was a randomized controlled trial that compared 10% povidone iodine and 4% chlorhexidine gluconate as surgical scrubs. Our primary end point was the proportion of contaminated specimens (defined as total bacterial colony counts of ≥5000 colony-forming units) per group found throughout the surgical procedures. All patients received standard infection prophylaxis that included preoperative intravenous antibiotics. Immediately before antibiotic administration baseline aerobic and anaerobic cultures of the vaginal flora were obtained, which were followed by cultures at 30 minutes after the surgical scrub and hourly thereafter throughout each patient's surgery.

Results.—A total of 50 patients were enrolled between October 2002 and September 2003. There were no differences between the povidone iodine (n = 27) and chlorhexidine (n = 23) groups with respect to age, race, exogenous hormone use, body mass index, gravity, parity, preoperative mean colony counts, or operative time. Among the first set of intraoperative specimens (which were obtained 30 minutes after the surgical scrub), 63% of the cultures (17/27) from the povidone iodine group and 22% of the cultures (5/23) from the chlorhexidine group were classified as contaminated ($P = .003$; relative risk, 6.12; 95% CI, 1.7, 21.6). Subsequent cultures failed to demonstrate significant differences.

Conclusion.—Chlorhexidine gluconate was more effective than povidone iodine in decreasing the bacterial colony counts that were found in the operative field for vaginal hysterectomy.

▶ Most physicians would agree that bacterial contamination of the vagina can be temporarily reduced but not eliminated. Reducing the vaginal colony count for as long as possible has significant implications in vaginal surgery. In this study, the authors have shown that chlorhexidine reduces the incidence of vaginal contamination (defined as >5000 colonies) compared with povidone iodine up to 150 minutes after vaginal prep. Although chlorhexidine had a lower proportion of contaminated specimens at all time points tested, only the levels at 30 minutes were statistically significant. This article presents an interesting hypothesis that chlorhexidine is a superior vaginal prep than the traditional povidone-iodine prep. Unfortunately, the authors were unable to show that the reduced colony counts resulted in decreased infection rates. As noted by the authors, to achieve a statistical power of 80% to detect a reduction in infection rate from 6% to 3% would take 813 patients in each arm. Of note, the Centers for Disease Control and Prevention has recommended the use of chlorhexidine over other skin preps for peripheral catheter insertion for several years.[1] However, no convincing data exist in this regard for other types of surgical incisions.

V. A. M. Givens, MD

Reference

1. O'Grady NP, Alexander M, Dellinger EP, et al: Guidelines for the prevention of intravascular catheter-related infections. *MMWR Morb Mortal Wkly Rep* 51(RR-10):1-29, 2002.

NovaSure Impedance Controlled System for Endometrial Ablation: Three-Year Follow-up on 107 Patients
Gallinat A (Tagesklinik Altonaer Straße, Hamburg, Germany)
Am J Obstet Gynecol 191:1585-1589, 2004   30–6

Objective.—This study was undertaken to assess the safety, efficacy, and data durability of the NovaSure ablation at 3 years after the procedure in women with menorrhagia secondary to dysfunctional uterine bleeding (DUB).

Study Design.—A prospective, single-arm, observational pilot study (Canadian Task Force classification II-1) was carried out at a specialized center for gynecologic endoscopy with 107 premenopausal women with menorrhagia secondary to DUB. NovaSure ablation was performed in 107 patients. Pictorial Blood loss Assessment Chart diary sampling was used to assess menstrual blood loss. Ablation was performed without any type of endometrial pretreatment.

Results.—No intraoperative or postoperative complications were observed. Treatment time averaged 94 seconds; 65% of the patients reported amenorrhea. Hysterectomy was avoided in 97.2% of patients at 3-year follow-up.

Conclusion.—Long-term clinical results demonstrate that the NovaSure system is a safe and effective method for treatment of women with menorrhagia secondary to DUB, yielding high amenorrhea and success rates, with low re-treatment rates.

▶ Because of the ease of use, global endometrial ablation techniques have become more popular than the more classic neodymium:yttrium-aluminum-garnet (Nd:YAG) laser or rollerball ablation methods. Many different global methods are now approved for endometrial methods, but it remains uncertain which method is the most appropriate for any particular patient.

The reviewed study is an observation study of 107 women treated with the NovaSure device and followed up for 3 years. All patients were treated for menorrhagia unresponsive to medical therapy, although the type and duration of medical therapy was undefined in the article. Menorrhagia was defined as a pictorial blood loss assessment chart (PBAC) score of greater than 150. All patients had a uterine cavity of 10 cm or less and underwent hysteroscopy to rule out abnormalities of the uterine cavity. Four patients were classified as failures, but 2 of these who were failures based on PBAC scores were satisfied with their bleeding. Three patients underwent hysterectomy (1 for menorrhagia, 1 for posttreatment hematometra, and 1 for a rapidly enlarging fibroid) and 1 patient required retreatment. Overall, 96.3% of patients avoided any additional treatment or surgery.

These data would suggest that in carefully selected patients, the NovaSure device produces excellent results in patients with menorrhagia. Ultimately, randomized trials between the various devices will be available to allow physicians to truly evaluate the most appropriate endometrial ablation device for a particular subset of patients.

G. H. Lipscomb, MD

31 Cervix

Screening, HPV, Vaccine

Current Cervical Neoplasia Screening Practices of Obstetrician/Gynecologists in the US
Saint M, Gildengorin G, Sawaya GF (Kaiser Permanente Northern California; Univ of California, San Francisco)
Am J Obstet Gynecol 192:414-421, 2005   31–1

Objective.—The purpose of this study was to determine cervical cancer screening practices of obstetrician/gynecologists in the US after recent revised guidelines.

Study Design.—Questionnaires were mailed to 355 randomly selected US obstetrician/gynecologists. Questions were structured as clinical vignettes.

Results.—Questionnaires were returned by 60% (213/355) of recipients; 185 were eligible. Seventy-four percent would begin screening virginal girls at age 18. Sixty percent would continue annual screening in a 35-year-old woman with 3 or more normal tests. Frequent screening is common in women after total hysterectomy for symptomatic fibroids and no history of dysplasia, and in 70-year-old women with a 30-year history of previous normal tests. Most (82%) use liquid-based cytology; 78% of female respondents would prefer it for themselves. Most (64%) would not adopt triennial Pap/HPV DNA screening, although 58% of women would choose it for themselves.

Conclusion.—Most US obstetrician/gynecologists screen low-risk women often and indefinitely, despite national guidelines designed to minimize screening harms resulting from overtesting.

▶ The American Cancer Society and the American College of Obstetricians and Gynecologists have recently adopted new screening recommendations, endorsed cotesting for human papillomavirus (HPV), and recommended discontinuing screening in certain women. Despite these national screening guidelines, little is known regarding whether obstetricians/gynecologists have adopted these guidelines in their practice.

A questionnaire was sent to a randomly selected population of obstetrician/gynecologists currently in practice—those who are doing the most screening, and are most likely to be updated on the most recent guidelines. This study also examined these physicians' views on cervical cancer screening preferences, and patterns for female physicians. The questionnaire itself is unique as it consisted predominantly of clinical vignettes, a tool to measure actual clinical behavior.

The survey showed that most clinicians are not adhering to the recommended guidelines. The majority of the participants (75.3%) would screen an 18-year-old patient who is not sexually active, and 94.6% would screen an 18-year-old patient who became sexually active for the first time 1 month ago and presents for her first gynecologic exam. Most participants screen all patients annually, and 25% would screen more often than annually if a woman requested it. Most screen regularly in a 70-year-old patient with a prior 30-year normal Pap history. If a patient had difficulty with the exam and inquired about stopping screening, 60% would continue screening, and 47% would continue screening if her life expectancy was less than 5 years.

This survey demonstrates that resources are being spent on annual screening in low-risk populations. Further research is needed to ascertain why clinicians are not adhering to the guidelines, and to devise educational interventions that will modify screening behaviors.

The guidelines were based on the most up-to-date knowledge of the natural history and outcome of HPV and cervical dysplasia in conjunction with expert opinion. They were designed with the intent to maximize benefit and and minimize harm. Adherence to the guidelines will help prevent overdiagnosis of lesions that will regress spontaneously, that would lead to increased referral for colposcopy, overtreatment, and increased health care costs.

M. E. App, MD, MPH

The Utility of HPV DNA Triage in the Management of Cytological AGC
Irvin W, Evans SR, Andersen W, et al (Univ of Virginia, Charlottesville)
Am J Obstet Gynecol 193:559-567, 2005   31–2

Objective.—Given the demonstrated utility of human papilloma virus DNA triage in the management of atypical squamous cells of undetermined significance, this study sought to evaluate the potential role of human papilloma virus DNA testing in the evaluation and management of cytological atypical glandular cells.

Study Design.—Following institutional review board approval, 28 women presenting with cytological atypical glandular cells underwent repeat thin-prep cytology, Hybrid Capture 2 human papilloma virus DNA testing, colposcopic evaluation, Fisher electrosurgical conization, and endometrial sampling. Human papilloma virus test results in each patient were then correlated with histologic lesions, if present.

Results.—Sixteen of the 28 study patients had pathologic lesions (11/28 high-grade squamous intraepithelial lesion, 3/28 low-grade squamous intraepithelial lesion, 1/28 adenocarcinoma in situ, 1/28 simple endometrial hyperplasia). Human papilloma virus DNA testing was available in 24 of 28 subjects (86%). The sensitivity of human papilloma virus positivity to predict the presence of cervical intraepithelial neoplasia was 100% (confidence interval 77% to 100%), specificity 64% (confidence interval 35% to 85%), positive predictive value 76%, and negative predictive value 100%. Women who tested human papilloma virus positive were 12 times more likely to have cervical intraepithelial neoplasia than women who were human papilloma virus negative (Fisher $P<.001$). Human papilloma virus positivity was not predictive of endometrial pathology; women who were human papilloma virus positive were less likely to have endometrial pathology than were women who were human papilloma virus negative (risk ratio 1.6, 95% confidence interval 0.01-1.7).

Conclusion.—Atypical glandular cells can represent a variety of lesions. The majority of the lesions will be squamous intraepithelial lesions of the cervix (50%), with high-grade squamous intraepithelial lesion present in 40% of subjects. Human papilloma virus DNA testing is a sensitive test for the presence of squamous intraepithelial lesion, with excellent negative predictive value for the absence of squamous intraepithelial lesion. The results of this study suggest human papilloma virus DNA testing might be an effective screening test in the initial evaluation and management of cytological atypical glandular cells.

▶ A study cohort of women who presented with an index smear of atypical glandular cells (AGC) underwent a thorough examination, including colposcopy, ectocervical/endocervical conization, and endometrial sampling. The goal of the study was to evaluate what utility, if any, human papillomavirus (HPV) testing results might have in predicting, prior to the examination, the location of disease in each patient, and hence the area on which subsequent evaluation should have focused.

Fifty percent of the patients were found to have squamous intraepithelial lesions, of which 80% were high grade. In 42% of the patients, no pathologic abnormality was detected. In terms of HPV testing in this small cohort, the positive predictive value was 76% for low-grade squamous intraepithelial lesions (LSIL) and 65% for high-grade squamous intraepithelial lesions (HSIL). The negative predictive value of a negative HPV test was 100%. No correlation was found between HPV typing and endometrial biopsy. In light of the demonstrated association of AGC with significant squamous and not glandular lesions, in this and other studies, HPV typing with AGC may be useful to screen for squamous lesions.

The current recommendations for AGC recommend colposcopy and endocervical sampling. If the workup is negative, conization is to be considered. The authors of this study recommend an alternative algorithm for the evaluation of AGC based on the negative and positive predictive value of HPV with AGC. However, much larger prospective studies would be needed to verify the utility of using an HPV result to determine the workup of AGC.

M. E. App, MD, MPH

Genital Tract Shedding of Herpes Simplex Virus Type 2 in Women: Effects of Hormonal Contraception, Bacterial Vaginosis, and Vaginal Group B *Streptococcus* Colonization

Cherpes TL, Melan MA, Kant JA, et al (Univ of Pittsburgh, Pa)
Clin Infect Dis 40:1422-1428, 2005   31–3

Background.—Genital infections due to herpes simplex virus type 2 (HSV-2) are characterized by frequent reactivation and shedding of the virus and by the attendant risk of transmission to sexual partners. We investigated the effects of vaginal coinfections and hormonal contraceptive use on genital tract shedding of HSV-2 in women.

Methods.—A total of 330 HSV-2–seropositive women were followed every 4 months for a year. At each visit, one vaginal swab specimen was obtained for detection of HSV-2 by polymerase chain reaction, a second vaginal swab specimen was obtained for detection of group B *Streptococcus* (GBS) organisms and yeast by culture, and a vaginal smear was obtained for the diagnosis of bacterial vaginosis by Gram staining.

Results.—HSV-2 DNA was detected in 88 (9%) of 956 vaginal swab specimens. Independent predictors of genital tract shedding of HSV-2 were HSV-2 seroconversion during the previous 4 months (adjusted odds ratio [aOR], 3.0; 95% confidence interval [CI], 1.3–6.8), bacterial vaginosis (aOR, 2.3; 95% CI, 1.3–4.0), high-density vaginal GBS colonization (aOR, 2.2; 95% CI, 1.3–3.8), and use of hormonal contraceptives (aOR, 1.8; 95% CI, 1.1–2.8).

Conclusions.—The present study identifies hormonal contraceptive use, bacterial vaginosis, and high-density vaginal GBS colonization as risk factors for genital tract shedding of HSV-2 in women. Because hormonal contraceptives are used by millions of women worldwide and because bacterial vaginosis and vaginal GBS colonization are common vaginal conditions, even modest associations with HSV-2 shedding would result in substantial attributable risks for transmission of the virus.

Safety and Immunogenicity of Glycoprotein D–Adjuvant Genital Herpes Vaccine

Bernstein DI, for the GlaxoSmithKline Herpes Vaccine Study Group (Univ of Cincinnati, Ohio; et al)
Clin Infect Dis 40:1271-1281, 2005   31–4

Background.—Two previous trials have suggested that a herpes simplex virus (HSV) type 2 glycoprotein D (gD) vaccine combined with the adjuvants alum and 3'-O-deacylated-monophosphoryl lipid A (MPL) is well tolerated and provides protection against genital herpes disease in women with no preexisting HSV antibody.

Methods.—The safety and immunogenicity of this vaccine were evaluated in a large, multicenter, double-blind, randomized, placebo-controlled trial. The effects of sex and preexisting HSV immunity were sought.

Results.—When solicited symptoms that continued after the initial 4 days of observation were excluded, the incidence of unsolicited symptoms occurring during the 7 months after vaccination (the primary analysis period) was 22.1% in vaccine recipients and 21.9% in placebo recipients. Significant increases in the number of local and systemic symptoms were found in vaccine recipients within 4 days after vaccination. However, most symptoms were mild to moderate in severity and were short lived. Women reported symptoms more frequently than did men, but preexisting immunity had little effect. The vaccine induced higher titers of HSV gD antibody on enzyme-linked immunosorbent assays than did natural infection with HSV.

Conclusion.—The vaccine was generally safe, well tolerated, and immunogenic.

▶ The impact of HSV-2 in obstetric and gynecologic practice is considerable. Accurate diagnosis, timely intervention and, optimally, prevention of genital tract shedding of HSV remains an important goal in women's health care. These 2 articles (Abstracts 31–3 and 31–4) assess different aspects of this endeavor. The article by Cherpes et al identifies several new factors that affect genital tract shedding of HSV-2 in women. The authors found that hormonal contraceptive use, bacterial vaginosis, and high-density vaginal GBS colonization were risk factors for genital tract shedding of HSV-2. Accordingly, the delineation of more accurate risk assessment is an important part of accurate diagnosis and more timely interventions for both obstetric and gynecologic patients. Antiviral drugs that suppress HSV are widely available, although all would agree that prevention of viral infection would likely eliminate most if not all adverse outcomes of HSV infections. To this end, the study by Bernstein et al reports on a study that demonstrated that a glycoprotein D–adjuvant genital herpes vaccine was found to be safe, well tolerated, and highly immunogenic. Better detection of women at risk for genital tract shedding of HSV-2 and the eventual availability of an effective vaccine to prevent genital herpes will considerably improve the health care of pregnant and nonpregnant women.

L. P. Shulman, MD

Preliminary Evaluation of a Cervical Self-Sampling Device With Liquid-Based Cytology and Multiparameter Molecular Testing
Knesel BW, Dry JC, Wald-Scott C, et al (Select Diagnostics, Greensboro, NC; Univ of Miami, Fla)
J Reprod Med 50:256-260, 2005   31–5

Objective.—To compare the collection of a liquid-based cell sample using a cervical self-sampling device and traditional sampling using cytologic and molecular-based tests.

Study Design.—This study evaluated the sampling efficiency of the Fournier Cervical Self-Sampling Device (BPG, LLC, Miami, Florida; Fig 1) with regard to overall cell volume of the sample, cytologic diagnoses

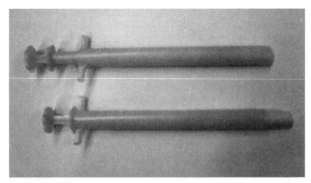

FIGURE 1.—Fournier Self-Sampling Device. (Courtesy of Knesel BW, Dry JC, Wald-Scott C, et al: Preliminary evaluation of a cervical self-sampling device with liquid-based cytology and multiparameter molecular testing. *J Reprod Med* 50:256-260, 2005.)

(SurePath, TriPath Imaging, Burlington, North Carolina) and molecular-based tests for *Chlamydia, Gonorrhoeae* and human papillomavirus (Hybrid Capture 2, Digene Corp., Gaithersburg, Maryland). Paired samples were blinded and prepared using the SurePath method.

Results.—The self-collected samples showed an overall increase in cellularity when compared to the cellularity of samples obtained from traditional sampling. Cytologic results were comparable for the 2 sampling methods. The self-sampling device showed greater sensitivity with regard to molecular-based human papillomavirus testing.

Conclusion.—The Fournier Device shows promise in the area of cytology and molecular diagnostics. The ability to perform cytology and molecular-based assays using a single sample obtained directly by the patient can lower the costs of screening and provide an efficient method of screening women in resource-poor countries or when cultural barriers exist to the use of traditional sampling methods.

▶ The goal of this study was to compare a new self-sampling method and to determine the feasibility of offering a liquid-based Pap test, and human papillomavirus (HPV), *Chlamydia trachomatis* (CT), and *Neisseria gonorrhoeae* (GC) DNA testing from one self-sampled, liquid-based specimen (Fig 1).

Sampled specimens from the traditional speculum collection device were compared with the results from the Fournier Device in regards to cytologic diagnosis, and diagnosis for *Trichomonas, Candida*, GC, CT, and HPV. Cytologic comparisons between cases yielded results within one cytologic diagnostic class. Equivalence was demonstrated in regards to *Trichomonas* and *Candida*. There was little difference in the number of CT and GC cases between the 2 methods. The Fournier Device demonstrated its ability to harvest more cells and identify more cases of HPV than the traditional method.

There are multiple barriers preventing women from being screened in countries with routine screening programs and, obviously, for those who do not have access to screening. In countries with routine screening, women may avoid being screened because of embarrassment, fear, pain, lack of knowledge, or lack of insurance. These women who choose not to or cannot seek medical attention until the disease is advanced require further intervention and cost. In resource-poor areas, health care personnel and facilities are not readily accessible, and if available, extended transportation times may lead to specimen deterioration.

The importance of this body of work is the development of a device that is less expensive, comfortable, private, and just as secure as conventional methods. Further work is needed to optimize this or other devices, as well as studies to demonstrate its strength as compared with traditional collection systems. Such a device is sorely needed in resource-poor countries and in medically underserved areas in our own country to increase the number of women screened, detecting disease and helping prevent the high cost associated with advanced disease.

M. E. App, MD, MPH

Papanicolaou Screening in an Urgent Care Setting
Dunn TS, Jazbec A, Awad R, et al (Univ of Colorado, Denver)
Am J Obstet Gynecol 192:1084-1086, 2005   31–6

Objective.—This study was undertaken to determine the efficacy of Papanicolaou (Pap) screening in an urgent care setting, and to compare the rates of cervical intraepithelial neoplasia (CIN), and follow-up in patients with and without established primary care.

Study Design.—All patients presenting with a complaint warranting pelvic examination between December 2000 and September 2001 underwent Pap screening. All patients were scheduled an appointment or follow-up visit when an abnormal Pap test was found. Charts were reviewed for cytologic interpretation, age, chief complaint, ethnicity, history of prior Pap smear in the institution, total visit history (includes urgent care and primary care clinics). SAS 8.1 was used for statistical analysis with the use of the Fisher exact test.

Results.—A total of 673 Pap smears were performed. Of those, 660 were analyzed and 13 were discarded because of inadequate slides. The mean age was 29.6 years; the ethnic distribution was 0.2% Native American, 1.2% Asian, 17% black, 62.4% Hispanic, 18.2% white, and 1.1% other. In the study population, only 40.6% of the patients had a prior Pap screen and 59.4% had not. There were 318 (48.2%) patients who had accessed care only through the urgent care clinic, and 342 (51.8%) patients who had established some kind of primary care in the past. The overall follow-up rate was 56% for any abnormal Pap smear, regardless of visit history.

Conclusion.—Patients accessing medical care through an urgent care clinic exclusively had identical rates of CIN and follow-up when compared with patients with established care (Table 2). Therefore, when a system ex-

TABLE 2.—Pap Screening in an Urgent Care Setting:
Cytology Results

Pap Result	Study/Urgent Care Setting	DHMC 2001 all Paps
WNL	85%	85%
ASCUS	7.0%	8.3%
LGSIL	5.0%	4.6%
HGSIL	0.3%	0.94%
AGCUS	0.8%	0.4%
SC cancer	0.3%	0.02%

Abbreviations: DHMC, Denver Health Medical Center; *WNL*, within normal limits; *ASCUS*, atypical squamous cells of undetermined significance; *LSIL*, low-grade squamous intraepithelial lesions; *HSIL*, high-grade squamous intraepithelial lesions; *AGCUS*, atypical glandular cells of undetermined significance; *SC*, squamous cell.
(Courtesy of Dunn TS, Jazbec A, Awad R, et al: Papanicolaou screening in an urgent care setting. *Am J Obstet Gynecol* 192:1084-1086, 2005. Copyright 2005 by Elsevier. Reprinted by permission.)

ists to centrally process and triage cervical cytology, it is efficacious to screen for CIN in an urgent care setting.

▶ Though cervical cytology screening has made cervical cancer almost entirely preventable, there are still women diagnosed and dying of cervical cancer every year in the United States. This is directly related to access to health care and poor follow-up. Patients who do not have a primary care physician or do not frequent their physician on an annual basis are those patients being missed for screening. These same patients, however, do present to clinics with other gynecologic complaints. This may be the opportunity to capture these patients for screening who would otherwise be missed.

This study focused on how efficacious it would be to do Pap smears in an urgent care setting, and whether the rates of cervical dysplasia in this setting would be comparable to those of patients who present for annual screening.

The patients presented with multiple gynecologic complaints, the most common being pelvic pain. Fifty-nine percent of these patients had not had a Pap smear within the last 5 years at that institution. It is also noteworthy that of the 151 patients who presented with the complaint of vaginal bleeding, only 7 (4.64%) Pap smears were interpreted as "obscured by blood" and deemed unsatisfactory.

Table 2 compares those Pap smears done in the urgent care clinic versus those done during annual screening, and shows that the rates of abnormal Pap smears for each class were similar. Follow-up rates were also compared and found not to be significantly different.

Many patients only use the urgent care setting as their site of health care. Given that, if a tracking and follow-up system is set in place, this is an excellent opportunity to screen for cervical dysplasia. This study demonstrates that the rates of dysplasia and follow-up in patients accessing medical care exclusively through an urgent care clinic are similar to those found in patients who seek annual screening.

M. E. App, MD, MPH

A Comparison of Modified MonoPrep2 of Liquid-Based Cytology With ThinPrep Pap Test

Nam J-H, Kim H-S, Lee J-S, et al (Chonnam Natl Univ, Gwangju, South Korea; Armed Forces Capital Hosp, Gyung-gi, South Korea; Deaconess Hosp, Oklahoma City, Okla)

Gynecol Oncol 94:693-698, 2004   31–7

Objective.—The purpose of this study is to evaluate a modified MonoPrep2™ (MP) of liquid-based cytology (LBC) to search for a less expensive alternative technique usable for screening of cervical cancers.

Study Design.—Cervicovaginal direct-to-vial samples from 1218 consecutive patients were processed with the modified MP technique and the results were compared with those of currently popular ThinPrep® Pap test (TP) technique.

Results.—Both MP and TP methods provide uniformly spread thin layers of cells without cellular overlap or significant obscuring elements. The diameter of the circular area was 20 mm in MP and 22 mm in TP. Obscuring factors were slightly more frequent in MP but not enough to affect interpretation. Thirteen specimens were excluded from the study because of poor specimen quality in MP (Table 2). In 1205 patients, there was an absolute agreement in results (the Bethesda diagnosis system) between the two methods, and discordances were observed in only 18 (1.5%) in 1187 cases (98.5%). Furthermore, there was no significant difference in diagnostic accuracy in histopathologic correlation between the two methods (Table 4). The sensitivity of MP was slightly lower than that of TP, and the specificity of MP was higher than that of TP. A human papillomavirus (HPV) test with polymerase chain reaction (PCR) using broad-spectrum probes has yielded good results in both MP and TP samples.

TABLE 2.—Comparisons of the Cytologic Diagnosis Between MonoPrep2™ and ThinPrep® Pap Test

	MonoPrep2™		ThinPrep® Pap Test	
	Frequency	Percentage	Frequency	Percentage
Negative	1052	86.4	1046	85.9
ASC-US	21	1.7	24	2.0
ASC-H	9	0.7	6	0.5
Low-grade SIL	33	2.7	38	3.1
High-grade SIL	58	4.8	63	5.2
Squamous cell carcinoma	21	1.8	20	1.6
AGC	3	0.2	5	0.4
Adenocarcinoma in situ	1	0.1	1	0.1
Adenocarcinoma	7	0.6	8	0.7
Unsatisfactory	13	1.1	7	0.6
Total	1218	100	1218	100

Abbreviations: ASC-US, Atypical squamous cells of undetermined significance; *ASC-H,* atypical squamous cells cannot exclude high-grade squamous intraepithelial lesion; *SIL,* squamous intraepithelial lesion; *AGC,* atypical glandular cells.

(Courtesy of Nam J-H, Kim H-S, Lee J-S, et al: A comparison of modified MonoPrep2 of liquid-based cytology with ThinPrep Pap test. *Gynecol Oncol* 94:693-698. Copyright 2004 by Elsevier Science Inc.)

TABLE 4.—Correlation of Histologic and Cytologic Diagnoses Between MonoPrep2™ and ThinPrep® Pap Test

Biopsy Diagnosis	Negative	ASC-US	ASC-H	LSIL	HSIL	Carcinoma	Total
MonoPrep2™ cytologic diagnosis							
Negative	49	1	1	2	3	0	56
CIN I[a]	6	8	1	16	2	0	33
CIN II or III[b]	4	2	3	5	43	1	58
Carcinoma	1	0	1	0	2	18	22
Total	60	11	6	23	50	19	169
ThinPrep® Pap test cytologic diagnosis							
Negative	48	4	2	2	3	0	59
CIN I[a]	5	7	1	19	2	0	34
CIN II or III[b]	4	2	2	6	44	1	59
Carcinoma	1	0	0	0	4	17	22
Total	58	13	5	27	53	18	174

[a]Includes human papilloma virus/condylomatous change and mild dysplasia.
[b]Includes moderate/severe dysplasia and carcinoma in situ.
Abbreviations: ASC-US, Atypical squamous cells of undetermined significance; *ASC-H,* atypical squamous cells cannot exclude HSIL; *LSIL,* low-grade squamous intraepithelial lesion; *HSIL,* high-grade squamous intraepithelial lesion; *CIN,* cervical intraepithelial neoplasia.
(Courtesy of Nam J-H, Kim H-S, Lee J-S, et al: A comparison of modified MonoPrep2 of liquid-based cytology with ThinPrep Pap test. *Gynecol Oncol* 94:693-698. Copyright 2004 by Elsevier Science Inc.)

Conclusions.—The modification of the MP method gave comparable results to those of TP in terms of smear quality, cytologic diagnostic evaluation, and biopsy correlation with much less cost. The modified MP offers a cost-effective alternative to the currently popular expensive techniques of liquid-based cytology practical for cervical cancer screening.

▶ LBC is quickly becoming the preferred technique over conventional Pap smears because of its improved quality of smears, fewer unsatisfactory specimens, and ability to test for HPV, chlamydia, and other viral studies. However, it is much more expensive than the routine Pap smear because of its instrumentation and preparation costs. This prohibits its use in the routine screening of the general population.

This study evaluated an alternative liquid-based technique using a manual filtration system as compared with the TP to see whether it provides a comparable quality of smears and comparable diagnostic results while at the same time being simpler and more cost-efficient. Table 2 demonstrates that the MP system delivered cytology results that were very comparable to those of the TP. The cytology from both systems were then compared with the histologic results gained from either clinical punch biopsy or cone biopsy. Table 4 demonstrates the ability of the MP system to correlate cytology with histology as well as the TP. The MP also was shown to test for HPV as well as did the TP.

A limitation of this study is that it did not do a cost analysis between these 2 systems. The MP does appear promising. These results would need to be duplicated in other studies and demonstrate its cost-effectiveness before such an alternative system would be adopted. However, a less expensive LBC system would be very welcome in routine screening for public health purposes, particularly in low-income, high-risk populations.

M. E. App, MD, MPH

Altered Recognition of Reparative Changes in ThinPrep Specimens in the College of American Pathologists Gynecologic Cytology Program
Snyder TM, for the Cytopathology Resource Committee, College of American Pathologists (Methodist Hosp, Houston; et al)
Arch Pathol Lab Med 129:861-865, 2005   31–8

Context.—Previous studies have shown that the diagnosis of reparative changes in conventional smears in the College of American Pathologists Interlaboratory Comparison Program in Gynecologic Cytology is one of the least reproducible diagnoses. Indeed, the diagnosis of reparative changes consistently yields the highest false-positive rate of any negative for intraepithelial lesions and malignancy (NILM) cytodiagnostic category. It is unknown whether cytologists recognize reparative changes in ThinPrep specimens as well, or less often, as in conventional smears.

Objective.—To assess and compare the ability of cytologists to recognize reparative changes in conventional and ThinPrep preparations.

Design.—We compiled performance data from the College of American Pathologists Interlaboratory Comparison Program in Gynecologic Cytology from the 2000-2003 program years. More than 400 slides with a reference diagnosis of reparative changes met our study criteria, representing a total of 11,200 individual responses for conventional cases and 1155 individual responses for ThinPrep specimens. We evaluated the results of both individual and laboratory participants using 2 performance criteria: the false-positive discordancy rate and the exact match error rate (any response that does not exactly match the reference diagnosis of 120 [reparative changes]).

Results.—Cases with a reference diagnosis of reparative changes made up 1.2% of all ThinPrep slides and 3.7% of all conventional slides in circulation. The false-positive discordancy rate of individual responses on educational slides for conventional smears was significantly higher than the corresponding false-positive discordancy rate for ThinPrep specimens (15.7% for conventional vs 7.1% for ThinPrep specimens, $P < .001$). Laboratory responses on educational conventional smears and ThinPrep slides showed a similar trend (14.2% for conventional smears vs 2.4% for ThinPrep slides, $P = .002$). The exact match error rate on educational conventional slides was 41.4% for individual responses, while on educational ThinPrep slides, the overall error rate was 57.5% ($P < .001$). For laboratory responses, the exact match error rate was 40.5% for educational conventional smears versus 58.9% for educational ThinPrep smears ($P < .001$). Characteristic features of reparative changes were identified in ThinPrep specimens.

Conclusions.—In the College of American Pathologists Interlaboratory Comparison Program in Gynecologic Cytology, ThinPrep slides with a reference diagnosis of reparative changes have a lower false-positive discordancy rate than conventional slides. Responses to ThinPrep cases with a reference diagnosis of reparative change show a higher exact match error rate than conventional smears. Since reparative changes in gynecologic cytology are recognized as indicating an increased risk of significant lesions, the clinical significance of these altered patterns of recognition of reparative changes in ThinPrep specimens warrants further investigation.

▶ Reparative changes, whether typical or atypical, have been shown in prior studies to be associated with an increased risk of squamous and other clinically significant lesions. It is also one of the least reproducible diagnoses.

The hypotheses of this study was that the ThinPrep slides with reparative changes were associated with a relatively low false-positive rate (high specificity) as compared with the conventional Pap smear. The data from the College of American Pathologists (CAP) Interlaboratory Comparison Program in Gynecologic Cytology (PAP) program for both conventional and ThinPrep specimens with reparative changes for the last 4 years were reviewed. The PAP program is a quarterly, mailed, glass slide quality improvement program utilized by cytology laboratories of all types.

Analysis of these data show that cases from Thin Prep with a diagnosis of reparative change were performing differently from conventional smears with the same diagnosis. This study suggests that the interpretation of reparative change in ThinPrep specimens is different than that in conventional smears. This would be important in light of the knowledge that with conventional Pap smears, reparative changes are associated with an increased risk of squamous intraepithelial lesions. It may be with the ThinPrep, reparative change may be associated with a decreased risk of squamous intraepithelial lesions. Thus, a diagnosis of reparative change from a ThinPrep specimen may not share the same clinical significance as the conventional Pap smear.

In light of these findings, further investigation is needed to confirm whether reparative changes with the ThinPrep is associated with a lower risk of squamous intraepithelial lesions.

M. E. App, MD, MPH

Vaccines Against Human Papillomavirus and Cervical Cancer: Promises and Challenges
Mahdavi A, Monk BJ (Univ of California, Orange)
Oncologist 10:528-538, 2005   31–9

Abstract.—Cervical cancer and precancerous lesions of the genital tract are major threats to the health of women worldwide. The introduction of screening tests to detect cervical cancer precursor lesions has reduced cervical cancer rates in the developed world, but not in developing countries. Human papillomavirus (HPV) is the primary etiologic agent of cervical cancer

TABLE 1.—Preventing HPV Infection: Comparison of Monovalent (Merck) and Bivalent (GlaxoSmithKline) L1 VLP Prophylactic Vaccines

Study	Koutsky et al. [19] (Merck Study)	Harper et al. [21] (GlaxoSmithKline Study)
Design	Randomized double-blind controlled trial	Randomized double-blind controlled trial
Age (years)	16-25	15-25
No. of enrollees	2,392	1,113
Location	16 sites in the U.S.	32 sites in North America and Brazil
Antigen	40µg HPV-16L1 VLP	20 µg HPV-16 L1 VLP 20 µg HPV-18L1 VLP
Adjuvant	225 µg aluminum hydroxyphosphate sulfate	500 µg aluminum hydroxide and 50 µg 3-deacylated monophosphoryl lipid (ASO4)
Vaccination schedule	0, 2, and 6 months	0, 1, and 6 months
Follow-up	Mean of 17.4 months	Up to 27 months
Specific titers compared with natural infection	60 times greater	50 times greater for HPV-16; 80 times greater for HPV-18
Clinical outcome	100% efficacy preventing persistent HPV-16 infection. No cytologic or histologic abnormalities.	100% efficacy preventing persistent HPV-16/18 infection. 93% efficacy preventing cytological abnormalities.
Adverse effects	Nonsignificant	Nonsignificant

Abbreviations: HPV, human papillomavirus; VLP, virus-like particle.
(Courtesy of Mahdavi A, Monk BJ: Vaccines against human papillomavirus and cervical cancer: Promises and challenges. *Oncologist* 10:528-538, 2005.)

and dysplasia. Thus, cervical cancer and other HPV-associated malignancies might be prevented or treated by HPV vaccines. Two vaccine strategies have been developed (Table 1). First, prevention of HPV infection through induction of capsid-specific neutralizing antibodies has been studied in clinical trials. However, because the capsid proteins are not expressed at detectable levels by infected basal keratinocytes or in HPV-transformed cells, a second approach of developing therapeutic vaccines by targeting nonstructural early viral antigens has also been developed. Because two HPV oncogenic proteins, E6 and E7, are critical to the induction and maintenance of cellular transformation and are coexpressed in the majority of HPV-containing carcinomas, most therapeutic vaccines target one or both of these gene products. A variety of approaches is being tested in therapeutic vaccine clinical trials, whereby E6 and/or E7 are administered in live vectors, as peptides or protein, in nucleic acid form, or in cell-based vaccines. The paradigm of preventing HPV infection through vaccination has been tested, and two vaccines are currently in phase III clinical trials. However, current therapeutic vaccine trials are less mature with respect to disease clearance. A number of approaches have shown significant therapeutic benefit in preclinical papillomavirus models and await testing in patient populations to determine the most effective curative strategy (Table 2).

TABLE 2.—Characteristics of Therapeutic HPV Vaccines

	Advantages	Drawbacks
Vector-based: viral/bacterial	Highly immunogenic	Safety concerns, previous immunization
Peptide-based	Safety, easy to produce	Weakly immunogenic, requires HLA compatibility
Protein-based	Safety, no HLA restriction	Weak activator of cell-mediated immunity
DNA	Easy to produce, store, and transport; sustained antigenic expression	Weakly immunogenic
DC-based	Highly immunogenic	Difficult to produce and biodeliver

Abbreviations: DC, dendritic cell; HPV, human papillomavirus.
(Courtesy of Mahdavi A, Monk BJ: Vaccines against human papillomavirus and cervical cancer: Promises and challenges. *Oncologist* 10:528-538, 2005.)

▶ The authors compare and contrast the 2 industry-funded approaches to prophylactic vaccines for HPV. Clinical results from these randomized trials are expected within the next year, potentially leading to FDA approval of a prophylactic VLP HPV vaccine. The Merck vaccine will target HPV types 6, 11, 16, and 18, while the GlaxoSmithKline vaccine will target HPV types 16 and 18.[1,2] The authors also review 2 promising therapeutic vaccines. The first vaccine is an encapsulated HPV vaccine and contains DNA-encoded fragments derived from E6 and E7 of HPV 16 and 18. These biodegradable particles have been shown to cause regression of CIN II and CIN III among young women.[3] In addition, the authors review another promising peptide vaccine. This vaccine uses a fusion protein consisting of heat shock proteins and E7 (HspE7). This vaccine has been shown in preliminary studies to also be associated with regression of CIN and anal dysplasia in men.[4]

Clearly, vaccination is the ultimate prevention and cure of cervical carcinoma. Exciting strategies are under way and will hopefully soon be widely available.

B. J. Monk, MD

References

1. Koutsky LA, Ault KA, Wheeler CM, et al: A controlled trial of a human papillomavirus type 16 vaccine. *N Engl J Med* 347:1645-1651, 2002.
2. Harper DM, Franco EL, Wheeler C, et al: Efficacy of a bivalent L1 virus-like particle vaccine in prevention of infection with human papillomavirus types 16 and 18 in young women: A randomized controlled trial. *Lancet* 364:1757-1765, 2004.
3. Garcia F, Petry KU, Muderspach L, et al: ZYC101a for treatment of high-grade cervical intraepithelial neoplasia: A randomized controlled trial. *Obstet Gynecol* 103:317-326, 2004.
4. Einstein MH, Kadish AS, Burk RD, et al: HSP-based immunotherapy (HspE7) for treatment of CIN 3. *Gynecol Oncol* 96:912a-913a, 2005.

Prophylactic Quadrivalent Human Papillomavirus (Types 6, 11, 16, and 18) L1 Virus-Like Particle Vaccine in Young Women: A Randomised Double-Blind Placebo-Controlled Multicentre Phase II Efficacy Trial

Villa LL, Costa RLR, Petta CA, et al (Ludwig Inst for Cancer Research, Sao Paulo, Brazil; Instituto Brasileiro de Controle do Cancer, Sao Paulo, Brazil; Universidade Estadual de Campinas, Brazil; et al)

Lancet Oncol 6:271-278, 2005   31–10

Background.—A randomised double-blind placebo-controlled phase II study was done to assess the efficacy of a prophylactic quadrivalent vaccine targeting the human papillomavirus (HPV) types associated with 70% of cervical cancers (types 16 and 18) and with 90% of genital warts (types 6 and 11).

Methods.—277 young women (mean age 20.2 years [SD 1.7]) were randomly assigned to quadrivalent HPV (20 µg type 6, 40 µg type 11, 40 µg type 16, and 20 µg type 18) L1 virus-like-particle (VLP) vaccine and 275 (mean age 20.0 years [1.7]) to one of two placebo preparations at day 1, month 2, and month 6. For 36 months, participants underwent regular gynaecological examinations, cervicovaginal sampling for HPV DNA, testing for serum antibodies to HPV, and Pap testing. The primary endpoint was the combined incidence of infection with HPV 6, 11, 16, or 18, or cervical or external genital disease (ie, persistent HPV infection, HPV detection at the last recorded visit, cervical intraepithelial neoplasia, cervical cancer, or external genital lesions caused by the HPV types in the vaccine). Main analyses were done per protocol.

Findings.—Combined incidence of persistent infection or disease with HPV 6, 11, 16, or 18 fell by 90% (95% CI 71-97, p<0.0001) in those assigned vaccine compared with those assigned placebo.

Interpretation.—A vaccine targeting HPV types 6, 11, 16, 18 could substantially reduce the acquisition of infection and clinical disease caused by common HPV types.

▶ The study was done to determine the efficacy of an HPV vaccine targeting HPV types 16 and 18, which are responsible for most cervical cancers, and types 6 and 11, which are associated with genital warts. The study looked at a group of young women receiving the vaccine in Europe, Brazil, and the United States. The subjects enrolled were healthy, not pregnant, had no history of prior abnormal Pap smears, and reported a lifetime history of 4 or fewer sex partners. It did not exclude women with prior HPV infection.

This is a randomized, double-blinded, placebo-controlled study of 1158 women recruited within the ages of 16 to 23 years. Fifty-two women were also enrolled in a dose-escalation safety assessment (Part A). The data presented in this article are from Part B, which is a fully blinded, dose-ranging assessment of immunogenicity and efficacy. From Part B, 552 subjects were enrolled in the "low-dose" group. From this group, 277 women were randomly assigned to receive the quadravalent (6, 11, 16, and 18) HPV vaccine, and 275 women were randomly assigned to receive placebo (control group). The groups were followed up for 36 months, undergoing regular Pap smears, gynecologic exams, and testing for HPV (serum antibodies as well as cervical sampling). The outcome measured was combined incidence of HPV infection, and cervical or external genital disease. The authors found that the combined incidence of the 4 types of HPV infection fell by 90% in those given the vaccine as compared with the control group.

The study adds to a growing body of evidence favoring the implementation of this vaccine in helping prevent HPV infection. It has shown that the vaccine substantially reduces the risk of acquiring disease with common HPV types that subsequently lead to morbidity of cervical and genital disease. Further studies need to be conducted to determine the long-term effectiveness of the vaccine. Acceptability of patients and parents of vaccines preventing sexually transmitted infections has been favorable in studies done.[1] Further steps need to be taken to study the safety and efficacy of the HPV vaccine in the adolescent age group.

E. A. Iglesias, MD

Reference

1. Zimet GD, Perkins SM, Sturm LA, et al: Predictors of STI vaccine acceptability among parents and their adolescent children. *J Adolesc Health* 37:179-186, 2005.

Comparison of Pap Smear, Visual Inspection With Acetic Acid, Human Papillomavirus DNA-PCR Testing and Cervicography

De Vuyst H, Claeys P, Njiru S, et al (Ghent Univ, Belgium; Univ of Nairobi, Kenya; Free Univ of Brussels, Belgium; et al)
Int J Gynecol Obstet 89:120-126, 2005   31–11

Objective.—To assess the test qualities of four screening methods to detect cervical intra-epithelial neoplasia in an urban African setting.

Method.—Six hundred fifty-three women, attending a family planning clinic in Nairobi (Kenya), underwent four concurrent screening methods: pap smear, visual inspection with acetic acid (VIA), PCR for high risk human papillomavirus (HR HPV) and cervicography. The presence of cervical intra-epithelial neoplasia (CIN) was verified by colposcopy or biopsy.

Result.—Sensitivity (for CIN2 or higher) and specificity (to exclude any CIN or cancer) were 83.3% (95% CI [73.6, 93.0]) and 94.6% (95% CI [92.6, 96.5]), respectively, for pap smear; 73.3% (95% CI [61.8, 84.9]) and 80.0% (95% CI [76.6, 83.4]) for VIA; 94.4% (95% CI [84.6, 98.8]) and 73.9% (95% CI [69.7, 78.2]) for HR HPV; and 72.3% (95% CI [59.1, 85.6]) and 93.2% (95% CI [90.8, 95.7]) for cervicography (Table 4).

Conclusion.—The pap smear had the highest specificity (94.6%) and HPV testing the highest sensitivity (94.4%). The visual methods, VIA and

TABLE 4.—Sensitivity and Specificity of the Four Screening Tests

| Disease Threshold | Pap Smear | | VIA | | HPV (Any Type) | | HPV HR | | Cervicography | |
	Sensitivity %, 95% CI %	Specificity %, 95% CI %	Sensitivity %, 95% CI %	Specificity %, 95% CI %	Sensitivity %, 95% CI %	Specificity %, 95% CI %	Sensitivity %, 95% CI %	Specificity %, 95% CI %	Sensitivity %, 95% CI %	Specificity %, 95% CI %
CIN1+	68.1, 59.4-76.9	94.6, 92.6-96.5	60.5, 51.4-69.6	80.0, 76.6-83.4	86.3, 79.5-93.1	59.4, 54.7-64.2	83.3, 76.0-90.7	73.9, 69.7-78.2	52.6, 42.4-62.9	93.2, 90.8-95.7
CIN2+	83.3, 73.6-93.0	90.3, 87.9-92.8	73.3, 61.8-84.9	77.6, 74.2-80.9	96.3, 87.3, 99.6	55.8, 51.3-60.4	94.4, 84.6, 98.8	69.3, 65.0-73.5	72.3, 59.1-85.6	90.5, 87.8-93.1

Abbreviations: VIA, Visual inspection with acetic acid; *HPV,* human papillomavirus; *HPV HR,* high-risk HPV; *CI,* confidence interval; *CIN,* cervical intraepithelial neoplasia.
(Courtesy of De Vuyst H, Claeys P, Njiru S, et al: Comparison of Pap smear, visual inspection with acetic acid, human papillomavirus DNA-PCR testing and cervicography. *Int J Gynecol Obstet* 89:120-126, 2005.)

cervicography, were similar and showed an accuracy in between the former two tests.

▶ The Pap smear has reduced the incidence of cervical cancer up to 80% in countries with organized screening and treatment programs. However, in the developing world, the incidence of cervical cancer remains high, particularly in sub-Saharan Africa, where cervical cancer is the most common cancer in women. The lack of organized cervical cancer control programs is the main reason for this. Effective cytologic screening programs are difficult to implement in low-resource settings because of high cost, training requirements, and competing health priorities. In addition, colposcopy and colposcopy-directed biopsy to confirm a positive test is cumbersome, costly, and requires highly trained personnel. Thus, the prospect of having one test sensitive enough for screening and specific enough to direct treatment in this poor resource environment is appealing.

The purpose of this cross-sectional study was to investigate the sensitivity and specificity of alternative screening methods that could be used in poor resource regions. The methods compared were the conventional Pap smear, HPV testing, cervicography (photographs of the cervix with a specially designed camera), and visual inspection of the transformation zone after application of acetic acid. Two groups were compared: those attending the clinic for family planning services (screening group) and those referred for an abnormal Pap smear or other clinical reasons (referral group). Lesions were more prevalent in the referred group.

Table 4 demonstrates the sensitivity and specificity of the 4 screening tests. Pap smear had the highest specificity, and HPV had the highest sensitivity. Cervicography and VIA were intermediate. The limitations of this study were that a number of HPV tests and cervicography are missing or noninterpretable, which only highlights the difficulty in using these screening methods with poor resources. This study also did not examine the cost-effectiveness of these methods. However, VIA was demonstrated to be cost saving in South Africa.[1]

A simple, widely applicable screening test for cervical dysplasia and cancer is desperately needed in poor resource countries, and VIA should be considered as a primary screening tool.

M. E. App, MD, MPH

Reference

1. Goldie SJ, Kuhn L, Denny L, et al: Policy analysis of cervical cancer screening strategies in low-resource settings: Clinical benefits and cost-effectiveness. *JAMA* 285:3107-3115, 2001.

Cervical Intraepithelial Neoplasia (CIN)

Cervical Intraepithelial Neoplasia: Prognosis by Combined LOH Analysis of Multiple Loci

ELhamidi A, Hamoudi RA, Kocjan G, et al (Univ College London)
Gynecol Oncol 94:671-679, 2004   31–12

Objective.—Cervical intraepithelial neoplasias (CIN) show markedly variable clinical behavior. Clinically, it is important to distinguish CIN lesions with different behaviors and identify those likely to persist and progress. The purpose of this study is to explore whether CIN lesions with different clinical behaviors can be stratified by analysis of loss of heterozygosity (LOH) at multiple loci.

Methods.—One hundred sixty-four cases of CIN (54 CIN1, 59 CIN2 and 51 CIN3) were screened for LOH at 12 microsatellite markers including 10 from 3p14, 3p21-22, 6p21 and 11q23. LOH was correlated with clinical follow-up data and high-risk HPV infection.

Results.—In a pilot study of 71 cases of CIN, screening of 12 microsatellite markers identified four (D3S1300, D3S1260, D11S35, and D11S528) at which LOH was significantly associated with disease persistence/progression. These four markers were further investigated in a larger cohort, which brought the total number of cases examined to 164. Combined analysis of LOH at the above four loci permitted the identification of 22-47% of CIN lesions depending on the histological grade, which showed disease persistence/progression. LOH at these loci was significantly associated with HPV16 infection. Bioinformatic analysis identified several candidate genes including the fragile histidine triad gene and progesterone receptor gene that may be the target of deletions.

Conclusions.—LOH at D3S1300, D3S1260, D11S35 and D11S528 was significantly associated with CINs that showed persistence/progression, and combined LOH analyses at these loci could be used to identify such cases.

▶ It has been shown that at least 5% of CIN will show disease recurrence despite treatment. It is not known at this time how to identify those CIN lesions that are likely to persist and progress despite treatment, making clinical management of such patients difficult.

Infection with high-risk human papillomavirus (HPV) alone is insufficient to cause cancer. Identifying factors that facilitate HPV oncogenesis can be important for early detection, therapeutic intervention, and monitoring the response to therapy. Genetic changes may play a crucial role in the transformation of HPV-infected cells and may account for the irreversible clinical behavior of CIN.

The aim of this study was to examine whether chromosomal regions associated with LOH could be used as a prognostic marker for CIN lesions and their clinical behavior. Four of 12 markers associated with LOH were found to be significantly associated with the clinical behavior of CIN. The combination of these 4 markers could predict at least one third of the CIN lesions that persist despite treatment.

Though this combination only predicts one third of such lesions, it may be that with the addition of other markers associated with LOH, the sensitivity would increase. In theory, a prognostic test using these markers could be created to predict which patients may have persistence of CIN after treatment, and aid in management of these patients.

M. E. App, MD, MPH

The Role Treatment for Cervical Intraepithelial Neoplasia Plays in the Disappearance of Human Papilloma Virus

Aschkenazi-Steinberg SO, Spitzer BJ, Spitzer M (North Shore Univ, Manhasset, NY)
J Low Genit Tract Dis 9:19-22, 2005   31–13

Objective.—To explore the role played by excision of the transformation zone in women diagnosed with cervical intraepithelial neoplasia (CIN) in the disappearance of human papillomavirus (HPV).

Material and Methods.—In a retrospective, cohort study, women with CIN who were treated by loop electrosurgical excision procedure of the transformation zone were compared with another group of women with CIN who were managed expectantly. The decision to treat or manage expectantly was made by one of the authors on clinical grounds. All patients were evaluated with cervical cytologic analysis, pathologic examination of excised tissue, and HPV DNA testing, which was considered positive when high-risk HPV types were detected. Among women treated with loop electrosurgical excision procedure, the median lag time was calculated from diagnosis of CIN to treatment. The median time for conversion from HPV-positive to HPV-negative status in both groups was compared, as well as the 1- and 2-year cure rates (defined as converting to HPV-negative status) in the treated and untreated groups.

Results.—In the treated group, 12% had CIN 1, 83% had CIN 2,3, 2% had cancer, and 3% had normal pathologic results. In the untreated group, 82% had CIN 1, 16% had CIN 2,3, and 2% had normal pathologic results ($p < 0.0001$). The lag time from the initial diagnosis of CIN to treatment was less than 1 month. The median follow-up time was 7 months (range, 1-121 months) in the treated group and 13 months (range, 1-70 months) in the untreated group. The 1-year rates of conversion to HPV-negative status, defined as the cure rates in the treated and untreated groups, were 65% ($\pm$ 6%) and 23% ($\pm$ 7%), respectively, and the 2-year cure rates in the treated and untreated groups were 90% ($\pm$ 4%) and 56% ($\pm$ 11%), respectively ($p < 0.0001$). Median time to conversion to a negative HPV status was 7.7 months for the treated patients compared with 19.4 months in the untreated patients ($p < 0.0001$).

Conclusions.—Women treated by loop electrosurgical excision procedure are more likely convert to HPV-negative status at 1 and 2 years and do so significantly sooner than those managed expectantly.

▶ Several studies have found that HPV DNA is cleared after effective treatment for CIN 0 and that persistence of HPV DNA predicts recurrence of CIN. However, this retrospective study followed the HPV status of women with CIN not treated and compared them to the HPV status of treated women.

The limitations of this study are that it is a retrospective study, has a small sample size, a wide age range of patients, and varying degrees of CIN between groups, and that the untreated patients with CIN 2 were almost all adolescents or in their early 20s, nulliparous patients who declined treatment after counseling, and some older patients in the midst of fertility treatment who refused treatment after counseling.

However, the difference of conversion time of the HPV status between treated and untreated women is worth further study as it may change the current recommended guidelines for HPV screening for both groups. In the 2001 consensus guidelines, one of the acceptable guidelines for follow-up after treatment of CIN is HPV testing 6 months after treatment, and follow-up of CIN 1 is either with a Pap at 6 and 12 months or HPV testing at 12 months. Given these study results, HPV testing after treatment at 6 months would be futile if the median time to conversion is 7.7 months, so delaying HPV testing to 12 months seems reasonable. Likewise, given the longer conversion time for the untreated patient, delaying HPV testing to 24 months rather than 12 months also should be considered.

Given these results, it would be worthwhile to do a prospective, randomized trial with longitudinal follow-up with HPV testing of treated and untreated women with CIN, with more narrow inclusion and exclusion criteria.

M. E. App, MD, MPH

Colposcopically Directed Biopsy, Random Cervical Biopsy, and Endocervical Curettage in the Diagnosis of Cervical Intraepithelial Neoplasia II or Worse
Pretorius RG, Zhang W-H, Belinson JL, et al (Southern California Permanente Med Group, Fontana; Chinese Academy of Med Sciences, Beijing; Cleveland Clinic Found, Ohio)
Am J Obstet Gynecol 191:430-434, 2004   31–14

Objectives.—The purpose of this study was to determine the relative importance of colposcopically directed biopsy, random biopsy, and endocervical curettage (ECC) in diagnosing ≥cervical intraepithelial neoplasia (CIN) II.

Study Design.—During a screening study, 364 women with satisfactory colposcopy and ≥CIN II were diagnosed. All colposcopically detected lesions were biopsied. If colposcopy showed no lesion in a cervical quadrant, a

TABLE 1.—Method of Diagnosing Cervical Intraepithelial
Neoplasia II or Worse in 364 Women
With Satisfactory Colposcopy

CIN II or Worse Diagnosed by	Number/Total	Percent	95% CI
Colposcopically directed biopsy	208/364	(57.1%)	52.1-62.2
With negative ECC	151/364	(41.5%)	36.4-46.6
With positive ECC	57/364	(15.7%)	11.9-19.4
Random biopsy	136/364	(37.4%)	32.4-42.3
With negative ECC	115/364	(31.6%)	26.8-36.4
With positive ECC	21/364	(5.8%)	26.8-36.8
Positive ECC only	20/364	(5.5%)	3.4-8.2
Total	364/364	(100.0%)	

Abbreviations: CIN, Cervical intraepithelial neoplasia; CI, confidence interval;
ECC, endocervical curettage.
(Courtesy of Pretorius RG, Zhang W-H, Belinson JL, et al: Colposcopically directed
biopsy, random cervical biopsy, and endocervical curettage in the diagnosis of cervical
intraepithelial neoplasia II or worse. *Am J Obstet Gynecol* 191:430-434, 2004. Copyright
2004 by Elsevier. Reprinted with permission.)

random biopsy was obtained at the squamocolumnar junction in that quadrant. ECC was then performed.

Results.—The diagnosis of ≥CIN II was made on a colposcopically directed biopsy in 57.1%, random biopsy in 37.4%, and ECC in 5.5% of women (Table 1). The yield of ≥CIN II for random biopsy when cytology was high grade (17.6%) exceeded that when cytology was low grade (2.8%). One of 20 women diagnosed solely by ECC had invasive cancer.

Conclusion.—Even when colposcopy is satisfactory, ECC should be performed. If cytology is high grade, random biopsies should be considered.

▶ Two techniques in the colposcopy procedure—ECC and random cervical biopsies—were the focus of this study. The value of ECC in the diagnosis of cervical dysplasia has been widely argued, whereas the use of random cervical biopsies when no overt lesions are visualized has not been adequately studied.

The hypothesis of this study was that the addition of random cervical biopsy and ECC with colposcopic-directed biopsy would improve the diagnosis of severe dysplasia.

Table 1 shows the method of diagnosing CIN II or worse in all the women with a satisfactory colposcopy. Fifty seven percent (57.1%) of women with CIN II or worse were diagnosed by directed biopsy. Of particular importance, 37.4% were diagnosed solely by random biopsies, and 5.5% were diagnosed solely by ECC. When these histologic specimens were compared with the preceding cytology outcomes, the yield of CIN II was 17% with high-grade squamous intraepithelial lesions (HSIL) but only 3.6% and 1.7% with low-grade squamous intraepithelial lesions (LSIL) and atypical squamous cells of uncertain significance (ASCUS) with high-risk human papillomavirus. In contrast to random biopsies, the yield of CIN II or worse is appreciable even with LSIL and ASCUS HRHPV+ (14.8%-15.6%).

The strength of the study was that the evaluation for each woman was uniform, with diagnosis based on at least 4 cervical biopsies and ECC performed by trained and experienced colposcopists. This trial demonstrates that random biopsies are warranted for those patients with Pap smears of HSIL or cancer and a negative colposcopy, and that ECC increases detection of CIN II or greater regardless of the Pap smear. These findings should be incorporated into one's practice of routine colposcopy.

M. E. App, MD, MPH

Efficacy of Cone Biopsy of the Uterine Cervix During Frozen Section for the Evaluation of Cervical Intraepithelial Neoplasia Grade 3

Gu M, Lin F (Univ of California, Orange)
Am J Clin Pathol 122:383-388, 2004   31–15

Abstract.—We retrospectively selected 22 cases in which patients with a biopsy-proven diagnosis of cervical intraepithelial neoplasia grade 3 underwent cervical conization for frozen section (FS) evaluation followed by hysterectomy at the University of California Irvine Medical Center, Orange, during the August 1995 to September 9, 2001. All slides from FS and permanent section (PS) and hysterectomy specimens were reviewed. FS diagnoses were compared with those of previous biopsies, PS, and hysterectomy specimens. The PS correlated with FS in all cases but 1. Appropriate surgery was performed for all patients based on FS diagnosis. The McNemar test was used to compare the results of FS and PS, with a 2-sided P value of 1.0 and a κ coefficient of 0.7755 with a 95% confidence level, indicating that the 2

TABLE 1.—Summary of Literature on Frozen Section Evaluation of Cervical Conization

		No. and Type of Cervical Lesions				
Reference	No. of Cases	Benign	Dysplasia	CIS	Invasive	Accuracy (%)
Rutledge and Ibanez,[3] 1962	70	0	0	70	0	100
Kaufman et al,[4] 1962	52	9	26	15	2	94.2
Dutra et al,[5] 1962	166	99	0	56	11	85.5
Greenberg and Kaufman,[6] 1963	117	18	56	38	5	97.4
Guerriero et al,[7] 1964	148	42	49	52	5	83.4
Kaufman et al,[8] 1965	210	29	105	63	13	93.3
DiMusto,[9] 1970	249	29	48	146	26	92.0
Woodruff et al,[10] 1970	40	4	10	17	9	NA
Holt and Armstrong,[11] 1970	210	4	90	99	17	93
Gupta,[12] 1971	150	0	50	100	0	92
Torres et al,[13] 1983	43	0	14 (CIN 2)	29	0	93
Fletcher et al,[14] 1985	282	NA	NA	NA	NA	NA
Hannigan et al,[15] 1986	96	13	36 (CIN 1/2)	45	2	95
Woodford et al,[16] 1986	80	11	13 (CIN 1/2)	49	7	80
Neiger et al,[17] 1991	43	0	38 (CIN 1/2/3)	NA	5	100
Hoffman et al,[18] 1993	128	23	24 (CIN 1/2)	62	19	See text

Abbreviations: CIN, Cervical intraepithelial neoplasia; CIS, carcinoma in situ; NA, not available.

groups were not significantly different. FS evaluation of cervical conization is as efficacious and accurate as evaluation of regular specimens in providing information for the appropriateness of same-day surgery. We recommend that entire tissue be submitted for FS to avoid sampling errors and to increase diagnostic accuracy (Table 1).

▶ It is standard practice to perform a cone biopsy to rule out invasive cervical carcinoma before definitive treatment. The comparison of FS to PS evaluation dates has been reviewed several times, starting in the 1960s and through the early 1990s. However, FS has not been widely accepted despite encouraging results. In light of the present managed care environment, the authors of this study decided to readdress the issue of same-day hysterectomy guided by FS to decrease costs and patient anxiety and to gain the advantages associated with same-day surgery.

The authors reviewed the past literature on this subject as well as conducted a retrospective review of their institutional experience of cervical intraepithelial neoplasia (CIN 3), comparing frozen and nonfrozen specimens. The retrospective review of the cone biopsies showed no discrepancies between the diagnoses between FS and PS except for one case, but appropriate operations were performed in all cases. The literature review of this comparison was interesting and enlightening. Table 1 summarizes the literature and shows that FS evaluation of cervical cone biopsies is reliable.

The authors discuss and review the advantages as well as disadvantages of FS. To counteract the disadvantages, they recommend guidelines to avoid erroneous diagnosis. These include having good equipment and experienced technicians, examining the entire tissue specimen, and working with an operating surgeon that is cooperative and willing to wait an average of 30 to 45 minutes for a result.

By their own institutional experience and review of the literature, the authors show that FS evaluation provides accurate guidance in same-day operations, and is efficient and cost-effective for a same-day hysterectomy procedure. These results should be strongly considered in the current managed care environment.

M. E. App, MD, MPH

32 Leiomyoma

Outcome of Uterine Embolization and Hysterectomy for Leiomyomas: Results of a Multicenter Study
Spies JB, Cooper JM, Worthington-Kirsch R, et al (Georgetown Univ, Washington, DC; Women's Health Research, Phoenix, Ariz; Roxborough Mem Hosp, Philadelphia; et al)
Am J Obstet Gynecol 191:22-31, 2004   32–1

Objective.—The purpose of this study was to estimate the outcomes of uterine embolization and hysterectomy for uterine leiomyomas.

Study Design.—This was a multicenter prospective study of patients who were treated with embolization (n = 102 patients) and hysterectomy (n = 50 patients) for leiomyomas. Changes in symptoms, complications, and quality of life were measured. The data analysis included linear and logistic regression, the Student *t* and paired *t* test, Fisher's exact test, and chi-squared test.

Results.—For patients who underwent embolization, there were marked reductions in blood loss scores ($P < .001$) and menorrhagia questionnaire scores ($P < .001$) compared with baseline. At 12 months, a larger proportion of the patients who had undergone hysterectomy experienced improved pelvic pain ($P = .021$). Both groups had marked improvement in other symptoms and quality of life scores, with no difference between groups. Complications were more frequent in patients who underwent hysterectomy (50% vs 27.5%; $P = .01$).

Conclusion.—Both procedures substantially improved symptoms for most patients, with an advantage for hysterectomy at 12 months for pelvic pain. Serious complications were infrequent in both groups.

▶ Symptomatic uterine leiomyomas remain a common indication for hysterectomy. The use of uterine artery embolization as an alternative to hysterectomy has become increasingly popular. This study attempts to compare the outcomes and complications in individuals undergoing either abdominal hysterectomy or uterine artery embolization. Both groups had substantial improvement in symptoms. Although a larger proportion of patients with pelvic pain had improvement with hysterectomy, the quality-of-life scores were no different between the groups.

The greatest criticism of this study is that patients were not randomized to therapy. Since patients self-selected treatment, this potentially introduces a bias into the study. Patients selecting embolization were also more likely to have had myomectomy of curettage than those selecting hysterectomy, potentially indicating a stronger desire to avoid hysterectomy. Until randomized studies are available, this study is the best evidence to date that uterine artery embolization is comparable to hysterectomy for symptom relief caused by leiomyomas.

G. H. Lipscomb, MD

Predictive Factors for Fibroids Recurrence After Uterine Artery Embolisation

Marret H, Cottier JP, Alonso AM, et al (Bretonneau Univ Hosp, Tours, France)
BJOG 112:461-465, 2005   32–2

Objectives.—To assess clinical failure and symptom recurrence after uterine artery embolisation (UAE) and to define predictive factors.

Design.—Prospective study of a case series.

Setting.—Gynaecology and radiology departments of a French University Hospital.

Population.—Eighty-five women who underwent embolisation for the treatment of uterine fibroids.

Method.—Vascular access was obtained via the right common femoral artery. Free-flow embolisation was performed using 150-250 µm polyvinyl alcohol particles and an absorbable particle sponge.

Main Outcome Measures.—Clinical failure was defined as persistence of symptoms at three months of follow up and recurrence as return of symptoms. The main outcome measure was the need for further treatment after UAE.

Results.—Results are available for 81 patients. Median follow up was 30 months. There were 15 clinical failures and recurrences requiring further treatment (eight hysterectomies, five hysteroscopic resections for submucous fibroids, one second embolisation and one woman refusing further treatment). Recurrence-free survival rate at 30 months (no clinical failure, no recurrence) was 82.8% (95% CI 73.7-91.8%). Multivariate analysis identified two predictive factors: dominant fibroid size on ultrasound imaging (each 1 cm increase: HR = 1.68, 95% CI 1.10-2.69) and number of fibroids (each additional fibroid: HR = 1.34, 95% CI 1.08-1.66).

Conclusions.—Symptom recurrence rate 30 months after fibroid embolisation was 17.2%. Fibroid size and number were predictive factors for recurrence. As most recurrences occurred after two years, we recommend that patients be monitored clinically and that imaging be for more than two years after UAE.

▶ Although UAE for symptomatic uterine fibroids has become a popular alternative to more traditional surgical methods, the long-tern success rate remains uncertain. This study examined a small number (85) of patients over a period of 30 months. Women with submucous or pedunculated fibroids were excluded. Four patients were lost to follow-up. Fifteen patients failed initial therapy (7 with symptoms not relieved after embolization and 8 with return of symptoms by 3 months). Menopause occurred in 21 patients during follow-up (all but 1 patient >49 years of age). By 30 months, 8 more patients had a return of symptoms. Recurrence-free survival rate at 30 months (no clinical failure, no recurrence) was quoted as 82.8%. However it is not clear exactly how this number was calculated, as the exact numerator and denominator for the calculation are not stated. Given the raw numbers above, one could argue that 23 patients either failed or recurred. Even including the patients lost to follow-up, this would give a recurrence-free rate of (85 − 23)/85 = 73%.

This confusion notwithstanding, this article emphases that UAE is not a "magic bullet" for fibroids. Further data are needed so patients and physicians can make an informed choice about treatment options for symptomatic uterine fibroids.

G. H. Lipscomb, MD

Predictors of Leiomyoma Recurrence After Myomectomy
Hanafi M (Saint Joseph's Hosp of Atlanta, Ga)
Obstet Gynecol 105:877-881, 2005   32–3

Objective.—The purpose of this study was to evaluate the factors associated with the recurrence of leiomyomata after myomectomy.

Methods.—One hundred forty-five consecutive cases of myomectomy by laparotomy were studied retrospectively. Leiomyoma recurrence, diagnosed by transvaginal ultrasonography, was evaluated by life-table analysis and log-rank tests according to clinical characteristics of patients.

Results.—The 5-year cumulative rates for leiomyoma recurrence and subsequent major surgery were 62% and 9%, respectively. At 5 years, the cumulative probability of recurrence was significantly lower in patients with a single leiomyoma removed (11%), compared with patients with multiple leiomyomata (74%) ($P = .011$); it was also lower in patients with intraoperative uterine size 10 menstrual weeks or less (46%), compared with more than 10 menstrual weeks (82%) ($P = .032$). However, there was a strong association of uterine size with the number of leiomyomata removed ($P = .009$). Childbirth after myomectomy was associated with a lower recurrence rate; the 5-year cumulative probability of recurrence was 26% in patients with subsequent parity, compared with 76% in those without subsequent parity ($P = .010$).

Conclusion.—Solitary myomectomy and smaller intraoperative uterine size are associated with lower rates of leiomyoma recurrence after myomectomy; the significance of uterine size may be affected by its correlation with the number of leiomyomata removed. Subsequent parity is associated with a lower probability of recurrence, but the cause and effect relationship between these two variables is unclear.

▶ As a counterpoint to the previous article on leiomyomata recurrence after uterine artery embolization (Abstract 32–2), this study dealt with recurrence of myomectomy by laparotomy. A recurrence rate of 62% at 5 years was noted. Not noted in the abstract was a menorrhagia recurrence rate of 50%. The abstract implies that this was based on US examinations of 145 patients. However, the body of the article noted that 13 patients were lost to follow-up, and only 61% of those had US follow-up. Recurrence in the article was defined as either US-diagnosed fibroids 2 cm or larger, or surgical findings including hysteroscopy, repeat myomectomy, or hysterectomy. This must be taken into account when comparing other studies using different criteria for recurrence. Of note, that recurrence was lower for patients with solitary fibroids or a uterus less than 10 weeks' gestational size. Although by 5 years, 9% of patients had subsequent major surgery (not necessarily for fibroid), 17% had minor surgery, presumably some being hysteroscopy or curettage, or both.

This article demonstrates the high recurrence rate of fibroids after surgical myomectomy. It is reassuring that the majority of patients were able to avoid repeat major surgery during the 5 years after the initial myomectomy. This figure is of particular importance to patients choosing myomectomy to preserve fertility.

G. H. Lipscomb, MD

The Effect of 1-Month Administration of Asoprisnil (J867), a Selective Progesterone Receptor Modulator, in Healthy Premenopausal Women

Chwalisz K, Elger W, Stickler T, et al (TAP Pharmaceutical Products, Inc, Lake Forest, Ill; EnTec GmbH, Jena, Germany)
Hum Reprod 20:1090-1099, 2005 32–4

Background.—Asoprisnil (J867) is a novel selective progesterone receptor modulator (SPRM) that exhibits partial agonist and antagonist activities and tissue selective effects. This double-blind, dose-escalation study was conducted to evaluate the effects of asoprisnil in 60 regularly cycling premenopausal women.

Methods.—Asoprisnil or placebo was administered orally for 28 days starting at the beginning of the menstrual cycle in doses of 5 mg once daily (QD), 5 mg twice daily (BID), 10 mg QD, 25 mg QD, 25 mg BID and 50 mg BID. Within each dose group, two women were randomized to placebo and eight to asoprisnil. Progesterone concentrations indicative of luteinization were defined as at least one progesterone measurement during the luteal phase exceeding 3.5 ng/ml.

Results.—Asoprisnil consistently prolonged the menstrual cycle at doses ≥10 mg QD. However, the effects on luteal phase progesterone indicative of luteinization were inconsistent and lacked dose dependency. Asoprisnil suppressed periovulatory estradiol but not below follicular phase levels. No significant changes were observed in cortisol and prolactin. Asoprisnil was well tolerated.

Conclusions.—Asoprisnil reversibly suppressed menstruation at doses ≥10 mg QD irrespective of the effect on luteal phase progesterone concentrations indicative of luteinization. It induces amenorrhea primarily by targeting the endometrium in the absence of estrogen deprivation.

▶ SPRMs are a relatively new class of drug that have been shown to have potential benefit for a variety of gynecologic conditions. Asoprisnil (J867) is an SPRM that exhibits partial agonist and partial antagonist activities in mammals and human beings. Combination of effects may have considerable benefits for a variety of conditions, including menstrual regulation, treatment of fibroids, and endometriosis. The current study demonstrates that asoprisnil reversibly suppressed menstruation at doses greater than 10 mg and induced amenorrhea primarily by targeting the endometrium in the absence of estrogen deprivation. Further work will be needed to determine the efficacy and clinical application of asoprisnil as well as the safety of this and other SPRM drugs.

L. P. Shulman, MD

33 Endometriosis

Genomewide Linkage Study in 1,176 Affected Sister Pair Families Identifies a Significant Susceptibility Locus for Endometriosis on Chromosome 10q26
Treloar SA, Wicks J, Nyholt DR, et al (Walter and Eliza Hall Inst, Melbourne; Queensland Inst of Med Research, Brisbane, Australia; Oxagen, Abingdon, England; et al)
Am J Hum Genet 77:365-376, 2005   33-1

Abstract.—Endometriosis is a common gynecological disease that affects up to 10% of women in their reproductive years. It causes pelvic pain, severe dysmenorrhea, and subfertility. The disease is defined as the presence of tissue resembling endometrium in sites outside the uterus. Its cause remains uncertain despite >50 years of hypothesis-driven research, and thus the therapeutic options are limited. Disease predisposition is inherited as a complex genetic trait, which provides an alternative route to understanding the disease. We seek to identify susceptibility loci, using a positional-cloning approach that starts with linkage analysis to identify genomic regions likely to harbor these genes. We conducted a linkage study of 1,176 families (931 from an Australian group and 245 from a U.K. group), each with at least two members—mainly affected sister pairs—with surgically diagnosed disease. We have identified a region of significant linkage on chromosome 10q26 (maximum LOD score [MLS] of 3.09; genomewide P = .047) and another region of suggestive linkage on chromosome 20p13 (MLS = 2.09). Minor peaks (with MLS > 1.0) were found on chromosomes 2, 6, 7, 8, 12, 14, 15, and 17. This is the first report of linkage to a major locus for endometriosis. The findings will facilitate discovery of novel positional genetic variants that influence the risk of developing this debilitating disease. Greater understanding of the aberrant cellular and molecular mechanisms involved in the etiology and pathophysiology of endometriosis should lead to better diagnostic methods and targeted treatments.

▶ This is the first major breakthrough regarding the identification of a susceptibility locus for familial endometriosis. We anxiously wait for the report of a susceptibility gene soon.

S. E. Bulun, MD

Oral Contraceptive Use, Reproductive History, and Risk of Epithelial Ovarian Cancer in Women With and Without Endometriosis
Modugno F, Ness RB, Allen GO, et al (Univ of Pittsburgh, Pa; Duke Univ, Durham, NC; Univ of Illinois at Chicago; et al)
Am J Obstet Gynecol 191:733-740, 2004   33–2

Objective.—Women with endometriosis may be at an increased risk of ovarian cancer. It is not known whether reproductive factors that reduce the risk of ovarian cancer in general also reduce risk in women with endometriosis. We investigated whether the odds ratios for ovarian cancer that were associated with oral contraceptive use, childbearing, hysterectomy, and tubal ligation differ among women with and without endometriosis.

Study Design.—We pooled information on the self-reported history of endometriosis from 4 population-based case-controlled studies of incident epithelial ovarian cancer, comprising 2098 cases and 2953 control subjects. We obtained data on oral contraceptive use, childbearing, breastfeeding, gynecologic surgical procedures, and other reproductive factors on each woman. Multivariable unconditional logistic regression was used to calculate odds ratios and 95% CI for ovarian cancer among women with endometriosis compared with women without endometriosis. Similar methods were used to assess the frequencies of risk factors among women with and without endometriosis. Adjustments were made for age, parity, oral contraceptive use, tubal ligation, family history of ovarian cancer, and study site.

Results.—Women with endometriosis were at an increased risk of ovarian cancer (odds ratio, 1.32; 95% CI, 1.06-1.65) (Table 3). Using oral contraceptives, bearing children, and having a tubal ligation or hysterectomy were associated with a similar reduction in the odds ratios for ovarian cancer among women with and without endometriosis. In particular, the use of oral contraceptives for >10 years was associated with a substantial reduction in risk among women with endometriosis (odds ratio, 0.21; 95% CI, 0.08-0.58).

Conclusion.—Women with endometriosis are at an increased risk of epithelial ovarian cancer. Long-term oral contraceptive use may provide substantial protection against the disease in this high-risk population.

▶ In counter distinction to the uncertainty of the effect of postmenopausal hormonal therapy for the development of ovarian cancer, the use of oral contraceptives remains a well-accepted approach to the reduction of ovarian cancer in low- and high-risk patients. The study by Modugno et al from Duke University shows that the use of oral contraceptives reduced the risk of ovarian cancer among women with and without endometriosis. Of interest is that women with endometriosis were found to have a higher risk of developing ovarian cancer and that the use of oral contraceptives served to substantially reduce the risk in all study groups. It is perhaps time to reconsider the language that oral contraceptives present with regard to ovarian cancer risk reduction and to encourage regulatory agencies to consider more strong lan-

TABLE 3.—Multivariable-Adjusted ORs for Epithelial Ovarian Cancer by Reproductive and Gynecologic Factors, Stratified by History of Endometriosis

Variable	All Women Control Subjects (%)	All Women Cases (%)	All Women OR (95% CI)	Endometriosis Control Subjects (%)	Endometriosis Cases (%)	Endometriosis OR (95% CI)	No Endometriosis Control Subjects (%)	No Endometriosis Cases (%)	No Endometriosis OR (95% CI)
Births (M)									
0	14.3	28.6		18.6	42.6		14	27.3	
1-2	46.1	41.8	0.46** (0.39-0.54)†	55.7	40.3	0.31‡ (0.18-0.54)†	45.5	41.9	0.48‡ (0.41-0.57)†
≥3	39.6	29.7	0.36* (0.30-0.43)† trend P <.001	25.7	17	0.22‡ (0.11-0.45)† trend P <.001	40.5	30.8	0.38‡ (0.31-0.45)† trend P <.001
P interaction #	.37								
OC duration									
Never	37	48.2		20.8	34.1		38.1	49.4	
<10 Y	53.4	45.9	0.69§ (0.60-0.79)†	68.9	61.4	0.58|| (0.33-1.03)	52.4	44.5	0.70|| (0.60-0.80)†
≥10 Y	9.6	6	0.45§ (0.35-0.57)† trend P <.001	10.4	4.5	0.21|| (0.08-0.58)¶ trend P = .003	9.5	6.1	0.47|| (0.37-0.61)† trend P <.001
P interaction#	.51								
Tubal ligation									
No	71.9	83.8		67.8	83		72.2	83.8	
Yes	28.1	16.2	0.68** (0.54-0.73)†	32.2	17	0.7†† (0.41-1.25)	27.8	16.2	0.63†† (0.54-0.73)†
P interaction#	.92								
Hysterectomy									
No	85.8	85.6		76.5	80.7		86.5	86.1	
Yes	14.2	14.4	0.99‡‡ (0.83-1.18)	23.5	19.3	0.69§§ (0.38-1.24)	13.5	13.9	1.02§§ (0.86-1.23)
P interaction#	.24								

All models adjusted for study site, age (continuous), family history of ovarian cancer (dichotomous). See Footnotes for additional information
* OC duration (continuous); endometriosis and tubal ligation (dichotomous).
†*P* < .001.
‡OC duration (continuous); and tubal ligation (dichotomous).
§Parity (continuous); endometriosis and tubal ligation (dichotomous).
||Parity (continuous) and tubal ligation (dichotomous).
¶*P* < .002.
#Interaction between risk factor and reported history of endometriosis.
** OC duration and parity (continuous); endometriosis (dichotomous).
††OC duration and parity (continuous).
‡‡OC duration and parity (continuous); endometriosis, tubal ligation (dichotomous).
§§OC duration and parity (continuous); tubal ligation (dichotomous).
(Courtesy of Modugno F, Ness RB, Allen GO, et al: Oral contraceptive use, reproductive history, and risk of epithelial ovarian cancer in women with and without endometriosis. *Am J Obstet Gynecol* 191:733–740. Copyright 2004 by Elsevier.)

guage supporting the use of oral contraceptives to reduce the risk of ovarian cancer in women of all risk categories.

L. P. Shulman, MD

A Prospective, Randomized Study Comparing Laparoscopic Ovarian Cystectomy Versus Fenestration and Coagulation in Patients With Endometriomas

Alborzi S, Momtahan M, Parsanezhad ME, et al (Shiraz Univ of Med Sciences, Iran)

Fertil Steril 82:1633-1637, 2004   33–3

Objective.—To determine the difference between two laparoscopic methods for the management of endometriomas with regard to recurrence of signs and symptoms and pregnancy rate.

Design.—Prospective, randomized clinical trial.

Setting.—Infertility and gynecologic endoscopy units of two medical university hospitals.

Patient(s).—One hundred patients with endometriomas who had either infertility or pelvic pain.

Intervention(s).—Patients were randomly divided into two groups; one group underwent cystectomy (group 1), and fenestration and coagulation were performed for the other (group 2).

Main Outcome Measure(s).—A comparison of recurrence of signs and symptoms of endometriomas and pregnancy rates in two groups.

Result(s).—Fifty-two patients were studied in group 1 and 48 in group 2. The recurrence of symptoms, such as pelvic pain and dysmenorrhea, was 15.8% in group 1 and 56.7% in group 2 after 2 years (Table 3). The rate of reoperation was 5.8% in group 1 and 22.9% in group 2 and these differences were statistically significant. The cumulative pregnancy rate was significantly higher in group 1 (59.4%) than in group 2 (23.3%) at 1-year follow-up.

Conclusion(s).—Laparoscopic cystectomy of endometriomas is a better choice than fenestration and coagulation because the former technique leads

TABLE 3.—Recurrence of Signs and Symptoms of Endometriomas and Rate of Reoperation After 2 Years

	Cystectomy	Fenestration and Coagulation	*P*
Recurrence of cyst (%)	9/52 (17.3)	15/48 (31.3)	.16
Recurrence of symptoms (%)	6/38 (15.8)	17/30 (56.7)	.001
Reoperation (%)	3/52 (5.8)	11/48 (22.9)	.003

(Courtesy of Alborzi S, Momtahan M, Parsanezhad ME, et al: A prospective, randomized study comparing laparoscopic ovarian cystectomy versus fenestration and coagulation in patients with endometriomas. *Fertil Steril* 82:1633-1637. Copyright 2004 with permission from the American College of Surgeons.)

to a lower recurrence of signs and symptoms and a lower rate of reoperation and a higher cumulative pregnancy rate than the latter.

▶ This study of 100 women with an endometrioma of at least 3 cm randomized to cystectomy or fenestration and coagulation confirms the findings of a previous, smaller randomized trial.[1] In the current study, subjects undergoing a cystectomy were significantly less likely to have a recurrence of pain or a second surgery after 2 years of follow-up. The pregnancy rate 1 year after surgery and without other interventions was significantly greater in the cystectomy group than in the fenestration group (59 vs 23%). These 2 randomized trials confirm what I believe is the general opinion among laparoscopic surgeons—cystectomy is superior to fenestration and coagulation for the treatment of ovarian endometriomas.

R. Barnes, MD

Reference

1. Beretta P, Franchi M, Ghezzi F, et al: Randomized clinical trial of two laparoscopic treatments of endometriomas: Cystectomy versus drainage and coagulation. *Fertil Steril* 70:1176-1180, 1998.

Randomized Clinical Trial of a Levonorgestrel-Releasing Intrauterine System and a Depot GnRH Analogue for the Treatment of Chronic Pelvic Pain in Women With Endometriosis

Petta CA, Ferriani RA, Abrao MS, et al (Universidade Estadual de Campinas, Brazil; Universidade de São Paulo, Brazil)
Hum Reprod 20:1993-1998, 2005   33–4

Background.—The objective of this multicentre randomized, controlled clinical trial was to compare the efficacy of a levonorgestrel-releasing intrauterine system (LNG-IUS) and a depot-GnRH-analogue in the control of endometriosis-related pain over a period of six months.

Methods.—Eighty-two women, 18 to 40 years of age (mean 30 years), with endometriosis, dysmenorrhoea and/or CPP, were randomized using a computer-generated system of sealed envelopes into either LNG-IUS ($n =$ 39) or GnRH analogue ($n = 43$) treatment groups at three university centres. Daily scores of endometriosis-associated CPP were evaluated using the Visual Analogue Scale (VAS), daily bleeding score was calculated from bleeding calendars, and improvement in quality of life was evaluated using the Psychological General Well-Being Index Questionnaire (PGWBI). The pain score diary was based on the VAS in which women recorded the occurrence and intensity of pain on a daily basis. A monthly score was calculated from the result of the sum of the daily scores divided by the number of days in each observation period.

Results.—CPP decreased significantly from the first month throughout the six months of therapy with both forms of treatment and there was no difference between the groups ($P > 0.999$) (Fig 2). In both treatment groups,

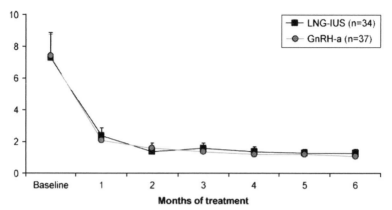

FIGURE 2.—Changes in the visual analogue score pain scores between the two treatment groups. Values are mean ± SEM. P-value: not significant between both groups. (Courtesy of Petta CA, Ferriani RA, Abrao MS, et al: Randomized clinical trial of a levonorgestrel-releasing intrauterine system and a depot GnRH analogue for the treatment of chronic pelvic pain in women with endometriosis. *Hum Reprod* 20:1993-1998, 2005. Reproduced by permission of Oxford University Press/Human Reproduction.)

women with stage III and IV endometriosis showed a more rapid improvement in the VAS pain score than women with stage I and II of the disease ($P < 0.002$). LNG-IUS users had a higher bleeding score than GnRH-analogue users at all time points of observation with 34% and 71% of patients in the LNG-IUS and GnRH-analogue groups, respectively, reporting no bleeding during the first treatment month, and 70% and 98% reporting no bleeding during the sixth month. No difference was observed between groups with reference to improvement in quality of life.

Conclusions.—Both, the LNG-IUS and the GnRH-analogue were effective in the treatment of CPP-associated endometriosis, although no differences were observed between the two treatments. Among the additional advantages of the LNG-IUS is the fact that it does not provoke hypoestrogenism and that it requires only one medical intervention for its introduction every 5 years. This device could therefore become the treatment of choice for CPP-associated endometriosis in women who do not wish to conceive.

▶ There has been much interest in the treatment of chronic pelvic pain associated with endometriosis with a levonorgestrel-releasing intrauterine device (LNG-IUD). The IUD is inexpensive compared with most other medical therapies and can be left in place for up to 5 years. In uncontrolled trials, the LNG-IUD has significantly improved symptoms and reduced lesion size in rectovaginal endometriosis[1] and in mild to moderate endometriosis,[2,3] and is reasonably well tolerated.

The present study is the first randomized clinical trial comparing the LNG-IUD and a gonadotropin-releasing hormone (GnRH) agonist (depot leuprolide). Women were treated for 6 months with either the LNG-IUD (n = 39) or depot leuprolide (n = 43). Pain relief was identical for the 2 treatments; however, the LNG-IUD users had significantly more bleeding than the leuprolide users. Although not evaluated in this study, the LNG-IUD has the potential advantage over GnRH agonist therapy in avoiding the consequences of hypoestrogenism such as vasomotor symptoms and loss of bone mineral content. It has the potential advantage over oral progestins in having fewer systemic side effects and a higher rate of amenorrhea. It should be considered as an important addition to our armamentarium of medical therapies for endometriosis-associated pain.

R. Barnes, MD

References

1. Fedele L, Bianchi S, Zanconato G, et al: Use of a levonorgestrel-releasing intrauterine device in the treatment of rectovaginal endometriosis. *Fertil Steril* 75:485-488, 2001.
2. Lockhat FB, Emembolu JO, Konje JC: The evaluation of the effectiveness of an intrauterine-administered progestogen (levonorgestrel) in the symptomatic treatment of endometriosis and in the staging of the disease. *Hum Reprod* 19:179-184, 2004.
3. Lockhat FB, Emembolu JO, Konje JC: The efficacy, side-effects and continuation rates in women with symptomatic endometriosis undergoing treatment with an intra-uterine administered progestogen (levonorgestrel): A 3 year follow-up. *Hum Reprod* 20:789-793, 2005.

34 Urogynecology

Laparoscopic Sacral Colpopexy Approach for Genito-Urinary Prolapse: Experience With 363 Cases
Rozet F, Mandron E, Arroyo C, et al (Université René Descartes, Paris; Clinique du Pré, Le Mans, France)
Eur Urol 47:230-236, 2005   34–1

Objective.—To evaluate the surgical outcome, complications and benefits of laparoscopic double promonto-fixation for patients with pelvic prolapse.

Methods.—Women with genito-urinary prolapse underwent a transperitoneal placement of a 100% polyester mesh on the anterior vaginal wall and a posterior mesh on the levator ani muscle. Both of these were anchored to the sacral promontory. A TVT was placed simultaneously in patients who had concurrent stress urinary incontinence.

Results.—A total of 363 patients were operated upon between 1996 and 2002. Their mean age was 63 (range 35–78), average follow-up was 14.6 months, the mean operating time was 97 minutes. There were 8 conversions due to anesthetic or surgical difficulties. Follow up was done by a postal questionnaire and physical examination at 6 months and then yearly. 96% were satisfied with the results of their operation and no patients complained of sexual dysfunction. There was a 4% recurrence rate of prolapse, 3 vaginal erosions, 2 urinary retentions that required TVT section, 1 bowel incarcerations, 1 spondylitis and 2 mesh infection.

Conclusions.—Laparoscopic promonto-fixation is feasible and highly effective technique that offers good long-term results with complication rates similar to open surgery, with the added benefits of minimally invasive surgery.

▶ The development of less-invasive surgical approaches to urogynecologic conditions is an ongoing and critically important process that serves to expand therapeutic options and improve the overall care of mature women who tend to suffer from these problems. In this report the authors found that a laparoscopic approach to sacral promontory fixation in women with genitourinary prolapse was not only feasible but highly effective, with good long-term outcomes and complication rates similar to conventional (open) surgical procedures. However, the ability to perform this procedure with minimally invasive laparoscopy provided benefits not obtainable by longer, open surgical procedures. Such studies provide important clinical information for clinicians and patients seeking to choose the optimal surgical approach for genitourinary prolapse.

S. A. Grochmal, MD

Tension Free Vaginal Tape: A Procedure for All Ages

Allahdin S, McKinley CA, Mahmood TA (Forth Park Hosp, Kirkcaldy, Scotland)
Acta Obstet Gynecol Scand 83:937-940, 2004   34–2

Objective.—To assess the success and complications of the tension free vaginal tape (TVT) procedure in different age groups.

Patients and Methods.—This prospective long-term study of 179 consecutive cases of urodynamically confirmed urinary incontinence that had had the TVT procedure was conducted from March 1999 to December 2002 at a District General Hospital. To assess whether outcome was influenced by the patient's age, the patients were divided into three age groups: group A (30–49 years old), group B (50–69 years old) and group C (70–90 years old). Operative details and early and late complications were recorded, and patients were followed up with clinic visits at 6 weeks and 6 months and a quality of life questionnaire was completed at 1 year.

Results.—Of the 179 patients included in the study, 53 (29.6%) were in group A, 91 (50.8%) in group B and 35 (19.5%) in group C. The subjective cure rate for the patients was 84.9%, 81.3% and 85.3% in groups A, B and C, respectively. A significant improvement in symptoms was reported by 3.8%, 14.3% and 8.6% women, respectively. The failure rate was 11.3%, 4.4% and 5.7%, respectively. The intraoperative complication rate was 5.6%. The overall postoperative complication rate was 29.6%. A total of 86.2% of the patients were treated as day cases. Patients who had intraoperative complications or initial voiding difficulties (i.e. those patients requiring "in/out" catheterization before spontaneous voiding was established) were in hospital for 1–2 days.

Conclusions.—Our data showed better subjective cure rates and substantial improvement rates without any significant increase in intraoperative complications with increasing age. Postoperative complications of urgency and vaginal wall erosion were more common in the older aged patients but were easily resolved. Hospital stay and recovery period were short, making TVT a suitable procedure for all ages.

▶ The use of TVT has revolutionized surgical intervention for stress urinary incontinence. The procedure is minimally invasive and is characterized by high efficacy and few serious adverse events. This study showed that increasing age of women undergoing TVT procedures was associated with better subjective cure rates and substantial improvement rates without significant increases in intraoperative complications. Although certain postoperative complications (eg, urgency, vaginal wall erosion) were more common in older patients, most of these problems resolved within a short period. As hospital stays and recovery periods are relatively brief for women undergoing TVT, this procedure can be considered a suitable procedure for women of all ages with stress urinary incontinence.

S. A. Grochmal, MD

Pelvicol™ Pubovaginal Sling Versus Tension-Free Vaginal Tape for Treatment of Urodynamic Stress Incontinence: A Prospective Randomized Three-Year Follow-up Study
Abdel-Fattah M, Barrington JW, Arunkalaivanan AS (Torbay Hosp, Torquay, Devon, England)
Eur Urol 46:629-635, 2004   34–3

Objectives.—The aim of this study was to compare the long-term success rates, complication rates and patient satisfaction rates for Pelvicol™ pubovaginal sling (Bard) versus TVT™ (Gynecare) in surgical treatment of urodynamic stress incontinence (USI) in women.

Design.—Prospective randomized cohort trial.

Setting.—District General Hospital, South West of England.

Methods.—One hundred and forty-two women with urodynamic stress incontinence were randomized to either surgical procedure (Pelvicol™ = 74, TVT™ = 68) with median follow-up of 36 months. A postal questionnaire was sent to all women and the response rate was excellent at approximately 90% in both groups.

Results.—Cure of incontinence, as identified by a quality of life improvement >90%, and/or patient-determined continent status as dry, were comparable in both groups. When the cure rates were adjusted assuming the non-respondents as failures the figures were almost identical ($p > 0.05$). Preoperative continence pad usage was similar for both groups. Overall, a postoperative significant decrease in pad score was noted in both groups ($p = 0.01$) but there was no significant difference between the groups ($p > 0.05$). Statistical analysis failed to detect significant differences between both groups as regards complication rates such as frequency, nocturia, de-novo urgency or dyspareunia.

Conclusion.—Pelvicol™sling is a safe procedure in the surgical management of USI with similar success rate and patient satisfaction rate to TVT™ up to three years of follow-up.

Effect of Transobturator Tape Procedure on Proximal Urethral Mobility
Minaglia S, Özel B, Hurtado E, et al (Univ of Southern California, Los Angeles; Washington Univ, St Louis)
Urology 65:55-59, 2005   34–4

Objectives.—To assess prospectively the degree of urethral mobility in the preoperative and postoperative periods after the transobturator tape procedure and correlate the findings with surgical outcome.

Methods.—Thirty-six consecutive patients with stress urinary incontinence underwent the transobturator tape procedure. A cotton-swab test was performed before the procedure and at the 6-week postoperative follow-up visit to evaluate proximal urethral mobility. Cure was defined as the absence of leak during cough stress testing at cystometric capacity.

Results.—Of the 36 patients, 26 were available for the complete follow-up evaluation. The mean preoperative and postoperative resting cotton-swab test values were 11.7° and 13.6°, respectively ($P = 0.347$). The mean preoperative and postoperative straining cotton-swab test values were 57.3° and 48.4°, respectively ($P = 0.047$). Of the 36 patients, 21 had a straining cotton-swab test result of 30 degrees or greater after surgery, and 19 (90.4%) of these 21 patients were objectively cured by the procedure. Overall, 21 patients (84%) were objectively cured of stress urinary incontinence. Four patients had urinary leakage during stress testing at cystometric capacity. Three of these patients reported subjective cure and one noted improvement. Of the 5 patients with a negative cotton-swab test after surgery, 2 were cured (50%), 2 were not cured, and 1 did not undergo cough stress testing at cystometric capacity because of urgency at 200-mL limiting bladder filling.

Conclusions.—The cure of urodynamic stress incontinence using the transobturator tape procedure does not require the correction of proximal urethral mobility.

▶ With the vaginal sling procedure being the most widely used surgical approach for women with SUI, investigators continue to evaluate a wide spectrum of materials and approaches that would improve clinical outcomes in women undergoing the procedure. This ongoing search has evaluated a variety of synthetic and allogenic materials. The development and use of the synthetic tension-free vaginal tape (TVT) in a minimally invasive sling procedure has led to increased interest in sling procedures by gynecologists, urogynecologists, and urologists. In the first study, the authors evaluated the use of an allogenic substance (Pelvicol) for sling procedures. The authors found that the Pelvicol sling procedure was characterized by a similar success rate for the treatment of SUI to that associated with the TVT procedure and that outcomes for women undergoing both procedures were similar through 3 years of follow-up. The second study by Minaglia et al prospectively evaluated urethral mobility preoperatively and postoperatively with a transobturator TVT procedure in 36 women with SUI. The authors found that reduction and elimination of SUI symptoms did not require correction of proximal urethral mobility, despite urethral mobility being a common feature of most women who undergo sling procedures. Further studies, and hopefully randomized comparison studies, of these products and procedures as well as other surgical approaches will be needed to provide strong evidence to physicians seeking to choose the optimal surgical procedure for a woman undergoing a sling procedure. Indeed, the demonstration of another safe and reliable surgical approach for women with SUI can only be of benefit to women seeking effective treatment.

S. A. Grochmal, MD

Efficacy of a Vaginal Sling Procedure in a Rat Model of Stress Urinary Incontinence

Hijaz A, Daneshgari F, Cannon T, et al (Cleveland Clinic Found, Ohio; Denver; Loyola Univ, Maywood, Ill)
J Urol 172:2065-2068, 2004   34–5

Purpose.—We validated the efficacy of the vaginal sling procedure for the restoration of leak point pressure (LPP) in the rat model of stress urinary incontinence (SUI).

Materials and Methods.—SUI was created in 10 female Sprague-Dawley rats by bilateral pudendal nerve transection (PNT) under urethane anesthesia. Vaginal dissection was performed, followed by placement of a 2×0.3 cm strip of Prolene (Ethicon, Somerville, New Jersey) mesh at the mid urethral level. LPP was measured before and after PNT through a suprapubic tube using a Credé maneuver. It was also measured after vaginal dissection (sham sling) and after true sling placement. All procedures and measurements were done at the same experimental setting. In each animal LPP was measured 4 or 5 times and the mean was taken. Pairwise differences in LPP between the true and sham slings were calculated using the Wilcoxon signed rank test with $p < 0.05$ considered significantly different.

Results.—Mean LPP at baseline in all rats was 65.1 ± 6.0 cm water. LPP decreased to 42.7 ± 3.7 cm water after PNT. The sham sling further decreased LPP to 26.5 ± 2.2 cm water, whereas the true sling restored LPP to 56 ± 4.8 cm water. LPP after true sling placement was not different from baseline ($p = 0.16$), whereas LPP after sham sling placement was significantly different from baseline ($p = 0.002$).

Conclusions.—This rat vaginal sling model represents a valid surgical method for LPP restoration in the rat model of SUI. This animal model could be used for future studies related to SUI and its treatment relevant to sling surgery.

▶ Surgical and medical interventions continue to be evaluated for the treatment of urinary incontinence. Approximately 165,000 surgical procedures are performed each year for SUI, with the sling procedure being one of the most commonly performed procedures. Despite the considerable success associated with the sling procedure, it is associated with considerable morbidity and high complication rates. To reduce the morbidity associated with this procedure, the authors sought to develop modifications to this procedure that would maintain the high success rate while reducing the complication rate. Using a previously validated rat model, the authors demonstrated that this model could be used as a valid surgical method for LPP restoration and thus contribute to the development of safer and effective surgical approaches to urinary incontinence.

S. A. Grochmal, MD

Lower Urinary Tract Symptoms (LUTS) and Sexual Function in Both Sexes

Hansen BL (Univ of Southern Denmark, Odense)
Eur Urol 46:229-234, 2004   34–6

Objectives.—It has been stated that lower urinary tract symptoms (LUTS) do not affect sexual function to any significant degree, but a recent study has suggested that there might be an association in men. The present study was conducted to investigate the relationship between LUTS and sexual problems in both men and women aged 40–65 years.

Methods.—The survey was conducted in Denmark between May and June 2003. Detailed questionnaires were mailed to a random sample of 15,000 men and women aged 40–65 years. LUTS and sexual function were assessed by validated symptom scales. Multivariate regression analysis was performed using logistic regression for dichotomous dependent variables of sexual function. The independent variables for both sexes were age, LUTS, partner status, body mass index (BMI), alcohol consumption and co-morbidities.

Results.—A total of 15,000 questionnaires were mailed out, 8491 were completed and returned, and 7741 were deemed valuable and included in the analysis. LUTS and sexual dysfunction were common in both men and women. Logistic regression analysis of items related to erection problems and satisfaction with sex life in men and sexual function in women showed that LUTS are an independent risk factor for sexual dysfunction in both men and women aged 40–65 years. Significant effects on sexual function were also found for the independent variables of partner status and co-morbidities.

Conclusions.—The presence of LUTS is an independent risk factor for sexual dysfunction in men and women. These results highlight the clinical importance of evaluating LUTS in patients with sexual dysfunction, and the need to consider sexual issues in the management of patients with LUTS.

Urinary Complications and Sexual Function After the Tension-Free Vaginal Tape Procedure

Mazouni C, Karsenty G, Bretelle F, et al (Salvator Hosp, Marseille, France; Conception Hosp, Marseille, France)
Acta Obstet Gynecol Scand 83:955-961, 2004   34–7

Objective.—The purpose of this prospective study was to evaluate urinary and sexual function after the tension-free vaginal tape (TVT) support procedure for stress urinary incontinence (SUI).

Methods.—Between January 1999 and July 2002 a total of 71 patients underwent comprehensive examination including urodynamics and a mailed self-administered questionnaire for assessment of voiding and sexual function before and after treatment of SUI by TVT.

Results.—Based on objective findings TVT was considered as curative in 48 patients (87.3%). Comparison of preoperative and postoperative urodynamic evidence demonstrated a significant outflow obstruction (<12 ml/s) in 19 patients (34.5%). A significant decrease in peak urinary flow during voiding ($p < 0.001$) was also observed. Of the 55 women (78.5%) who responded to the questionnaire before and after TVT, 42 (76.3%) reported satisfaction with the outcome. Postoperatively, 60% of patients reported voiding difficulty, 47.2% complained of urgency, and 32.7% of frequency. Regarding sexual function 20% reported impairment after surgery including dyspareunia in 14.5% (none preoperatively vs. eight postoperatively, <0.01) and loss of libido in 5.4%.

Conclusion.—The TVT procedure is an effective treatment for SUI. However, it can lead to postoperative voiding and sexual impairment.

Sexual Function in Women Before and After Suburethral Sling Operation for Stress Urinary Incontinence: A Retrospective Questionnaire Study

Glavind K, Tetsche MS (Aalborg Sygehus, Denmark)
Acta Obstet Gynecol Scand 83:965-968, 2004   34–8

Background.—The aim of this questionnaire study dealing with women with stress urinary incontinence was to find out what influence incontinence and operation for incontinence in the form of tension-free vaginal tape (TVT) or intravaginal slingplasty operation (IVS) had on the patient's sexuality and if there were any adverse effects on sexuality after the operation.

Methods.—Eighty-four patients were operated on from April 1998 to September 2002. A questionnaire was sent to all patients with questions concerning their sexuality before and after the operation.

Results.—Sixty-seven patients (81%) answered the questionnaire. Before the operation 53 patients (79%) were sexually active and 26 patients (49%) experienced incontinence during intercourse. Only one patient (0.01%) stated the incontinence as the reason for not being sexually active. No patients developed de novo incontinence during intercourse after the operation. Half of the patients who were cured of their incontinence during intercourse experienced a better sexual life. Five patients (7%) cited reduced libido after the operation and two patients (3%) felt the operation to be the cause.

Conclusion.—Among sexually active women with stress urinary incontinence referred for suburethral sling operation 49% experienced incontinence during intercourse and half of the cured patients in this group experienced a better sexual life after the operation. Incontinence affects sexual life to a great extent. Two patients (4%) experienced less libido after the operation and found the operation to be the cause of this. The risk of deterioration of sexual life after the operation is very small. Further investigation into this subject is needed.

▶ Urinary tract symptoms and disorders often create a considerable adverse impact on a woman's quality of life and can lead to other morbidities by forcing affected women to change their normal activities in response to the specific urogynecologic condition. One quality of life aspect that is commonly affected by urologic conditions is sexual function. These 3 articles address different urologic conditions that adversely affect sexual function. Hansen et al show that the presence of LUTS is an independent risk factor for sexual dysfunction in women as well as men. This report highlights the critical need for gynecologic clinicians to evaluate LUTS in women with sexual problems as well as for those clinicians to use their clinical skills and acumen to ascertain the presence of sexual problems in their patients. The second article from 2 centers in Marseille, France, reports on the urinary and sexual problems in women who have undergone successful TVT procedures for SUI. The authors found that although close to 80% of women undergoing the TVT procedure reported satisfaction with their clinical outcomes, significant outflow obstruction was demonstrated in approximately one third of patients, and 20% reported sexual impairment after the procedure, including dyspareunia and loss of libido. On the contrary, the third article from the Aalborg Sygehus in Denmark showed considerable improvement in sexual function and enjoyment among half the women who experienced improvement in incontinence during sex after having undergone a suburethral sling procedure. Approximately 5% of cured women reported reduced libido after surgery, similar to the frequency reported in the study by Manzouni et al.

Several selections in this 2006 YEAR BOOK highlight the use of TVT and other sling procedures. These 3 articles (Abstracts 34–6, 34–7, and 34–8) provide important information that should be included in the counseling of women who are considering such procedures for SUI therapy. As with any surgical intervention, adverse effects and secondary clinical outcomes are a part of the postoperative course; a frank discussion of these issues and other potential complications and benefits must be a part of the preoperative counseling process so that women can make a truly informed decision about which therapeutic option is best for them.

S. A. Grochmal, MD

The Effect of Botulinum-A Toxin on Patients With Severe Urge Urinary Incontinence
Flynn MK, Webster GD, Amundsen CL (Duke Univ, Durham, NC)
J Urol 172:2316-2320, 2004   34–9

Purpose.—We determined the effect of 150 units of botulinum-A toxin (Botox, Allergan, Irvine, California) on subjects with severe urge urinary incontinence (UUI).

Materials and Methods.—This was an open label uncontrolled clinical trial. Subjects were recruited from the female urology and urogynecology clinics at Duke University. Inclusion criteria included evidence of UUI on 3-day bladder diary, a 24-hour pad weight of 100 gm or greater, absent or minimal stress leakage, absent detrusor dysfunction, and a history of failed anticholinergic and physical therapies. Exclusion criteria included evidence of a urinary tract infection, or other correctable or neurological etiology for UUI. The detrusor of each subject was injected with 150 units of botulinum-A toxin. Evaluations were performed at 2 weeks, 6 weeks, 3 months and 6 months after injection. Outcome measures included daily incontinence episodes, Urogenital Distress Inventory and the Incontinence Impact Questionnaire, 24-hour pad weights, daily pad usage and urinalysis at all visits. Urodynamic studies were performed at the 6-week and 3-month visits.

Results.—Three subjects had uncomplicated urinary tract infections during followup. No other adverse effects occurred. Statistically and clinically significant decreases greater than 50% were seen in virtually all outcome measures at all visits up to 3 months. Most subjects showed signs of recurrent UUI by 6 months. All subjects reported remarkable subjective improvement in incontinence. No significant changes in maximal cystometric capacity, maximal detrusor pressure, peak flow or post-void residual volumes were seen.

Conclusions.—Botulinum-A toxin can significantly decrease urge urinary incontinence and improve quality of life for 3 months after injection. Additional studies are needed to determine ideal doses, dosing intervals, safety and cost-effectiveness of this therapy.

Botulinum Toxin A Has Antinociceptive Effects in Treating Interstitial Cystitis

Smith CP, Radziszewski P, Borkowski A, et al (Baylor Coll of Medicine, Houston; Warsaw School of Medicine; Univ of Pittsburgh, Pa)
Urology 64:871-875, 2004   34–10

Objectives.—To present clinical evidence with botulinum toxin A (BTX-A) suggesting an antinociceptive role in patients with interstitial cystitis (IC). Intriguing evidence in a somatic pain model has suggested that BTX-A injection may have an antinociceptive effect on both acute and chronic (inflammatory) pain.

Methods.—Thirteen female patients (6 in the United States and 7 in Poland) with IC according to the criteria of the National Institute of Diabetes, Digestive and Kidney Disease were included. Under short general anesthesia or sedation, 100 to 200 U of Dysport (Polish patients) or Botox (U.S. patients) was injected through a cystoscope into 20 to 30 sites submucosally in the trigone and floor of the bladder. Patients were evaluated with the O'Leary-Sant validated IC questionnaire or with voiding charts and a visual analog pain scale 1 month postoperatively and at subsequent 3-month intervals. The Polish patients also underwent pretreatment and post-treatment urodynamic evaluations.

Results.—Overall, 9 (69%) of 13 patients noted subjective improvement after BTX-A treatment. The Interstitial Cystitis Symptom Index and Interstitial Cystitis Problem Index mean scores improved by 71% and 69%, respectively (*P* <0.05). Daytime frequency, nocturia, and pain by visual analog scale decreased by 44%, 45%, and 79%, respectively (*P* <0.01). The first desire to void and maximal cystometric capacity increased by 58% and 57%, respectively (*P* <0.01).

Conclusions.—Our results suggest that BTX-A has an antinociceptive effect on bladder afferent pathways in patients with IC, producing both symptomatic and functional (ie, urodynamic) improvements.

Single-Institution Experience in 110 Patients With Botulinum Toxin A Injection into Bladder or Urethra

Smith CP, Nishiguchi J, O'Leary M, et al (Univ of Pittsburgh, Pa; Okayama Univ, Japan)

Urology 65:37-41, 2005   34–11

Objectives.—To detail, in a review, one institution's 6-year experience using botulinum toxin A (BTX-A) in the bladder and urethra in 110 patients for a variety of lower urinary tract disorders.

Methods.—A total of 110 patients (35 men and 75 women, age range 19 to 82 years) received injections of BTX-A into the bladder (n = 42) or urethra (n = 68). Voiding dysfunction included neurogenic detrusor overactivity and/or detrusor sphincter dyssynergia, overactive bladder, bladder neck obstruction, and interstitial cystitis. Under light sedation in most cases, patients were treated with either 100 to 200 U of BTX-A in 4 mL divided in equal doses into the four quadrants of the external sphincter or by injection into the bladder base using 100 to 300 U of BTX-A diluted in approximately 10 to 30 mL of sterile saline. At last follow-up, 27 patients had received additional injections (up to six) at intervals of 6 months or longer.

Results.—All patients who underwent bladder BTX-A injection had preoperative evidence of involuntary detrusor contractions during urodynamic testing. Analysis of the 110 patients indicated that 67.3% reported a decrease or absence of incontinence. Diaries indicated a decrease in both daytime and nighttime voiding symptoms. Maximal efficacy occurred between 7 and 30 days and lasted for at least 6 months. Condition-specific quality-of-life symptom scores also demonstrated improvement. No long-term complications had occurred at last follow-up. Two women with multiple sclerosis and mild baseline stress urinary incontinence reported increased leakage with stress after BTX-A external sphincter injection, and one woman with multiple sclerosis noted new onset stress urinary incontinence after external sphincter injection. However, they all reported significant improvement in their detrusor sphincter dyssynergia with decreased postvoid residual urine volume, improved uroflow, decreased urge incontinence, and decreased daytime and nighttime frequency. One woman with multiple sclerosis who underwent bladder injection had increased postvoid residual urine volume from 78 to 155 mL. She did not have to perform intermittent catheterization. *Conclusions.*—BTX-A injection is a safe and promising treatment modality for a variety of lower urinary tract dysfunctions for both skeletal and smooth muscle dysfunction. In our series, BTX-A is equally effective in women as it is in men. When injected into the sphincter, the risk of stress incontinence is low. Bladder injections with BTX-A are effective for not only neurogenic detrusor overactivity, but also overactive bladder. BTX-A can even be considered for interstitial cystitis.

Success of Repeat Detrusor Injections of Botulinum A Toxin in Patients With Severe Neurogenic Detrusor Overactivity and Incontinence
Grosse J, Kramer G, Stöhrer M (Berufsgenossenschaftliche Unfallklinik Murnau, Germany)
Eur Urol 47:653-659, 2005   34–12

Objectives.—Detrusor injections with botulinum toxin type A are an effective treatment for neurogenic detrusor overactivity, lasting for 9–12 months. When the patients develop botulinum resistance, subsequent injections might be less effective. Repeat injections in patients with severe neurogenic detrusor overactivity and incontinence were studied.

Methods.—Patients received Botox® (300 UI) or Dysport® (750 UI) injections. Clinical variables: satisfaction, anticholinergics use, mean and maximum bladder capacity, continence volume. Cystometric parameters: compliance, cystometric capacity, reflex volume. Statistics: Anova, χ^2-tests; *t*-tests and paired *t*-tests ($p = 0.05$).

Results.—Forty-three men and 23 women (mean age 38.3 years; mean duration of lesion 9.2 years) were included. The interval between subsequent injections (on average 9–11 months) did not change significantly ($p = 0.5594$). The satisfaction was high and anticholinergics use decreased substantially ($p = 0.0000$). Significant improvements were found in clinical parameters and in cystometric capacity, for compliance only at the second treatment. The incidence of reflex contractions was significantly reduced. Four patients had transient adverse events after Dysport®.

Conclusions.—Repeat injections with botulinum toxin type A are as effective as the first one. The cause for repeat treatment is relapse of overactive bladder symptoms.

▶ BTX-A is best known as an important therapeutic modality in facial cosmetic procedures. These articles (Abstracts 34–9 through 34–12) demonstrate the potential use of BTX-A for women with urologic conditions. Urinary incontinence remains a common and challenging clinical problem for reproductive-age and menopausal women. The prevalence of urinary incontinence in the United States ranges from 3% to 14% and may be as high as 40% in elderly women. Diagnosis remains difficult as disparate etiologies involving structural, hormonal, and neurologic pathophysiologic processes can separately or, in combination, lead to incontinence. Flynn et al evaluated the effect of BTX-A in women with severe UUI. The authors found this regimen to be highly effective for reducing UUI for up to 3 months after injection. Although further studies are needed to better delineate the efficacy, safety, and cost effectiveness of this regimen, this study presents important initial data concerning a potentially effective and facile approach for reducing the symptoms associated with UUI. The second study reports on 13 women with IC who had BTX-A cytoscopically injected into 20 to 30 submucosal sites in the trigone and floor of the bladder. Nine of the 13 women reported subjective improvement, with IC scores improving an average of 70% in the treated cohort. This same group reports on the successful use of BTX-A for a variety of urologic conditions in the third article. Finally, Grosse et al report on the successful use of BTX-A for men and women with severe neurogenic detrusor overactivity and incontinence. The authors found high levels of satisfaction and a considerably reduced need for anticholinergics among the treated patients. Although adverse events were reported in this cohort, the authors found that the average interval between injections was 9 to 11 months and that the need for repeat treatments was primarily attributable to relapse of overactive bladder symptoms.

Further studies will be needed to better assess the efficacy and safety of BTX-A for the variety of urologic conditions reported herein; however, new nonsurgical therapeutic options for women with urogynecologic conditions represent important options for women with conditions that have not been generally amenable to easy diagnosis or universally successful management options.

S. A. Grochmal, MD

Use of Urethral Plugs for Urinary Incontinence Following Fistula Repair
Goh JTW, Browning A (Gold Coast Hosp, Queensland, Australia; Addis Ababa Fistula Hosp, Ethiopia)
Aust N Z J Obstet Gynaecol 45:237-238, 2005   34–13

Abstract.—A common complication following anatomical closure of obstetric genito-urinary fistula is urinary incontinence. Management is often suboptimal with lack of urodynamic equipment in most fistula centres in developing countries. Surgical interventions have been described with varying success. The aim of this paper is to describe the use of urethral plugs as an alternative management for women with postfistula incontinence, in a developing country. A pilot study was undertaken to assess the effectiveness of the urethral plugs in these women. The use of urethral plugs appear to be an effective short-term management of women with postfistula incontinence, with minimal complications. Longer follow-up and in larger numbers are required.

▶ Prolonged obstructed labor is the most common cause of genitourinary fistula worldwide. The authors describe the initial successful use of urethral plugs for the treatment of ongoing incontinence after the closure of genitourinary fistula. Such a facile and potentially highly effective approach to reducing the morbidity of genitourinary fistula can provide important care for the tens of thousands of women worldwide who suffer considerable organic and emotional trauma after the detection and initial treatment of fistula.

S. A. Grochmal, MD

Hyperbaric Oxygen for the Treatment of Interstitial Cystitis: Long-term Results of a Prospective Pilot Study
van Ophoven A, Rossbach G, Oberpenning F, et al (Universitätsklinikum Münster, Germany; Ctr for Hyperbaric Medicine, Münster, Germany; Universitätsklinikum Bonn, Germany)
Eur Urol 46:108-113, 2004   34–14

Objective.—We conducted a prospective pilot study to assess the safety and efficacy of hyperbaric oxygen (HBO) for the treatment of interstitial cystitis (IC).

Methods.—Six patients underwent 30 sessions of 100% oxygen inhalation in a hyperbaric chamber and were followed up over 15 months. The measures of efficacy were changes in pain and urgency (visual analog scales), alteration in the patient's assessment of overall change in his well-being (Patient Global Assessment Form), and changes in frequency and functional bladder capacity (48-hours voiding log). Evaluation of symptom severity regarding pain and voiding problems was done using the O'Leary-Sant index.

Results.—Four patients rated the therapeutic result as either excellent or good and assessed their well-being after HBO treatment as improved. Two patients showed only short-term amelioration of some of their symptoms. At 12 months follow-up the baseline functional bladder capacity increased from 37–161 ml (range) to 160–200 ml in the responder group. The 24-hour voiding frequency decreased from 15–27 to 6–11 voids per day, a pain scale improvement from 20–97 mm at baseline to 3–30 mm at 12 months follow-up and an urgency scale improvement from 53–92 mm to 3–40 mm, respectively was observed at 12 month follow-up. The symptom and pain index score decreased from 23–35 at baseline to 3–17 at 12 months follow-up.

Conclusion.—HBO appears to be effective to treat IC patients. Treatment was well tolerated and resulted in a sustained decrease of pelvic pain and urgency, improvement of voiding patterns and increase of functional bladder capacity for at least 12 months.

▶ IC is a chronic and debilitating condition characterized by difficulties in diagnosis and suboptimal therapeutic interventions. HBO treatments for a variety of urologic disorders have gained recognition over the past 2 decades. In this regard, the authors sought to determine whether HBO is a safe and reliable approach for patients with IC. They found, in this prospective pilot study, that HBO was effective in reducing or eliminating the symptoms associated with IC. Indeed, 4 of the 6 patients rated the therapeutic result to be excellent or good. Further study will be needed to determine the efficacy (short- and long-term) and safety of this approach; nonetheless, this study serves to present a potentially effective therapeutic option for the treatment of IC, and this can only be of benefit for the thousands of women seeking effective care and a return to a normal lifestyle.

S. A. Grochmal, MD

Prevention of Recurrent Bacterial Cystitis by Intravesical Administration of Hyaluronic Acid: A Pilot Study
Constantinides C, Manousakas T, Nikolopoulos P, et al (Univ of Athens)
BJU Int 93:1262-1266, 2004   34–15

Objectives.—To assess the effect of bladder instillations of hyaluronic acid (HA) on the rate of recurrence of urinary tract infection (UTI).

Patients and Methods.—Forty women (mean age 35 years) with a history of recurrent UTI received intravesical instillations of HA (40 mg in 50 mL phosphate-buffered saline) once weekly for 4 weeks then once monthly for 4 months. The UTI status was assessed over a prospective follow-up of 12.4 months and compared with the rates of UTI before instillation, determined by a retrospective review of patient charts covering 15.8 months.

Results.—After HA treatment no patients had a UTI during the 5-month treatment phase and 28 (70%) were recurrence-free at the end of the follow-up. The mean (sd) rate of UTI per patient-year was 4.3 (1.55) before treatment and 0.3 (0.55) afterward ($P < 0.001$). The median time to recurrence after HA treatment was 498 days, compared with 96 days beforehand ($P < 0.001$). The tolerability was excellent, as side-effects were limited to nine patients who reported mild bladder irritation; no patient interrupted the treatment.

Conclusions.—In this preliminary study, bladder instillations of HA had a significant effect on the rate of UTI in women with a history of recurrent UTIs. The bladder instillation of HA is an acceptable and promising therapeutic alternative in patients with recurrent UTI. Expanded placebo controlled clinical trials examining this application of HA are currently underway.

▶ UTIs are among the most common problems managed by gynecologists and obstetricians. Although most UTIs are treated successfully with a variety of antimicrobial and supportive therapies, approximately one quarter to one third of initial UTI infections are followed by a recurrent infection within 3 to 6 months. The morbidity and cost of recurrent infections thus deserve important consideration in the development of more effective initial therapies and protocols to reduce the overall frequency of recurrence. This study evaluated the use of bladder instillations with HA on the rate of recurrence of UTI. Forty women with a history of recurrent UTI received a bladder instillation containing HA once a week for 4 weeks. None of the 40 women had a UTI for the initial 5 months after treatment, and only 30% had a recurrent infection within the 12.4-month follow-up period. This preliminary study demonstrates the efficacy of intravesicular HA for reducing the frequency of recurrent UTIs. Further study of this regimen, as well as evaluation of other less invasive and more facile approaches, are needed to provide effective and safe approaches for reducing the frequency, and thus the morbidity, of recurrent UTIs.

S. A. Grochmal, MD

35 Fecal Incontinence

Randomized Clinical Trial of Intra-anal Electromyographic Biofeedback Physiotherapy With Intra-anal Electromyographic Biofeedback Augmented With Electrical Stimulation of the Anal Sphincter in the Early Treatment of Postpartum Fecal Incontinence
Mahony RT, Malone PA, Nalty J, et al (Univ College Dublin; Mater Misericordiae Univ, Dublin; Natl Maternity Hosp, Dublin)
Am J Obstet Gynecol 191:885-890, 2004   35–1

Objective.—The purpose of this study was to compare intra-anal electromyographic biofeedback alone with intra-anal biofeedback that was augmented with electrical stimulation of the anal sphincter in the treatment of postpartum fecal incontinence. A secondary aim was to examine the impact of the treatment on continence-related quality of life.

Study Design.—Sixty symptomatic women were assigned randomly to receive intra-anal electromyographic biofeedback or electrical stimulation of the anal sphincter once weekly for 12 weeks and to perform daily pelvic floor exercises between treatments. Therapeutic response was evaluated with a symptom questionnaire to determine continence score, anal manometry, and endoanal ultrasound scanning. Quality of life was assessed before and after treatment with a validated questionnaire.

Results.—Fifty-four women completed the treatment; 52 women (96%) had ultrasonic evidence of an external anal sphincter defect. After the treatment, both groups demonstrated significant improvement in continence score ($P < .001$) and in squeeze anal pressures ($P < .04$). Resting anal pressures did not alter significantly. Quality of life improved after the completion of physiotherapy, but there were no differences in outcome between intra-anal electromyographic biofeedback and electrical stimulation of the anal sphincter.

Conclusion.—Intra-anal electromyographic biofeedback therapy was associated with improved continence and quality of life in women with altered fecal continence after delivery. The addition of electrical stimulation of the anal sphincter did not enhance symptomatic outcome.

▶ Altered fecal continence is a common condition among women after vaginal delivery, with approximately 1 in 4 reporting fecal continence problems and fecal incontinence issues in up to 50% of women who sustain a third-degree laceration during delivery. Despite widespread recognition of this problem by obstetrician-gynecologists, this common and often embarrassing and debilitating condition is underreported by patients and thus underrecognized by physicians. Current treatment for this condition centers on invasive and minimally invasive surgical interventions and physiotherapy; however, without adequate recognition by physicians, many affected women continue to suffer needlessly. In this multicenter study from Ireland, the authors found that intra-anal electromyographic biofeedback therapy was associated with improved fecal continence and a markedly improved quality of life. Discussion about fecal continence should be a core component of the gynecologic evaluation of all reproductive-age and menopausal women. Affected women should be informed that effective therapeutic interventions are available that can provide considerable symptom improvement and improved quality of life.

S. A. Grochmal, MD

Effect of Vaginal Distension on Anorectal Function: Identification of the Vagino-Anorectal Reflex

Shafik A, Shafik I, El-Sibai O (Cairo Univ; Menoufia Univ, Shebin El-Kom, Egypt)
Acta Obstet Gynecol Scand 84:225-229, 2005 35–2

Background.—Sexual stimulation produces not only reflex changes in the female external and internal reproductive organs but also extragenital reactions. A mention of the response of the anal sphincters and the rectum to penile thrusting could not be traced in the literature. We investigated the hypothesis that the anal sphincters and the rectum respond to penile thrusting in a way that prevents gas and fecal leakage during sexual intercourse.

Methods.—The response of the external anal sphincter (EAS) and the internal anal sphincter (IAS) and the rectum to vaginal balloon (condom) distension was recorded in 23 healthy women (age: 33.7 ± 7.3 years). The vaginal condom was inflated with air in increments of 50–300 ml, and the electromyographic (EMG) activity of the EAS and the IAS, as well as rectal pressure, was recorded. The test was repeated after separate anesthetization of the vagina, the rectum, the EAS and the IAS and after the use of normal saline instead of lidocaine.

Results.—Vaginal distension reduced the rectal pressure in the ratio of expansion of the vaginal volume up to a certain volume, beyond which the rectal pressure ceased to decline when more distending volume was added. Similarly, the internal sphincter EMG activity increased progressively on incremental vaginal distension increase until the 150-ml distension was reached after which more vaginal distension caused no further increase of the EMG activity; external sphincter EMG activity showed no response. Vaginal distension, while the vagina, the rectum, the EAS, and the IAS had been separately anesthetized, produced no significant change, but saline did.

Conclusions.—Vaginal balloon distension appears to effect rectal wall relaxation and increase of the internal sphincter tone. This seems to provide a mechanism to avoid rectal contents leakage during coitus. Rectal and internal sphincter response to vaginal distension is suggested to be mediated through a reflex we term 'vagino-anorectal reflex', which seems to be evoked by vaginal distension during penile thrusting. The reflex may prove of diagnostic significance in sexual disorders; further studies are needed in order to investigate this point.

▶ This article does not require much comment. It pretty well speaks for itself. The evolutionary advantage to those who possess this reflex is self-evident. Those who do not possess the reflex are less likely to reproduce successfully. The significance of the vagino-anorectal reflex as a test of sexual or anorectal function remains to be determined.

D. S. Miller, MD

36 Menopause

Heritability of Age at Natural Menopause in the Framingham Heart Study
Murabito JM, Yang Q, Fox C, et al (Natl Heart, Lung, and Blood Inst, Framingham, Mass; Boston Univ; Natl Heart, Lung, and Blood Inst, Bethesda, Md;
et al)
J Clin Endocrinol Metab 90:3427-3430, 2005   36–1

Background.—Twin registries and family history studies provide evidence that genetic factors contribute to the onset of menopause, but heritability estimates in population-based samples are limited. We sought to estimate heritability of age at natural menopause in women participating in the
multigenerational Framingham Heart Study, a community-based epidemio-
logical study.

Methods.—A total of 1500 original cohort and 932 offspring cohort
women from 1296 extended families reported a natural menopause defined
as the natural cessation of menses for 1 yr or more. Correlation coefficients
were calculated using family correlations in Statistical Applications for Genetic Epidemiology for mother-daughter, sister-sister, and aunt-niece pairs.
Heritability was estimated using variance-components methods in the Sequential Oligogenic Linkage Analysis Routines (SOLAR) computer pack-

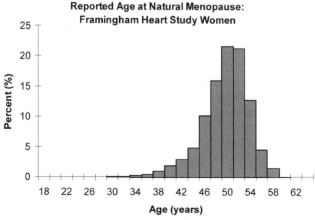

FIGURE 1.—Distribution of age at natural menopause in the study sample. (Courtesy of Murabito JM,
Yang Q, Fox C, et al: Heritability of age at natural menopause in the Framingham Heart Study. *J Clin Endocrinol Metab* 90:3427-3430, 2005, copyright The Endocrine Society.)

age. Covariates in the multivariable models included generation, number of cigarettes smoked, body mass index, and parity.

Results.—The mean age at natural menopause was 49.1 and 49.4 yr in original cohort and offspring women, respectively (Fig 1). The multivariable-adjusted correlation coefficients for mother-daughter, sister-sister, and aunt-niece pairs were 0.21, 0.22, and 0.12, respectively. The crude and multivariable-adjusted heritability estimates for age at natural menopause were 0.49 (0.37, 0.61) and 0.52 (0.35, 0.69).

Conclusions.—Our data suggest that at least 50% of the interindividual variability in menopausal age appears to be attributable to genetic effects.

▶ The age of menopause influences many risk factors concerning quality and longevity of life for menopausal women. As the age of menopausal onset varies considerably (between 40 and 60 years of age), studies have shown that age of onset appears to be modulated by environmental and genetic factors. For example, smoking is an important factor, with smokers experiencing the onset of menopause an average of 1 to 2 years earlier than nonsmokers. The current study by Murabito et al used information from the Framingham Heart Study and evaluated the age of menopause onset among mother/daughter, sister/sister, and aunt/niece pairs. They found that at least 50% of the interindividual variability in menopausal age appears to be attributable to genetic factors. Menopause represents a "struggle" between genomics and environment, and clinicians must be prepared to recognize and utilize both camps for improved clinical outcomes for their patients.

L. P. Shulman, MD

Treatment of Menopausal Symptoms: What Shall We Do Now?

Hickey M, Davis SR, Sturdee DW (Univ of Western Australia, Subiaco; Monash Med School, Prahran, Victoria, Australia; Heart of England NHS Found Trust, Solihull, West Midlands, England)
Lancet 366:409-421, 2005   36–2

Abstract.—During the past few years, many women and doctors have revised their opinions of hormone replacement therapy (HRT) for menopausal symptoms, and a substantial number of individuals have discontinued its use because of concerns about side-effects. Numerous alternatives to HRT are promoted, and assessment of the quality of evidence about the safety and effectiveness of these compounds can be difficult. In this Review, we summarise the data from studies addressing the efficacy, risks, and benefits of frequently prescribed treatments, and offer evidence-based clinical guidelines for the management of menopausal symptoms. Although few comparative studies exist, oestrogen alone or combinations of oestrogen and progestagen are likely to be the most effective treatments for menopausal hot flushes and vaginal dryness. Tibolone is as effective as HRT, however, and might also improve libido. For those who wish to avoid hormonal treatments, there are few effective options. Selective serotonin reuptake inhibitors might be effective in the very short term (less than 12 weeks) and are well tolerated. There is not enough evidence that any of the complementary therapies available are any better than placebo for menopausal vasomotor symptoms, and few safety data exist.

▶ The authors provide a review on the treatment of menopausal symptoms based on a literature search using PubMed for peer-reviewed, randomized, controlled trials and observational studies published in English since 2000. The purpose of this review was to summarize the evidence and to offer evidence-based clinical guidelines for treatment of symptoms of menopause. They begin with a definition of the climacteric as the physiological events that accompany the onset of decline of ovarian function, both before and after the last menstrual period. Their summary of the data included the following important points. (1) The hot flush is the most characteristic manifestation of menopause; almost 80% of women are affected and 20% find this symptom intolerable. (2) Other accompanying symptoms include sweating, tachycardia, palpitations, anxiety, irritability, and even panic attacks. (3) Estrogen-only and combination estrogen plus progestagen HRT reduces vasomotor symptoms. (4) Vaginal estrogen can be used to treat vaginal dryness and atrophy and is safe for use by women with a uterus because there is minimum systemic absorption. (5) HRT does not improve urinary incontinence and can even make it worse. (6) The primary indication for systemic HRT is the relief of moderate-to-severe vasomotor symptoms, and vaginal estrogens are effective for urogenital symptoms. (7) Based on the Women's Health Initiative study, those treated with HRT for more than 5 years were significantly less likely than women on placebo to sustain a fracture. (8) Current guidelines recommend that HRT should only be considered as a first-line treatment for fracture prevention with vasomotor symptoms. (9) HRT appears to reduce the risk of colorectal cancer; however, HRT cannot be recommended to prevent colorectal cancer as a prophylactic measure. (10) More than 5 years' use of HRT conveys up to a 2-fold increased risk of breast cancer, but this risk is reduced if estrogen-only HRT is used. (11) All women about to take combined HRT should be advised of the small potential increased risk of breast cancer after 5 years of use. (12) Women who have a uterus should be cautioned against the use of estrogen-only HRT, which has been shown to increase the risk of endometrial hyperplasia and cancer. (13) HRT cannot be recommended for women with a history of breast cancer. (14) Continuous combined regimens protect the endometrium from endometrial cancer more efficiently than do sequential regimens. However, sequential HRT should not generally be continued for more than 5 years in postmenopausal women. (15) Women who take oral HRT face up to a 3-fold increased risk of venous thromboembolic events. (16) Increasing age and body mass index are additional risk factors. (17) HRT is contraindicated for those at high risk of venous thromboembolic events. (18) Estrogen-only and combined HRT are associated with an increased risk of stroke. (19) It is controversial whether HRT causes or prevents cardiovascular disease. (20) HRT should not be given for primary or secondary prevention of cardiovascular disease. (21) HRT is not recommended for the preservation of cognitive function or the prevention of dementia. (22) There is little evidence to support the effectiveness of complementary therapies for menopausal symptoms. Of note, however, is that long-term treatment with soy is associated with an increased incidence of endometrial hyperplasia. (23) Selective serotonin reuptake inhibitors are helpful and well tolerated for hot flushes, at least in the very short term.

Finally, because of the concerns about side effects of HRT and widespread publicity, a substantial number of women have discontinued the use of these medications. For many women, HRT remains as an important part of the management of vasomotor symptoms in perimenopause. It is critical that the physician individualize patient risks and benefits and obtain informed consent from women considering the use of HRT and their alternatives.

S. Elias, MD

Estrogen Therapy and Risk of Cognitive Decline: Results from the Women's Estrogen for Stroke Trial (WEST)
Viscoli CM, Brass LM, Kernan WN, et al (Yale Univ, New Haven, Conn; McGill Univ, Montreal; Case Western Reserve Univ, Cleveland, Ohio)
Am J Obstet Gynecol 192:387-393, 2005   36–3

Objective.—This study was undertaken to assess whether estrogen therapy (ET) reduces the risk of cognitive decline in women with cerebrovascular disease.

Study Design.—We conducted a randomized, double-blind trial of estradiol 17β versus placebo for secondary stroke prevention in 664 postmenopausal women with a recent stroke or transient ischemic attack. The Mini-Mental State Examination (MMSE) and 5 domain measures were obtained at baseline and exit.

Results.—Among 461 women withdrawn alive without stroke, ET did not have a significant effect on cognitive measures after an average of 3 years (relative risk of MMSE decline: 0.74, 95% CI, 0.49-1.13). In women with normal MMSE at entry, estrogen was associated with less decline (relative risk, 0.46, 95% CI, 0.24-0.87).

Conclusion.—In this study, estradiol did not have significant effects on cognitive measures. However, in women with normal function at baseline, there may be a benefit for ET in reducing the risk for cognitive decline.

▶ There have been suggestions for years that ET might prevent postmenopausal decline in female cognitive function. The recent Women's Health Initiative showed that neither conjugated estrogen plus medroxyprogesterone nor conjugated estrogen alone resulted in an improvement in global cognitive function compared with placebo, and was associated with a small increased risk of mild cognitive impairment and an increased risk for probable dementia.[1,2] However, when women with recurrent stroke were removed, the increased risk of dementia was not statistically significant.

In the reviewed study, women were placed on estrogen alone after a nondisabling ischemic stroke. While the study did not show improvement in cognitive function, those who had normal function at baseline and were given estrogen showed less decline in cognitive function than those who received placebo. Unfortunately, this study was powered to study recurrent stroke and death and not cognitive function. As a result, the statistical power of 30% to detect a difference in cognitive function of all women who completed the trial without a recurrent stroke was not achieved. Accordingly, the definitive answer on the effect of estrogen on cognitive function in postmenopausal women remains uncertain.

G. H. Lipscomb, MD

References

1. Shumaker S, Legault C, Kuller L, et al: Conjugated equine estrogens and incidence of probable dementia and mild cognitive impairment in postmenopausal women: Women's Health Initiative Memory Study. *JAMA* 291:2947-2958, 2004.
2. Espeland M, Rapp S, Shumaker S, et al: Conjugated equine estrogens and global cognitive function in postmenopausal women. *JAMA* 291:2959-2968, 2004.

Hormone Therapy and Sleep Quality in Women Around Menopause
Sarti CD, for the Gruppo di Studio IperAOGOI (Azienda Ospedaliera di Perugia, Italy; et al)
Menopause 12:545-551, 2005   36–4

Objective.—To obtain data on sleep quality in women attending menopause clinics in Italy.

Design.—A cross-sectional study was conducted on the sleep quality of postmenopausal women attending a network of first-level outpatient menopause clinics in Italy for general counseling about menopause or treatment of its symptoms. Eligible for the study were women observed consecutively during the study period with natural or spontaneous menopause. All participating centers enrolled women into the study who had never used hormone therapy (HT) (group 1, 819 women), current users of transdermal estrogens with or without progestins (group 2, 819 women), and current users of oral estrogens with or without progestins (group 3, 790 women). The women were asked about their quality of sleep using the Basic Nordic Sleep Questionnaire, their quality of life using the Short Form-12 questionnaire, and the intensity of hot flushes using a visual analogue scale.

Results.—Women in groups 2 and 3 tended to report difficulties in sleeping less often than those in group 1. For example, never users of HT more frequently reported sleeping poorly and needed more time to sleep or had problems falling asleep; these differences were significant ($P < 0.05$). Otherwise, no difference emerged from the Basic Nordic Sleep Questionnaire between women in groups 2 and 3.

Conclusions.—This study gives support to the suggestion that HT improves the quality of sleep. The effect was similar in women taking oral or transdermal therapy with or without progestins.

▶ The late Trudy Bush was one of the most influential epidemiologists and a leading force in the study of menopause. One of her most commonly used statements was that "no one study has a cornerstone on the truth." With the publication of the Women's Health Initiative studies, certain aspects of menopausal management have become confused because of the cohort (asymptomatic, older) followed in that study. In particular, some have called into question the ability of estrogen-containing hormone therapy to reduce estrogen-deprivation sleep problems. This study shows a clear benefit of estrogen therapy to reduce sleep-associated problems in menopausal women, whether or not the hormone therapy contained a progestin. We need to evaluate the entire literature when arriving at evidence-based therapeutic options and to recognize the limitations and biases of all studies.

L. P. Shulman, MD

Menopausal Hormones and Risk of Ovarian Cancer

Moorman PG, Schildkraut JM, Calingaert B, et al (Duke Univ, Durham, NC)
Am J Obstet Gynecol 193:76-82, 2005   36–5

Objective.—The objective of this study was to determine if use of menopausal hormones was associated with ovarian cancer and if risk varied by type of hormone used.

Study Design.—Data from a population-based, case-control study of ovarian cancer in North Carolina (364 cases, 370 controls, all postmenopausal) were analyzed to evaluate the relationship between menopausal hormones and ovarian cancer. Logistic regression analyses were used to calculate odds ratios (OR) and 95% CIs associated with various patterns of hormone use.

Results.—Ovarian cancer cases were more likely than controls to report long-term use (≥ 10 years) of unopposed estrogens (OR 2.2; 95% CI 1.2–4.1). No relationship was observed for estrogen always used with progestin.

Conclusion.—Hormone replacement therapy used according to current recommendations should not increase risk of ovarian cancer; however, clinicians should be aware of possible increased risk among women with a long history of estrogen replacement therapy (Table 3).

▶ The use of oral contraceptives has been consistently found to reduce the risk of developing ovarian cancer. However, the use of menopausal hormonal therapies has not been shown to have a consistent effect on ovarian cancer development, with studies showing an increased risk and others showing a slightly decreased or no effect on the risk of ovarian cancer. The authors, who are from Duke University, performed a population-based, case-control study in North Carolina. They found that those women who developed ovarian cancer

TABLE 3.—Odds Ratios for Ovarian Cancer by Hormone Regimen
Used and Duration of Use

	Cases (n = 364) n	Controls (n = 370) n	OR*	95% CI	OR†	95% CI
Never use	129	152	Referent		Referent	
Estrogen only						
Ever use	105	79	1.2	(0.7-2.0)	1.5	(0.9-2.3)
< 12 months	5	6	0.8	(0.2-2.9)	0.9	(0.3-3.2)
12-59 months	23	24	1.0	(0.5-1.8)	1.2	(0.6-2.3)
60-119 months	17	11	1.7	(0.7-3.7)	1.5	(0.6-3.5)
> 119 months	52	32	2.1	(1.2-3.4)	2.2	(1.2-4.1)
Missing duration	8	6				
Estrogen always with progestin						
Ever use	70	87	0.8	(0.6-1.3)	0.9	(0.6-1.4)
< 12 months	3	7	0.5	(0.1-1.8)	0.5	(0.1-2.0)
12-59 months	29	31	0.9	(0.5-1.7)	1.0	(0.6-1.9)
60-119 months	14	14	1.0	(0.4-2.2)	1.1	(0.5-2.6)
> 119 months	20	28	0.9	(0.5-1.7)	1.0	(0.5-2.0)
Missing duration	4	7				
Estrogen and progestin, not always used together						
Ever use	44	38	1.2	(0.7-2.0)	1.3	(0.8-2.2)
< 12 months	0	1	—		—	
12-59 months	9	4	1.8	(0.5-6.3)	2.2	(0.6-7.9)
60-119 months	10	14	0.7	(0.3-1.6)	0.7	(0.3-1.9)
> 119 months	22	14	1.9	(0.9-4.0)	2.4	(1.1-5.3)
Missing duration	3	5				
Progestin only						
Ever use	7	1	6.9	(0.8-57.3)	6.7	(0.8-57.9)
Testosterone						
Ever use	9	13	0.7	(0.3-1.6)	0.6	(0.3-1.6)

* ORs (odds ratios) adjusted for age and race using logistic regression modeling.

†ORs adjusted for age, race, parity, tubal ligation, hysterectomy, BMI 1 year before interview, 1st degree family history of breast or ovarian cancer, breastfeeding (yes/no), oral contraceptive use (yes/no), and educational level using logistic regression modeling.

(Courtesy of Moorman PG, Schildkraut JM, Calingaert B, et al: Menopausal hormones and risk of ovarian cancer. *Am J Obstet Gynecol* 193:76-82. Copyright 2005 by Elsevier.)

were more likely that the control population to report long-term use (defined as more than 10 years) of unopposed estrogen. And unlike earlier studies, no relationship was reserved for women using estrogen with a progestational agent. This article serves to provide more information concerning overall risks and benefits of hormone therapy for menopausal women. It serves to demonstrate the wide spectrum of outcomes in scientific studies evaluating benefits and risks of hormone therapy. Further studies will be needed to better delineate the risk of ovarian cancer among users of hormone therapy, and care should be taken to better describe the epidemiologic characteristics or the demographic characteristics of women who are entering such trials. It is clear that the discrepancies in clinical outcomes of these studies point to unknown study-based factors that have served to alter clinical outcomes among the studies of ovarian cancer in postmenopausal women.

L. P. Shulman, MD

Prevalence and Histologic Diagnosis of Adnexal Cysts in Postmenopausal Women: An Autopsy Study

Dørum A, Blom GP, Ekerhovd E, et al (Norwegian Radium Hosp, Oslo, Norway; Akershus Univ, Oslo, Norway; Sahlgrenska Univ, Göteborg, Sweden; et al)
Am J Obstet Gynecol 192:48-54, 2005   36–6

Objective.—The purpose of this autopsy study was to examine the prevalence and histologic condition of adnexal cysts in postmenopausal women. *Study Design.*—Adnexa of 234 postmenopausal women who had died from nongynecologic diseases were examined by the team pathologist. *Results.*—Ovarian cysts were found in 36 of the women (15.4%). Nine women (3.8%) had ovarian cysts with a diameter between 20 and ≤50 mm; 4 women (1.7%) had cysts that were >50 mm in diameter. Four women had bilateral ovarian cysts. Paraovarian cysts were found in 11 women (4.7%). All cysts were benign, except for 1 woman, who had bilateral serous cystadenoma of borderline type. Macroscopically, the borderline cysts were multilocular with mean diameters of 60 mm and 15 mm, respectively. *Conclusion.*—Because of the high prevalence of benign adnexal cysts, the identification of small unilocular cysts in postmenopausal women should be regarded as a normal finding.

▶ This study determined the prevalence of adnexal cysts in postmenopausal women (mean age, 73 years) who died of nongynecologic disease and had no history of gynecologic surgery. A high incidence of gynecologic cysts was noted. Although the majority were smaller than 2 cm (62.7%), 29.4% were between 2 and 5 cm and 7.8% were greater than 5 cm. Only 1 cyst was of borderline malignancy. Since these women were a select healthy group of women without previous gynecologic surgery, it could be hypothesized that the incidence of adnexal cysts may be even higher in the average population.

Before accurate and readily available US, postmenopausal adnexal cysts were considered uncommon and if found, necessitated removal to exclude malignancy. Since that time, many studies have noted the presence of adnexal cysts by US in as many as 14.6% of postmenopausal women.[1] The findings in this study confirm the previous US studies but also add reassurance that the majority of these cysts are histologically benign. This study further supports the concept that the postmenopausal ovary does not become quiescent after menopause and that with appropriate follow-up, most postmenopausal adnexal cysts can be managed conservatively.

G. H. Lipscomb, MD

Reference

1. Wolf SI, Gosink BB, Feldesman MR, et al: Prevalence of simple adnexal cysts in postmenopausal women. *Radiology* 180:65-71, 1991.

Estrogen Plus Progestin and Risk of Venous Thrombosis

Cushman M, for the Women's Health Initiative Investigators (Univ of Vermont, Burlington; et al)
JAMA 292:1573-1580, 2004   36–7

Context.—Postmenopausal hormone therapy increases the risk of venous thrombosis. It is not known whether other factors influencing thrombosis add to this risk.

Objective.—To report final data on incidence of venous thrombosis in the Women's Health Initiative Estrogen Plus Progestin clinical trial and the association of hormone therapy with venous thrombosis in the setting of other thrombosis risk factors.

Design, Setting, and Participants.—Double-blind randomized controlled trial of 16,608 postmenopausal women between the ages of 50 and 79 years, who were enrolled in 1993 through 1998 at 40 US clinical centers with 5.6 years of follow up; and a nested case-control study. Baseline gene variants related to thrombosis risk were measured in the first 147 women who developed thrombosis and in 513 controls.

Intervention.—Random assignment to 0.625 mg/d of conjugated equine estrogen plus 2.5 mg/d of medroxyprogesterone acetate, or placebo.

Main Outcome Measures.—Centrally validated deep vein thrombosis and pulmonary embolus.

Results.—Venous thrombosis occurred in 167 women taking estrogen plus progestin (3.5 per 1000 person-years) and in 76 taking placebo (1.7 per 1000 person-years); hazard ratio (HR), 2.06 (95% confidence interval [CI], 1.57-2.70). Compared with women between the ages of 50 and 59 years who were taking placebo, the risk associated with hormone therapy was higher with age: HR of 4.28 (95% CI, 2.38-7.72) for women aged 60 to 69 years and 7.46 (95% CI, 4.32-14.38) for women aged 70 to 79 years. Compared with women who were of normal weight and taking placebo, the risk associated with taking estrogen plus progestin was increased among overweight and obese women: HR of 3.80 (95% CI, 2.08-6.94) and 5.61 (95% CI, 3.12-10.11), respectively. Factor V Leiden enhanced the hormone-associated risk of thrombosis with a 6.69-fold increased risk compared with women in the placebo group without the mutation (95% CI, 3.09-14.49). Other genetic variants (prothrombin 20210A, methylenetetrahydrofolate reductase C677T, factor XIII Val34Leu, PAI-1 4G/5G, and factor V HR2) did not modify the association of hormone therapy with venous thrombosis.

Conclusions.—Estrogen plus progestin was associated with doubling the risk of venous thrombosis. Estrogen plus progestin therapy increased the risks associated with age, overweight or obesity, and factor V Leiden.

▶ As the data from the Women's Health Initiative are further analyzed, more information will emerge that will help clinicians and their patients make informed decisions about menopause management. In this study the authors present data that confirm earlier studies of the role of estrogen-progestin therapy for menopausal women. Of interest was that obesity and factor V Leiden mutation further increased the risk of thromboembolic events while other mutations did not further increase the risk. Accordingly, use of combination hormone therapies in women at increased risk for thromboembolic events may increase the risk for adverse clinical events above that observed among all users of combination hormonal therapies.

L. P. Shulman, MD

Different Effect of Hormone Replacement Therapy, DHEAS and Tibolone on Endothelial Function in Postmenopausal Women With Increased Cardiovascular Risk

Silvestri A, Gambacciani M, Vitale C, et al (Cardiovascular Research Unit, San Raffaele–Roma, Rome)
Maturitas 50:305-311, 2005   36–8

Abstract.—Menopause is associated with an increased cardiovascular risk and with a decrease in endothelial function. Hormone replacement therapy (HRT) improves endothelial function in post-menopausal women (PMW) without established atherosclerosis. New alternative treatments, among which tibolone (T) and DHEAS have been suggested to reduce postmenopausal cardiovascular risk. Although, in vitro animal studies have suggested that T and DHEAS improve endothelial function, their effect in humans has never been tested. The aim of the present study was to compare the effects of HRT (continuous combined 0.625 mg conjugated equine estrogen plus 2.5 mg/d medroxyprogesterone) DHEAS and T on endothelium-dependent flow-mediated vasodilatation (FMD), plasma nitrite, nitrate and endothelin-1 levels in 16 PMW with increased cardiovascular risk in a double-blinded, double-crossover study. Women were randomized and treated for 4 weeks with HRT, T or DHEAS. Brachial artery diameter, FMD, endothelin-1 and plasma nitrite and nitrate levels were measured at baseline and after each treatment phase.

Brachial artery diameters remained unchanged after each treatment phase. HRT significantly improved FMD compared to both baseline and to T and DHEAS therapies while no effect of T or DHEAS on FMD was noted.

In conclusion, HRT, but neither T nor DHEAS, improves endothelial function and reduces plasma levels of endothelin-1 in PMW at risk of CAD.

▶ Menopause is associated with an increased risk for adverse cardiovascular events and a decrease in endothelial function. Hormone therapy has been shown to improve endothelial function without increasing the risk of atherosclerosis. In this study, only HRT was associated with improved endothelial function, whereas tibolone and DHEAS had no impact on endothelial function. This study may provide critical information that explains the role and effects of hormones and selective estrogen receptor modulators in menopause management.

L. P. Shulman, MD

Postmenopausal Estrogen Use Affects Risk for Parkinson Disease

Currie LJ, Harrison MB, Trugman JM, et al (Univ of Virginia, Charlottesville)
Arch Neurol 61:886-888, 2004   36–9

Background.—Although estrogen therapy has been associated with improved cognitive functioning, a reduced risk of dementia in women with Parkinson disease (PD), and a decreased risk of Alzheimer disease, estrogen therapy has not affected the risk of PD per se.

Objective.—To determine whether postmenopausal women with PD differed from control subjects with regard to estrogen exposure.

Design, Setting, and Patients.—A case-control design was used, abstracting questionnaire data obtained via interview from 133 female PD cases and 128 female controls during routine outpatient clinic visits in 1999 at a mid-Atlantic tertiary care referral center. There were 140 subjects (68 PD cases and 72 controls) who met the inclusion criteria.

Main Outcome Measure.—Use of postmenopausal estrogen therapy.

Results.—More women in the control group than in the PD group took postmenopausal estrogen (36 [50%] of 72 women vs 17 [25%] of 68 women; $P<.003$), and women who had taken postmenopausal estrogen were less likely to develop PD than those who had not (odds ratio, 0.40 [95% confidence interval, 0.19-0.84]; $P<.02$). Among PD cases only, postmenopausal estrogen use was not associated with age of onset.

Conclusion.—Postmenopausal estrogen therapy may be associated with a reduced risk of PD in women.

▶ Despite widespread misgivings about the safety of hormone therapy, there is increasing recognition of benefits for women who choose to use postmenopausal estrogen for the relief of menopausal symptoms. This case-controlled study by Currie et al from the University of Virginia showed a reduced risk of PD among women taking postmenopausal estrogen therapy compared with those women who were taking no hormonal therapy. This preliminary study provides more tantalizing information as to the actual risks and benefits of hormone therapy for the symptomatic menopausal woman.

L. P. Shulman, MD

Endometrial Carcinoma Risks Among Menopausal Estrogen Plus Progestin and Unopposed Estrogen Users in a Cohort of Postmenopausal Women

Lacey JV Jr, Brinton LA, Lubin JH, et al (NIH, Bethesda, Md)
Cancer Epidemiol Biomarkers Prev 14:1724-1731, 2005   36–10

Background.—Because unopposed estrogen substantially increases endometrial carcinoma risk, estrogen plus progestin is one menopausal hormone therapy formulation for women who have not had a hysterectomy. However, endometrial carcinoma risks among estrogen plus progestin users and among former unopposed estrogen users are not firmly established.

Methods.—We evaluated endometrial carcinoma risks associated with estrogen plus progestin and unopposed estrogen therapies in 30,379 postmenopausal Breast Cancer Detection Demonstration Project follow-up study participants. We ascertained hormone therapy use and other risk factors during telephone interviews and mailed questionnaires between 1979 and 1998. We identified 541 endometrial carcinomas via self-report, medical records, the National Death Index, and state cancer registries. Poisson regression generated time-dependent rate ratios (RR) and 95% confidence intervals (95% CI).

Results.—Endometrial carcinoma was significantly associated with estrogen plus progestin only use ($n = 68$ cancers; RR, 2.6; 95% CI, 1.9-3.5), including both sequential (progestin <15 days per cycle; $n = 32$ cancers; RR, 3.0; 95% CI, 2.0-4.6) and continuous (progestin at least 15 days per cycle; $n = 15$ cancers; RR, 2.3; 95% CI, 1.3-4.0) regimens. The RR increased by 0.38 (95% CI, 0.20-0.64) per year of estrogen plus progestin use, and RRs increased with increasing duration of use for both regimens. The strong association with unopposed estrogen use declined after cessation but remained significantly elevated ≥10 years after last use (RR, 1.5; 95% CI, 1.0-2.1).

Conclusions.—Both estrogen plus progestin regimens significantly increased endometrial carcinoma risk in this study. Risks among unopposed estrogen users remained elevated long after last use. The prospect that all estrogen plus progestin regimens increase endometrial carcinoma risk deserves continued research.

▶ This study illustrates the perils of drawing conclusions about causation based on associations, particularly from epidemiologic studies for which the report does not involve one of the primary end points of the study. This study analyzed data from the National Cancer Institute Breast Cancer Detection Demonstration Project begun in 1979, which has queried a group of patients who were or thought they were at high risk for the development of breast cancer, a disease that shares many epidemiologic associations with endometrial cancer. Relatively unique in this trial, the authors reported an increased risk of developing endometrial cancer in patients who took estrogen and progestin therapy. Most other studies have shown no increased risk or a protective effect of estrogen and continuous progestin therapy. The discrepancy can likely be accounted for by 2 factors. First, prolonged progestin therapy in this study was defined as greater than 15 days but not every single day. Second, in most other trials where endometrial status is the primary outcome, such as the Women's Health Initiative, the endometrium was evaluated at the beginning of the study, thus eliminating patients with preexisting endometrial hyperplasia or cancer.[1]

D. S. Miller, MD

Reference

1. Anderson GL, Judd H, Kaunitz A, et al: Effects of estrogen plus progestin on gynecologic cancers and associated diagnostic procedures: The Women's Health Initiative randomized trial. *JAMA* 290:1739-1748, 2003. (2005 YEAR BOOK OF OBSTETRICS, GYNECOLOGY, AND WOMEN'S HEALTH, p 251-252.)

37 Botanicals

Polyunsaturated Fatty Acids (PUFAs) Might Reduce Hot Flushes: An Indication From Two Controlled Trials on Soy Isoflavones Alone and With a PUFA Supplement
Campagnoli C, Abbà C, Ambroggio S, et al (Ospedale Ginecologico Sant'Anna, Torino, Italy)
Maturitas 51:127-134, 2005   37–1

Objectives.—To investigate the effect on hot flushes of a soy isoflavone extract alone (Study A) and with the addition of a supplement of polyunsaturated fatty acids, PUFAs (Study B).

Methods.—Subjects were postmenopausal women (29 in Study A, 28 in Study B) with more than five troublesome hot flushes per day. Both studies were double-blind randomized placebo-controlled trials with cross-over design, of 24-week duration. After a 2-week observation period, they were randomized to receive two capsules per day providing 60 mg of isoflavones or placebo for 12 weeks; thereafter, women who had taken isoflavones were given placebo for a second 12-week period, and vice-versa. Women in the Study B were given also two capsules per day containing a PUFA supplement for the entire 24-week test period.

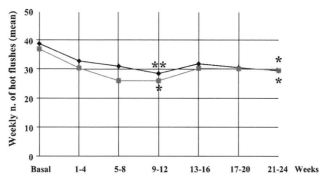

FIGURE 1.—Weekly number of hot flushes (mean) in women treated first with isoflavones (weeks 1–12) and then with placebo (weeks 13–24) (squares) and in women treated first with placebo (weeks 1–12) and then with isoflavones (weeks 13–24) (diamonds). Study A. Significantly different from basal value *$p<0.05$; **$p<0.01$. (Courtesy of Campagnoli C, Abbà C, Ambroggio S, et al: Polyunsaturated fatty acids (PUFAs) might reduce hot flushes: An indication from two controlled trials on soy isoflavones alone and with a PUFA supplement. *Maturitas* 51:127-134. Copyright 2005 by Elsevier Science Inc.)

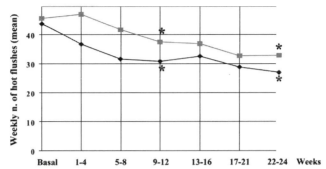

FIGURE 2.—Weekly number of hot flushes (mean) in women treated first with isoflavones + PUFA supplement (weeks 13–12) and then with placebo + PUFA supplement (weeks 13–24) (squares) and in women treated first with placebo + PUFA supplement (weeks 1–12) and then with isoflavones + PUFA supplement (weeks 13–24) (diamonds). Study B. Significantly different from basal value *$p<0.05$. (Courtesy of Campagnoli C, Abbà C, Ambroggio S, et al: Polyunsaturated fatty acids (PUFAs) might reduce hot flushes: An indication from two controlled trials on soy isoflavones alone and with a PUFA supplement. *Maturitas* 51:127-134. Copyright 2005 by Elsevier Science Inc.)

Results.—Both studies showed the isoflavone extract to have no greater efficacy on hot flushes than the placebo. During the 24 weeks of the Study B there was a progressive and highly significant reduction in the number of hot flushes, independent of whether the women had begun with isoflavones or with placebo (Figs 1, 2, and 3).

Conclusion.—In these two trials the isoflavone extract did not show greater efficacy on the hot flushes than the placebo. The reduction of hot flushes observed in the Study B might be due to the PUFA supplement. PUFAs, particularly Omega (Ω) 3-fatty acids, could reduce hot flushes through their influence on neuronal membranes and/or the modulation of the neurotransmitter function and the serotoninergic system. Studies specifi-

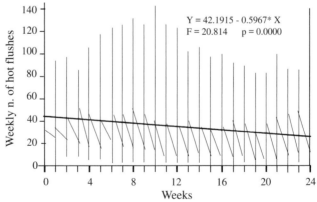

FIGURE 3.—Linear regression analysis of the weekly number of hot flushes in all the women treated with PUFA supplement for 24 weeks ($n = 28$) (Study B). (Courtesy of Campagnoli C, Abbà C, Ambroggio S, et al: Polyunsaturated fatty acids (PUFAs) might reduce hot flushes: An indication from two controlled trials on soy isoflavones alone and with a PUFA supplement. *Maturitas* 51:127-134. Copyright 2005 by Elsevier Science Inc.)

cally designed to document the action of PUFAs on hot flushes would be welcome.

The Effects of Flaxseed Dietary Supplement on Lipid Profile, Bone Mineral Density, and Symptoms in Menopausal Women: A Randomized, Double-blind, Wheat Germ Placebo-controlled Clinical Trial

Dodin S, Lemay A, Jacques H, et al (Laval Univ, Québec; Fred Hutchinson Cancer Research Ctr, Seattle)
J Clin Endocrinol Metab 90:1390-1397, 2005   37–2

Abstract.—Phytoestrogens are increasingly incorporated into the diet of menopausal women. However, there are limited data on the efficacy of flaxseed on the consequences of estrogen deficiency in menopausal women. The purpose of the study was to assess the effects of flaxseed incorporation into the diet of healthy menopausal women. One hundred and ninety-nine menopausal women were randomly assigned to consume 40 g flaxseed/d (n = 101) or wheat germ placebo (n = 98) for 12 months. At baseline and at month 12, serum levels of lipids, bone mineral density (BMD), and menopausal symptoms were evaluated. Statistical analysis was performed under the intention to treat principle. Flaxseed reduced serum total (-0.20 ± 0.51 mmol/liter; $P = 0.012$) and high-density lipoprotein (-0.08 ± 0.24 mmol/liter; $P = 0.031$) cholesterol concentrations compared with wheat germ placebo. BMD did not differ significantly between the two arms. Both flaxseed and wheat germ reduced ($P < 0.0001$) the severity scores of menopausal symptoms, but no statistical difference was found between the two arms. Our findings suggest that 1-yr incorporation of flaxseed into the diet produced a favorable, but not clinically significant, effect on blood cholesterol and caused no significant change in BMD or symptoms in healthy menopausal women.

▶ Studies of nonpharmacologic botanical products are currently under way to assess more rigorously the benefits and safety of these products for menopausal women. These 2 studies (Abstracts 37–1 and 37–2) evaluated 2 different products that have been widely believed to have a beneficial effect for the symptomatic menopausal woman. Study of PUFAs and a flaxseed dietary supplement both showed no significant benefit with regard to symptom relief for menopausal women. It is unfortunate that many women have been convinced that a variety of plant-based products may be beneficial and even preferred over proven pharmacologic agents. It will be studies such as these and other rigorous scientific trials that actually delineate benefits and, as importantly, risks of these products so that women can eventually make a truly informed decision about the type of therapeutic intervention that they may desire for the treatment of the symptomatic menopause.

L. P. Shulman, MD

Effects of a 2-Year Randomized Soy Intervention on Sex Hormone Levels in Premenopausal Women

Maskarinec G, Franke AA, Williams AE, et al (Cancer Research Ctr of Hawaii, Honolulu; Univ of Southern California, Los Angeles)
Cancer Epidemiol Biomarkers Prev 13:1736-1744, 2004   37–3

Objective.—Several epidemiologic studies have described protective effects of soy consumption against breast cancer. The goal of this trial among premenopausal women was to examine the effect of soy foods on menstrual cycle length and circulating sex hormone levels.

Methods.—This 2-year dietary intervention randomized 220 healthy premenopausal women. The intervention group consumed two daily servings of soy foods containing 50 mg of isoflavones; the control group maintained their regular diet. Five blood samples (obtained in months 0, 3, 6, 12, and 24) were taken 5 days after ovulation as determined by an ovulation kit. The serum samples were analyzed for estrone, estradiol, sex hormone binding globulin, androstenedione, and progesterone by immunoassay.

Results.—At baseline, both groups had similar demographic, anthropometric, and nutritional characteristics. The dropout rates of 15.6% (17 of 109) in the intervention group and 12.6% (14 of 111) in the control group did not differ significantly. According to soy intake logs, 24-hour recalls, and urinary isoflavone excretion, the women closely adhered to the study regimen. Menstrual cycles became slightly shorter in both groups but did not differ by group. Mixed general linear models indicated no significant intervention effect on any of the serum hormones. However, androstenedione and progesterone decreased significantly over time in both groups.

Conclusions.—The results of this study suggest that the preventive effects of soy on breast cancer risk in premenopausal women may not be mediated by circulating sex hormone levels. Different mechanisms of actions or effects of exposure earlier in life are alternate hypotheses that require further investigation.

Soy Intake and Blood Cholesterol Concentrations: A Cross-Sectional Study of 1033 Pre- and Postmenopausal Women in the Oxford Arm of the European Prospective Investigation into Cancer and Nutrition

Rosell MS, Appleby PN, Spencer EA, et al (Univ of Oxford, England)
Am J Clin Nutr 80:1391-1396, 2004   37–4

Background.—Clinical trials have suggested that the intake of soy protein reduces blood cholesterol. Few studies have explored this relation in subjects who consume soy as part of their regular diet.

Objective.—In this study, we investigated whether blood cholesterol concentrations are related to the intake of soyfoods in a cohort comprising subjects with a wide variation in soy intake.

Design.—This cross-sectional study included 1033 pre- and postmenopausal women selected from the Oxford arm of the European Prospective

Investigation into Cancer and Nutrition. The sample included 361 nonvegetarians, 570 vegetarians, and 102 vegans. Their dietary intake was assessed by using a food-frequency questionnaire. Anthropometric data, medical history, and lifestyle information were obtained with the use of a questionnaire, blood samples were obtained, and plasma total, LDL-, and HDL-cholesterol concentrations were measured.

Results.—Soy-protein intake was inversely associated with total and LDL-cholesterol concentrations and with the ratio of total to HDL cholesterol but not with HDL-cholesterol concentrations. Mean plasma LDL-cholesterol concentrations in women with a soy-protein intake ≥6 g/d was 12.4% lower than that in women who consumed <0.5 g/d ($P < 0.001$).

Conclusion.—Moderate intakes of soyfoods as part of a regular diet are associated with favorable blood cholesterol concentrations.

Dietary Soy Containing Phytoestrogens Does Not Activate the Hemostatic System in Postmenopausal Women

Teede HJ, Dalais FS, Kotsopoulos D, et al (Monash Univ, Clayton, Victoria, Australia; Dandenong Hosp, Australia; Monash Med Centre, Clayton, Victoria, Australia)
J Clin Endocrinol Metab 90:1936-1941, 2005　　　　　　　　　37–5

Abstract.—The soybean is rich in isoflavone phytoestrogens, which are ligands for estrogen receptors, but it is unknown whether soy/phytoestrogens have similar procoagulant effects to estrogen. In this randomized double-blind trial, 40 healthy postmenopausal women of age 50–75 yr received soy protein isolate (40 g soy protein, 118 mg isoflavones) (n = 19) or casein placebo (n = 21). Plasma markers of coagulation, fibrinolysis, and endothelial dysfunction were measured at baseline and 3 months. The baseline characteristics of the two groups were similar. Compared with casein placebo, soy decreased triglycerides ($P < 0.005$) and low-density lipoprotein/high-density lipoprotein ratio ($P < 0.001$) and increased lipoprotein (a) ($P < 0.05$). Activity of coagulation factor VII (VIIc) decreased similarly in both groups ($P < 0.005$). Prothrombin fragments 1 + 2 (a marker of thrombin generation) decreased in the soy group ($P < 0.005$), but the change was not different from the casein group. There was no effect of soy on soluble fibrin (a marker of fibrin production), plasminogen activator inhibitor-1 (a marker of fibrinolytic inhibitory potential), D-dimer (a marker of fibrin turnover), or von Willebrand factor (a marker of endothelial damage). In conclusion, the results of the current study do not support biologically significant estrogenic effects of soy/phytoestrogens on coagulation, fibrinolysis, or endothelial function.

▶ Phytoestrogens are a diverse group of nonsteroidal plant-derived compounds that are structurally similar to estrogenic steroids and have an affinity for estrogen receptors. In this regard, phytoestrogens have been considered as alternative therapeutic option for women seeking relief from menopausal symptoms. However, rigorous studies evaluating the safety and benefit of soy and phytoestrogens have, until recently, been lacking. These 3 studies (Abstracts 37–3 through 37–5) represent a diverse cross-section of the new literature concerning the impact of soy use in premenopausal, perimenopausal, and postmenopausal women. The study by Maskarinec et al shows that the physiologic impact of soy use may not be mediated by changes in circulating sex hormone levels. This change in the mechanism of soy use is postulated based on the impact of soy on breast cancer risk in premenopausal women. Rosell et al found that moderate intakes of food containing soy were associated with favorable blood-cholesterol alterations, comparable to those observed with the use of estrogen containing regimens. Finally, Teede et al found that use of soy-containing phytoestrogens in postmenopausal women did not activate the hemostatic system; accordingly, this study does not support a biologically significant estrogenic effect of soy and phytoestrogens on coagulation, fibrinolysis, or endothelial function. These studies serve to show the importance of performing rigorous scientific evaluations to determine physiologic and clinical outcomes rather than relying on surrogate markers conjecture and anecdote to assess the benefit and safety of new and novel therapeutic options.

L. P. Shulman, MD

NEOPLASIA

38 Surgical and Medical Oncology

Validation of Referral Guidelines for Women With Pelvic Masses
Im SS, Gordon AN, Buttin BM, et al (Univ of California, Orange; Baylor Univ,
Dallas; Barnes-Jewish Hosp, St Louis; et al)
Obstet Gynecol 105:35-41, 2005   38–1

Objective.—Guidelines for referring women with pelvic masses suspicious for ovarian cancers to gynecologic oncologists have been published jointly by Society of Gynecologic Oncologists (SGO) and the American College of Obstetricians and Gynecologists (ACOG). They are based on patient age, CA 125 level, physical findings, imaging study results, and family history. Although the guidelines are evidence-based, their predictive value in distinguishing cancers from benign masses is unknown.

Methods.—Chart review for factors included in the guidelines of surgically evaluated women with pelvic masses at 7 tertiary care centers during a 12-month interval was performed. This information was used to estimate the predictive values of the SGO and ACOG guidelines in identifying patients with malignant pelvic masses.

Results.—A total of 1,035 patients were identified, including 318 (30.7%) with primary malignancies of the ovary, fallopian tube, or peritoneum. Seventy-seven were younger than 50 years old (premenopausal group), and 240 were 50 years old or older (postmenopausal group). Fifty additional patients (4.8%) had cancers metastatic to the ovaries, and the remaining 667 (64.4%) had benign masses. The referral guidelines captured 70% of the ovarian cancers in the premenopausal group and 94% of the ovarian cancers in the postmenopausal group. The positive predictive value was 33.8% for the premenopausal group and 59.5% for the postmenopausal group, whereas the negative predictive values were more than 90% for both groups. Elevated CA 125 level was the single best predictor of malignancy in both groups.

Conclusion.—The SGO and ACOG referral guidelines effectively separate women with pelvic masses into 2 risk categories for malignancy. This distinction permits a rational approach for referring high-risk patients to a gynecologic oncologist for management.

▶ After much discussion, ACOG and SGO agreed on referral guidelines for women with pelvic masses for whom gynecologic oncology consultation would be appropriate.[1] Curiously, no US or other imaging characteristics of the mass were incorporated into these guidelines despite evidence to suggest that information could be helpful.[2] Nonetheless, the authors present their efforts to validate these guidelines, albeit in a retrospective evaluation. Utilizing these guidelines, 70% of premenopausal and 94% of postmenopausal women with ovarian cancer would have been correctly predicted. But this required referral of 31% of the premenopausal and 42% of the postmenopausal benign pelvic masses. Utilizing multiple regression models and discriminate analysis, the authors proposed a modified referral criteria that would have correctly predicated 85% of the premenopausal and 90% of the postmenopausal ovarian cancers while requiring referral of only 27% of benign masses in premenopausal women and 24% in postmenopausal women. Clearly, the use of simple imaging criteria could likely further improve these predictive criteria.

D. S. Miller, MD

References

1. ACOG: Committee Opinion number 280: The role of the generalist obstetrician-gynecologists in the early detect of ovarian cancer. *Obstet Gynecol* 100:1413-1416, 2002.
2. Twickler D, Forte T, Santos-Ramos R, et al: The ovarian tumor index predicts risk for malignancy. *Cancer* 86:2280-2290, 1999. (2001 YEAR BOOK OF OBSTETRICS, GYNECOLOGY, AND WOMEN'S HEALTH, p. 421.)

Ten-Year Experience With Laparoscopy on a Gynecologic Oncology Service: Analysis of Risk Factors for Complications and Conversion to Laparotomy

Chi DS, Abu-Rustum NR, Sonoda Y, et al (Mem Sloan-Kettering Cancer Ctr, New York; Harvard Med School, Boston; St Lukes-Roosevelt Hosp, New York)
Am J Obstet Gynecol 191:1138-1145, 2004   38-2

Background.—This study was conducted to assess the role of laparoscopy on a gynecologic oncology service at an academic institution over a 10-year period.

Methods.—The charts of all laparoscopic procedures from January 1991 through December 2000 were reviewed. The procedures were divided into 4 distinct levels based upon the degree of difficulty of the procedure. Level I consisted of diagnostic procedures, while level II represented procedures performed upon the uterus or adnexa, or both. Level III procedures consisted of second-look operations for malignancies, and level IV procedures were defined as lymphadenectomies or other complex cases. The grade of the complications was defined as 1 to 5, with 1 representing mild and 5 representing death.

Findings.—A total of 1451 procedures were identified during this 10-year period. A total of 129 complications occurred, representing 9% of the cases. Only 2.5% of the cases were associated with significant complications (grade 3-5). Multivariate analysis was performed to identify predictors of complications and showed that older age, prior radiation, and presence of malignancy were associated with an increased risk of significant morbidity. The rate of significant complications increased 4 times when malignancy was present. Conversion to laparotomy occurred in 7% of the cases secondary to technical difficulties. Predictors of conversion on multivariate analysis were previous abdominal surgery and performance of a more complex procedure.

Conclusions.—Simple and complex laparoscopic procedures can be performed on a gynecologic oncology service with a reasonable complication and laparotomy conversion rate.

▶ This study illustrates the growing acceptance of laparoscopy within the discipline of gynecologic oncology. The data heretofore have been limited in terms of global experiences describing complications.

Weaknesses of this article include the retrospective descriptive nature of this study, and the subjective scoring systems utilized by the authors to grade both procedure difficulty and degree of complications. In terms of complication grading, use of currently available and validated scoring systems would have been preferable. Furthermore, little has been learned from this study regarding the role of laparoscopy in obese patients, as nearly 95% of the patients had a body mass index of less than 35. Also, the total prevalence of laparoscopy and how this increased over time in this institution are not clearly stated.

Nonetheless, this article serves as a benchmark for defining the learning curve of the introduction of laparoscopy onto a gynecologic oncology service. Importantly, this particular experience reflects a program that is a major teaching program in that they have an approved gynecologic oncology fellowship. The identification of particular variables that predict an increased chance of complications or need for conversion to laparotomy is helpful. Use of this information can aide the clinician in proper patient selection for laparoscopic procedures.

T. J. Herzog, MD

Laparoscopic Modified Radical Hysterectomy: A Strategy for a Clinical Dilemma

Eisenkop SM, Spirtos NM, Lin WM, et al (Women's Cancer Ctr, Tarzana, Calif; Women's Cancer Ctr, Palo Alto, Calif; LAC/USC Med Ctr, Los Angeles)
Gynecol Oncol 96:484-489, 2005   38–3

Objective.—To investigate the role of laparoscopic modified radical (type 2) hysterectomy when cervical cancer cannot be excluded or documented preoperatively.

Methods.—Between 1996 and 2004, 50 patients with cervical intraepithelial neoplasia (CIN III) or adenocarcinoma in situ (AIS) involvement of cone endocervical margins and/or endocervical curettings, who were not candidates for observation or repeat conization, underwent laparoscopy to perform a modified radical hysterectomy.

Results.—Forty-nine (98.0%) modified radical hysterectomies were completed laparoscopically and one (2.0%) patient required a laparotomy. Of the overall group, 35 (70.0%) had residual pathology; 26 (52.0%) were precancerous lesions, and 9 (18.0%) had invasive disease (5 adenocarcinomas, 3 squamous lesions, and 1 adenosquamous carcinoma). Of the nine with cancer, one had stage IA1 disease, three had stage IA2 disease, and five had stage IB1 disease. Five (55.6%) invasive lesions were diagnosed intraoperatively (frozen section), and a laparoscopic pelvic and lower aortic lymph node dissection was performed. The median operative time was 96 min (range 58–185), blood loss 100 ml (50–450), and postoperative hospital stay 2.5 days (range 1–14). There were no incidences of prolonged urinary retention fistulas, or other serious complications. All patients with cancer remain disease-free (median follow-up 44.2 months, range 1–88.7 months).

Conclusions.—Laparoscopic modified radical hysterectomy is a treatment option for patients for whom cervical cancer cannot be definitively excluded, and can be completed with acceptable operative time, blood loss, and hospitalization.

▶ These authors report a large experience with a situation that most of us see only occasionally: patients who might have invasive cancer of the cervix but cannot or refuse to be further evaluated to rule out invasion. Eighteen percent were found to have invasive cancer, most of whom should have been treated with a radical type of hysterectomy. Only half of these cancers were identified at frozen section at the time of the laparoscopic modified radical hysterectomy. Presumably the remaining patients required either radiation or another procedure to assess their risk of lymph node metastasis. Fortunately, no significant complications were reported. Thus, at least 82% of patients did not benefit from this approach. Thus, laparoscopic modified radical hysterectomy appears to be feasible in this group of patients. It remains to be seen if it is indicated.

D. S. Miller, MD

FDG-PET for Management of Cervical and Ovarian Cancer
Havrilesky LJ, Kulasingam SL, Matchar DB, et al (Duke Univ, Durham, NC; Duke Ctr for Clinical Health Policy Research, Durham, NC; Dept of Veterans Affairs, Durham, NC)
Gynecol Oncol 97:183-191, 2005   38–4

Objective.—To assess the diagnostic performance of Positron Emission Tomography using fluorodeoxyglucose (FDG-PET) in comparison to conventional imaging modalities in the assessment of patients with cervical and ovarian cancer.

Methods.—Studies published between 1966 and 2003 were identified using an OVID search of the MEDLINE database. Inclusion criteria were use of a dedicated scanner, resolution specified, ≥12 human subjects, clinical follow-up ≥6 months or histopathology as reference standard, and sufficient data provided to construct a two-by-two table. Two reviewers independently abstracted data regarding sensitivity and specificity of PET.

Results.—25 studies (15 cervical cancer, 10 ovarian cancer) met inclusion criteria for full text review. For cervical cancer, pooled sensitivity and specificity of PET for aortic node metastasis are 0.84 (95% CI 0.68–0.94) and 0.95 (0.89–0.98). Pooled sensitivity and specificity for detection of pelvic node metastasis are: PET, 0.79 (0.65–0.90) and 0.99 (0.96–0.99); MRI, 0.72 (0.53–0.87) and 0.96 (0.92–0.98). Pooled sensitivity for CT is 0.47 (0.21–0.73) (pooled specificity not available). Pooled sensitivity and specificity of PET for recurrent cervical cancer with clinical suspicion are 0.96 (0.87–0.99) and 0.81 (0.58–0.94). For ovarian cancer, pooled sensitivity and specificity to detect recurrence with clinical suspicion are: PET, 0.90 (0.82–0.95) and 0.86 (0.67–0.96); conventional imaging, 0.68 (0.49–0.83) and 0.58 (0.33–0.80); CA-125, 0.81 (0.62–0.92) and 0.83 (0.58–0.96). When conventional imaging and CA-125 are negative, pooled sensitivity and specificity of PET are 0.54 (0.39–0.69) and 0.73 (0.56–0.87), respectively. When CA-125 is rising and conventional imaging is negative, the pooled sensitivity and specificity of PET are 0.96 (0.88–0.99) and 0.80 (0.44–0.97).

Conclusions.—There is good evidence that PET is useful for the pretreatment detection of retroperitoneal nodal metastasis in cervical cancer. There is fair evidence that PET is useful for the detection of recurrent cervical cancer. PET is less useful for the detection of microscopic residual ovarian cancer but has fair sensitivity to detect recurrence in the setting of a rising CA-125 and negative conventional imaging studies. Available studies are limited by low numbers of patients and wide confidence intervals.

▶ Cervical cancer spreads by direct extension in the lymphatics, with pelvic node metastases preceding aortic metastases in almost all cases. Hematogenous spread is less common. CT and MRI are fairly inaccurate for the detection of retroperitoneal nodal metastases. Calculated sensitivities range from 24% to 34% for CT and from 44% to 62% for MRI in studies that have accrued more than 20 patients. This review demonstrates that the sensitivity of detecting pelvic node metastases with PET is 79%. All imaging modalities, including

CT, MRI, and PET, are more specific than sensitive in the pretreatment evaluation of metastases. These findings have significant implications in the pretreatment evaluation of the patient with cervical carcinoma. Detecting aortic metastases may change radiation ports. It may lead to changing the primary treatment modality from radical surgery to chemoradiation. Clinicians treating patients with lesions greater than FIGO stage IB where metastases are common should consider PET scanning before treatment recommendations.

PET scanning appears to be substantially more sensitive than conventional imaging in detecting recurrent cervical cancer when there is clinical suspension of recurrent disease. The estimated sensitivity is approximately 96%, although the specificity is only 81%. In other words, PET is less specific in detecting persistent or recurrent disease than it is in detecting metastases before therapy. Importantly, PET can also be used to detect persistent disease after chemotherapy and radiation. Thus, patients with persistent metabolic activity in the cervix 3 months after chemotherapy and radiation should be evaluated for persistent disease. Taken together, these data suggest that PET is a useful adjunct to conventional imaging and may have a potential to hasten diagnosis of recurrent or persistent cervical cancer.

The evaluation of the patient with ovarian cancer differs from the evaluation of the patient with cervical cancer in 2 important ways. First, unlike cervical cancer, ovarian cancer is surgically staged. Because cervical cancer is clinically staged, imaging modalities are much more important in determining primary therapy. In addition, ovarian cancer differs from cervical cancer because ovarian cancer is frequently associated with an elevated tumor marker, CA-125. In contrast, no such tumor marker exists for cervical cancer.

Although recurrent ovarian cancer is almost never curable, early detection of recurrence theoretically affords a better chance at salvage when treatment might have an increased chance at prolonging remission or improving quality of life. Elevation in CA-125 after the primary therapy of ovarian cancer almost always is associated with persistent disease. Conventional imaging modalities often give nonspecific results and are suboptimal in the reliable detection of ovarian cancer in the peritoneal cavity. Unfortunately, some studies have shown that PET is also not sensitive in detecting microscopic recurrent disease. However, some studies demonstrate that PET has good sensitivity and specificity in the detection of recurrent ovarian cancer when there is clinical suspension of recurrence. Although the clinical usefulness of PET in this setting is unclear, PET may help localize the site of recurrence when CA-125 is elevated despite negative conventional imaging techniques. Thus, the use of PET in ovarian cancer is more controversial than in cervical cancer. It can only be recommended in women with negative conventional imaging and CA-125 testing. The pooled sensitivity and specificity in this setting are only 54% and 73%, respectively.

B. J. Monk, MD

The Use of Colorectal Stents for Palliation of Large-Bowel Obstruction Due to Recurrent Gynecologic Cancer

Pothuri B, Guirguis A, Gerdes H, et al (Mem Sloan-Kettering Med Ctr, New York; Rush Univ, Chicago)
Gynecol Oncol 95:513-517, 2004   38–5

Background.—Patients with gynecologic malignancies can present with acute large-bowel obstruction. Surgery has been the standard approach in treating these patients. Significant drawbacks can occur when surgery is utilized due to the associated morbidity. The use of colorectal stents in gynecologic oncology patients with large-bowel obstructions was explored.

Methods.—Data were obtained from a chart review of patients who underwent colorectal stent placement for validation of large-bowel obstruction over a 2-year period.

Findings.—A total of 6 patients were identified, of whom 5 had recurrent ovarian cancer and 1 had recurrent endometrial carcinoma. The mean age of the patients was 51.5 years. The length of bowel obstruction ranged from 2 to 10 cm. Four of the 6 patients had a successful procedure in terms of immediate relief with the ability to pass flatus after stent placement. The remaining 2 patients had unsuccessful stent placement and required a subsequent colostomy. Of those who underwent stent placement, the median survival was 120 days after the procedure. Of note, 1 patient had a sigmoid bowel perforation 12 days after the procedure that resolved with conservative observation.

Conclusion.—The use of colorectal stents for relief of large-bowel obstruction in recurrent gynecologic malignancies appears to be feasible.

▶ This study examines a very difficult management scenario in caring for patients with recurrent cancers, whose lifespan may be limited, but who then present with an acute large-bowel obstruction. These patients are obviously very symptomatic and require relief of the obstruction for quality-of-life preservation, as well as to prevent impending perforation, peritonitis, and sepsis. The stents were placed by gastroenterologists, who initially performed flexible endoscopy to the site of obstruction with the patient under sedation. A guidewire was placed, and it should be noted that all the patients had 2 mm or less of functional diameter in the colon. Also, for the patients who demonstrated a complete obstruction, balloon dilatation was necessary before placement of the stents. With long obstructions, 2 stents were placed as a precautionary measure. The mean hospital stay for stent placement was 15 days, and the mean survival was approximately 4 months.

The use of these colorectal stents did provide excellent symptom relief for this small series of patients. In addition, two thirds of the patients were able to avoid operative intervention in terms of an exploratory laparotomy or other procedure that would likely have resulted in the formation of an ostomy.

The only significant concerns with this particular study are, of course, the very small numbers examined in this series. The small number of patients enrolled precludes generalizations that verify the applicability of this technique in the palliation of gynecologic malignancies. An additional concern is the perforation that occurred in 1 patient. It is unclear whether this perforation resulted from progression of tumor or whether it was due to the stent placement itself.

Nonetheless, further study is indicated to establish an adequate safety profile for the placement of these stents, especially when balloon dilatation is required at the time of placement. Quality of life is an important factor to consider in these patients with recurrent cancer and an overall poor prognosis. Future studies of this technique are warranted based on these results and should include a formal quality-of-life assessment and a comparative cost analysis in order to establish this technique as a viable alternative option in patients with gynecologic malignancies and large-bowel obstructions.

T. J. Herzog, MD

Tumor-Specific Targeting of an Anticancer Drug Delivery System by LHRH Peptide

Dharap SS, Wang Y, Chandna P, et al (State Univ of New Jersey, Piscataway; Cancer Inst of New Jersey, New Brunswick; New Jersey Ctr for Biomaterials, Piscataway)
Proc Natl Acad Sci U S A 102:12962-12967, 2005   38–6

Abstract.—The central problem in cancer chemotherapy is the severe toxic side effects of anticancer drugs on healthy tissues. Invariably the side effects impose dose reduction, treatment delay, or discontinuance of therapy. To limit the adverse side effects of cancer chemotherapy on healthy organs, we proposed a drug delivery system (DDS) with specific targeting ligands for cancer cells. The proposed DDS minimizes the uptake of the drug

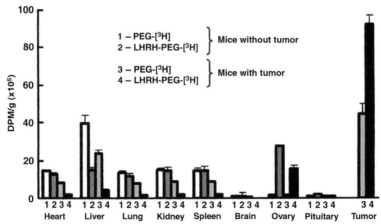

FIGURE 4.—Distribution of tritium-labeled PEG and LHRH-PEG conjugates in different tissues of mice without tumor and mice bearing xenografts of A2780 human ovarian carcinoma. Radioactivity is expressed in disintegrations per min (dpm) per g of tissue weight. Means ± SD from four independent measurements are shown. (Courtesy of Dharap SS, Wang Y, Chandna P, et al: Tumor-Specific Targeting of an Anticancer Drug Delivery System by LHRH Peptide. *Proc Acad Natl Sci U S A* 102:12962-12967, 2005. Copyright 2005 National Academy of Sciences, U.S.A.)

by normal cells and enhances the influx and retention of the drug in cancer cells. This delivery system includes three main components: (*i*) an apoptosis-inducing agent (anticancer drug), (*ii*) a targeting moiety-penetration enhancer, and (*iii*) a carrier. We describe one of the variants of such a system, which utilizes camptothecin as an apoptosis-inducing agent and poly(ethylene glycol) as a carrier. Luteinizing hormone-releasing hormone (LHRH) was used as a targeting moiety (ligand) to LHRH receptors that are overexpressed in the plasma membrane of several types of cancer cells and are not expressed detectably in normal visceral organs. The results showed that the use of LHRH peptide as a targeting moiety in the anticancer DDS substantially enhanced the efficacy of chemotherapy, led to amplified apoptosis induction in the tumor, and minimized the side effects of the anticancer drug on healthy organs. The LHRH receptor targeting DDS did not show *in vivo* pituitary toxicity and did not significantly influence the time course or the plasma concentration of luteinizing hormone and its physiological effects on the reproductive functions of mice (Fig 4).

▶ The human ovary is an endocrine organ and end organ. Hormones and their receptors have been associated with ovarian cancer and may be related to its causation. Ovarian cancer specimens have most commonly been shown to contain receptors for gonadotropins and steroid hormones. However, they also have receptors for luteinizing hormone–releasing hormone (LHRH). The role of these receptors in ovarian cancer is unclear. Its function in the hypothalamic pituitary axis to stimulate the release of gonadotropin is well known, but LHRH is not detectable in the peripheral circulation. There is considerable embryologic, epidemiologic, and in vivo evidence implicating gonadotropins in the initiation or promotion of epithelial ovarian cancers.[1] Yet treatment of epithelial ovarian cancer with gonadotropin-releasing hormone agonist is not effective.[2] However, targeting LHRH receptors with an LHRH chemotherapy conjugate appears to be feasible.

D. S. Miller, MD

References

1. Miller DS, Teng NNH, Ballon SC: Epithelial ovarian carcinoma in patients with intersex disorders: The role of pituitary gonadotropins in ovarian tumorigenesis. *Gynecol Oncol* 24:299-308, 1986.
2. Miller DS, Brady MF, Barrett RJ: A phase ii trial of leuprolide acetate in patients with advanced epithelial ovarian carcinoma: A Gynecologic Oncology Group study. *Am J Clin Oncol* 15:125-128, 1992.

Low-Molecular-Weight Heparin (Dalteparin) in Women With Gynecologic Malignancy

DeBernardo RL Jr, Perkins RB, Littell RD, et al (Massachusetts Gen Hosp, Boston)
Obstet Gynecol 105:1006-1011, 2005   38–7

Objective.—To compare the efficacy of dalteparin, a low-molecular-weight heparin, to unfractionated heparin (UFH) in the prevention of deep venous thrombosis (DVT) and pulmonary embolism in patients after surgery for gynecologic malignancy.

Methods.—The medical records of all patients undergoing major surgery on the Gynecologic Oncology Service at the Massachusetts General Hospital from July 2002 through April 2003 were reviewed. Patients with confirmed malignancy were included. Between July 1, 2002, and November 15, 2002, dalteparin (5,000 U subcutaneously each day) was used for postoperative prophylaxis for DVT and pulmonary embolus. After November 15, 2002, the method of prophylaxis was changed to UFH (5,000 U subcutaneously every 8 hours) exclusively. Patients were evaluated for DVT or pulmonary embolus based on clinical suspicion using computed tomographic angiography, ventilation and perfusion scan, or lower extremity doppler.

Results.—A total of 214 patients were identified who met study criteria. Dalteparin was administered to 103 patients, and UFH was administered to 111. The rates of clinically significant DVT or pulmonary embolus in patients receiving dalteparin and UFH were 8.9% and 1.2%, respectively ($P = .009$). Major risk factors for DVT or pulmonary embolus, including age, obesity, duration of surgery, and type of malignancy, did not differ between groups. There were no significant differences in bleeding complications or transfusion requirements between groups.

Conclusion.—The low-molecular-weight heparin dalteparin dosed 5,000 U daily is inadequate postoperative prophylaxis in women undergoing surgery for gynecologic cancer. In addition, heparin administered every 8 hours was not associated with increased bleeding complications. The use of dalteparin at the doses used in this study should be questioned until a large randomized trial shows efficacy in these high-risk patients.

▶ The development of postoperative venous thromboembolism, especially pulmonary embolism, can be a devastating complication of gynecologic surgery. Surgical trauma leads to endothelial injury and anesthetic immobilization leads to stasis. Patients with cancer also have the third limb of Virchow's triad: hypercoagulability. Our prevention interventions have been geared to addressing one or more aspects of Virchow's triad. For more than 30 years UFH has been shown to be useful in many studies for preventing venous thromboembolism in perioperative patients. However, heparin is not without its complications and the pharmaceutical industry has developed low-molecular-weight fragments of heparin, which reproduce many of the benefits of UFH with fewer side effects. But the hypercoagulability of cancer patients, particularly gynecologic cancer patients, is far more complex and the low-molecular-weight heparins may not address all these coagulation abnormalities. Presumably that is why, in this study, the new intervention was not as good as the old intervention.

D. S. Miller, MD

Duration of Human Chorionic Gonadotropin Surveillance for Partial Hydatidiform Moles
Lavie I, Rao GG, Castrillon DH, et al (Univ of Texas, Dallas)
Am J Obstet Gynecol 192:1362-1364, 2005   38–8

Objective.—Partial hydatidiform moles infrequently progress to gestational trophoblastic neoplasia. The purpose of this study was to determine the optimal duration of human chorionic gonadotropin surveillance.

Study Design.—We retrospectively reviewed the clinical follow-up of all women who were diagnosed with partial hydatidiform mole at our institution from 1983 to 2003.

Results.—One hundred sixty-three patients were identified with a median age of 23 years (range, 14-42 years). Seventy-four patients (45%) attained undetectable levels of human chorionic gonadotropin; none of the patients had gestational trophoblastic neoplasia. Forty patients completed the 6 months of recommended follow-up; 6 patients conceived during surveillance, and 28 patients did not return for any further office visits 1 to 5 months after achieving remission. Eighty-three patients (51%) were lost to follow-up before normalization of human chorionic gonadotropin. Six women (4%) had stage I gestational trophoblastic neoplasia during surveillance.

Conclusion.—Our results support the suggestion that a single undetectable human chorionic gonadotropin level after evacuation is sufficient follow-up to ensure remission in patients with partial hydatidiform moles.

▶ The detection of gestational trophoblastic disease initiates intensive diagnostic and therapeutic interventions. This group from the University of Texas Southwestern Medical Center sought to determine whether a subgroup of women with gestational trophoblastic disease, specifically those with partial hydatidiform moles, could obtain optimal surveillance with a protocol that differs somewhat from currently accepted management options. The authors retrospectively reviewed the clinical follow-up of all women who were diagnosed with partial hydatidiform moles and found that a single undetectable human chorionic gonadotropin level after uterine evacuation was sufficient to ensure remission in patients with partial hydatidiform moles. As a wide variety of patients may have difficulties in returning for regular evaluations after the detection and treatment of a partial hydatidiform mole, this study provides good evidence that optimal care can be obtained with the detection of a single undetectable human chorionic gonadotropin level after uterine evacuation.

L. P. Shulman, MD

39 Screening Modalities and Cancer Genetics

Screening for Familial Ovarian Cancer: Failure of Current Protocols to Detect Ovarian Cancer at an Early Stage According to the International Federation of Gynecology and Obstetrics System
Stirling D, Evans DGR, Pichert G, et al (Western Gen Hosp, Edinburgh, Scotland; Royal Infirmary of Edinburgh, Scotland; St Mary's Hosp, Manchester, England; et al)
J Clin Oncol 23:5588-5596, 2005   39–1

Purpose.—To assess the effectiveness of annual ovarian cancer screening (transvaginal ultrasound and serum CA-125 estimation) in detecting presymptomatic ovarian cancer in women at increased genetic risk.

Patients and Methods.—A cohort of 1,110 women at increased risk of ovarian cancer were screened between January 1991 and March 2004; 553 were moderate-risk individuals (4% to 10% lifetime risk) and 557 were high-risk individuals (> 10% lifetime risk). Outcome measurements include the number and stage of screen-detected cancers, the number and stage of cancers not detected at screening, the number of equivocal screening results requiring recall/repetition, and the number of women undergoing surgery for benign disease.

Results.—Thirteen epithelial ovarian malignancies (12 invasive and one borderline), developed in the cohort. Ten tumors were detected at screening: three International Federation of Gynecology and Obstetrics (FIGO) stage I (including borderline), two stage II, four stage III, and one stage IV. Of the three cancers not detected by screening, two were stage III and one was stage IV; 29 women underwent diagnostic surgery but were found not to have ovarian cancer.

Conclusion.—Annual surveillance by transvaginal ultrasound scanning and serum CA-125 measurement in women at increased familial risk of ovarian cancer is ineffective in detecting tumors at a sufficiently early stage to influence prognosis (Table 2). With a positive predictive value of 17% and a sensitivity of less than 50%, the performance of ultrasound does not satisfy the WHO screening standards. In addition, the combined protocol has a particularly high false-positive rate in premenopausal women, leading to unnecessary surgical intervention.

TABLE 2.—Performance of TVU and CA-125

Parameter	Sensitivity %	95% CI	Specificity %	95% CI	PPV %	95% CI	NPV %	95% CI
TVU	46.2	19.1 to 73.3	99.2	98.9 to 99.5	17.1	4.7 to 29.6	99.8	99.7 to 100
Serum CA-125	81.8	59.0 to 100	99.8	99.6 to 100	63.4	39.2 to 89.4	99.9	99.8 to 100

Abbreviations: TVU, transvaginal ultrasound; PPV, positive predictive value; NPV, negative predictive value.
(Courtesy of Stirling D, Evans DGR, Pichert G, et al: Screening for familial ovarian cancer: Failure of current protocols to detect ovarian cancer at an early stage according to the International Federation of Gynecology and Obstetrics system. *J Clin Oncol* 23:5588-5596, 2005. Reprinted with permission from the American Society of Clinical Oncology.)

▶ Ovarian cancer kills more women in developed countries than any other gynecologic malignancy. This is because most cases are not found until the cancer is spread far beyond the ovary. In spite of aggressive surgery and chemotherapy, to which most patients will respond for a while, most patients will then recur and succumb to their disease. While most patients with early ovarian cancer will have symptoms, they are nonspecific and easily overlooked.[1] Attempts at screening patients for ovarian cancer have been under way for decades. Most of the strategies to date have been based on various algorithms that involve identifying high-risk patients and screening them with various algorithms of transvaginal US and serum levels of CA-125. In this trial more than 1000 women were screened, and 29 women underwent surgery to find 2 stage I ovarian cancers. This study identifies another ineffective screening strategy that, like those before it, is characterized by low positive predictive values and sensitivities as well as a high false-positive rate.[2]

D. S. Miller, MD

References

1. Goff BA, Mandel LS, Melancon CH, et al: Frequency of symptoms of ovarian cancer in women presenting to primary clinics. *JAMA* 291:2705-2712, 2004. (2005 YEAR BOOK OF OBSTETRICS, GYNECOLOGY, AND WOMEN'S HEALTH, p 439)
2. Sato S, Yokoyama Y, Sakamoto T, et al: Usefulness of mass screening for ovarian carcinoma using transvaginal ultrasonography. *Cancer* 89:582-588, 2000. (2002 YEAR BOOK OF OBSTETRICS, GYNECOLOGY, AND WOMEN'S HEALTH, p 483)

The Role of Ultrasound Evaluation in the Detection of Early-Stage Epithelial Ovarian Cancer

Fishman DA, Cohen L, Blank SV, et al (New York Univ; Northwestern Univ, Evanston, Ill; Yale Univ, New Haven, Conn)

Am J Obstet Gynecol 192:1214-1222, 2005   39–2

Objective.—Epithelial ovarian cancer kills more women than all other gynecologic malignancies combined because of our inability to detect early-stage disease. Ultrasonography has demonstrated usefulness in the detection of ovarian cancer in asymptomatic women, but its value for the detection of early-stage epithelial ovarian cancer in women of increased risk is uncertain. We examined the usefulness of sonography in the detection of early-stage epithelial ovarian cancer in asymptomatic high-risk women who participated in the National Ovarian Cancer Early Detection Program.

Study Design.—Only asymptomatic women of increased risk for the development of ovarian cancer with initial normal gynecologic and ultrasound examinations were eligible to participate in the institutional review board-approved National Ovarian Cancer Early Detection Program. Participants underwent comprehensive gynecologic and ultrasound examinations every 6 months. Increased risk includes women with at least 1 affected first-degree relative with ovarian cancer; a personal history of breast, ovarian, or colon cancer; ≥1 affected first- and second-degree relatives with breast and or ovarian cancer; inheritance of a breast cancer mutation from an affected family member, or membership within a recognized cancer syndrome.

Results.—The average age of the 4526 women who were evaluated was 46 years; 2610 women were premenopausal, and 1916 women were postmenopausal. A total of 12,709 scans have been performed since 1990. Visualization of both ovaries was noted in 98% of premenopausal and in 94% of postmenopausal women. Fourteen women had undergone unilateral salpingo-oophorectomy. Recall rates at less than the routine 6-month interval were 0.4% in the premenopausal and 0.3% in postmenopausal women. A total of 98 women with persistent adnexal masses were identified, and 49 invasive surgical procedures were performed that diagnosed 37 benign ovarian tumors and 12 gynecologic malignancies. All cancers were detected in asymptomatic women who had normal ultrasound and physical examinations 12 and 6 months before the cancer diagnosis. The detected malignancies were fallopian tube carcinoma (stage IIIC; n = 4 women), primary peritoneal carcinoma (n = 4 women; stage IIIA, 1 woman; stage IIIB, 2 women; stage IIIC, 1 woman), epithelial ovarian cancer (stages IIIA and IIIB; n = 2 women), and endometrial adenocarcinoma (stage IA; n = 2 women). Additionally 37 primary and 12 recurrent breast carcinomas were detected by physical examination. A total of 184 women with genetic predisposition (breast cancer positive) have undergone a prophylactic bilateral salpingo-oophorectomy; 23% of these procedures found atypical hyperplasia, and unexpectedly, 2 women (1%) were found to have stage III (A and B) primary peritoneal carcinoma.

Conclusion.—This study demonstrates the limited value of diagnostic ultrasound examination as an independent modality for the detection of early-stage epithelial ovarian cancer in asymptomatic women who are at increased risk for disease.

▶ Women with early-stage ovarian cancer have an excellent prognosis. The long-term survival in women with early-stage disease approximates 90%, and in most cases adjuvant chemotherapy is not required. These data provide a strong rationale for the development of effective methods for the early detection of ovarian cancer.

Unfortunately, the low prevalence of ovarian cancer and the lack of highly specific screening tests have precluded the development of an effective screening method for the disease. The use of CA-125 has been associated with an unacceptably high false-positive rate. In addition, the predictive value of US for the detection of ovarian cancer has also been inadequate. In this study, a large number of women at increased risk for ovarian cancer were followed up for many years and underwent serial US screening as part of a comprehensive approach for the early detection of ovarian cancer. The data from the study fail to demonstrate the utility of diagnostic US as an independent modality for the early detection of ovarian cancer. Notably, the majority of women diagnosed with gynecologic malignancies while undergoing screening had advanced-stage disease at diagnosis.

G. Rodriguez, MD

Serum Protein Markers for Early Detection of Ovarian Cancer
Mor G, Visintin I, Lai Y, et al (Yale Univ, New Haven, Conn; George Washington Univ, Washington DC; Nevada Cancer Inst, Las Vegas)
Proc Natl Acad Sci U S A 102:7677-7682, 2005   39–3

Abstract.—Early diagnosis of epithelial ovarian cancer (EOC) would significantly decrease the morbidity and mortality from this disease but is difficult in the absence of physical symptoms. Here, we report a blood test, based on the simultaneous quantization of four analytes (leptin, prolactin, osteopontin, and insulin-like growth factor-II), that can discriminate between disease-free and EOC patients, including patients diagnosed with stage I and II disease, with high efficiency (95%). Microarray analysis was used initially to determine the levels of 169 proteins in serum from 28 healthy women, 18 women newly diagnosed with EOC, and 40 women with recurrent disease. Evaluation of proteins that showed significant differences in expression between controls and cancer patients by ELISA assays yielded the four analytes. These four proteins then were evaluated in a blind cross-validation study by using an additional 106 healthy females and 100 patients with EOC (24 stage I/II and 76 stage III/IV). Upon sample decoding, the results were analyzed by using three different classification algorithms and a binary code methodology. The four-analyte test was further validated in a blind binary code study by using 40 additional serum samples from normal and EOC cancer patients. No single protein could completely distinguish the cancer group from the healthy controls. However, the combination of the four analytes exhibited the following: sensitivity 95%, positive predictive value (PPV) 95%, specificity 95%, and negative predictive value (NPV) 94%, a considerable improvement on current methodology.

▶ This study reports on a serum-based blood test looking simultaneously at quantization of 4 proteins (leptin, prolactin, osteopontin, and insulinlike growth factor II), that can discriminate between patients with EOC and those who are disease free. The investigators used microarray analysis to determine the expression levels of 169 proteins in serum samples from untreated EOC patients and healthy age-matched control subjects. In the initial screen, 35 proteins were differentially expressed and differentiated by independent ELISA assays yielding the 4 proteins of interest.

These 4 proteins of interest were subsequently evaluated in a blind cross-validation study by using an additional 106 healthy women and 100 patients with EOC (25 stage I/II and 276 stage III/IV). The 4 proteins were further validated in a blind binary code study by using 40 additional serum samples from normal and EOC patients. The investigator found that no single protein could completely distinguish the cancer group from the healthy group, but the combination of the 4 proteins exhibited a sensitivity of 95% with a specificity of 95% and a PPV of 95% and an NPV of 94%.

There are many studies currently evaluating a number of serum biomarkers for early detection of EOC. There are also a number of serum-based assays that have become very popular recently, such as the analysis of serum samples by mass spectrometry. This approach analyzes the serum of patients to find a specific pattern of proteins or protein fragments that could be used in early detection of ovarian cancer. Analysis by mass spectrometry has come under severe criticism because the function and identity of the proteins are not known and, more importantly, reanalysis of the same patient serum samples in other laboratories has not yielded a reproducible and consistent result.

In this study, 4 proteins with known functions were identified from patient serum samples as potential markers of early disease. Because ovarian cancer is a rare disease in the general population, a screening test would require a specificity of 99.6% in the general population of postmenopausal women to yield a PPV of at least 10% while maintaining a sensitivity of at least 80% in every disease subtype. The investigators, in this select population of patients, identified a sensitivity and specificity of 95%, yielding a PPV and NPV of 95% and 94%, respectively. This is very encouraging and the investigators should be commended for their work. However, it should be noted that detection of EOC in its early stages has not yet been shown to change overall mortality rates. Furthermore, the molecular biology of ovarian cancer is not well known, and currently there is a paucity of data showing that early disease is a precursor of advanced disease. However, this is an important study that may provide further insight into the molecular biology of EOC as well as provide further data on the potential for an early-detection, serum-based assay.

J. A. Hurteau, MD

Proteomic Analysis of a Preneoplastic Phenotype in Ovarian Surface Epithelial Cells Derived From Prophylactic Oophorectomies
He Q-Y, Zhou Y, Wong E, et al (Univ of Hong Kong; Univ of British Columbia, Vancouver, Canada)
Gynecol Oncol 98:68-76, 2005   39–4

Objective.—To study the pattern of protein expression associated with a predisposition to develop ovarian cancer.

Methods.—Prophylactic oophorectomy is used to prevent ovarian carcinoma in high-risk populations who have a strong family history of breast/ovarian cancer. In ovarian specimens of these women, the ovarian surface epithelium (OSE), which is tissue of origin of epithelial ovarian cancer, often shows altered morphology, growth patterns and differentiation features that are believed to be preneoplastic. This study has used a proteomic approach, based on two-dimensional gel electrophoresis and mass spectrometry, to compare the protein profiles of OSE from women with a history of familial ovarian cancer (FH-OSE), i.e., at least two first-degree relatives with such cancer and/or testing positive for *BRCA1* mutations, to those without such history (NFH-OSE).

Results.—Of >1500 protein spots, there were 8 proteins whose levels were significantly altered in FH-OSE. Three were known ovarian tumor associated proteins, others were novel changes. A number of the alterations seen were accompanied with protein modifications and have not been previously reported. There was a predominance of sequences related to the stress response pathway. Differential expression of selected genes was confirmed by Western blotting and real-time reverse transcription polymerase chain reaction.

Conclusions.—Our findings define the OSE phenotype of women at a high risk of developing ovarian cancer. Protein alterations seen in these tissues may represent an early, irreversible, non-mutational step in ovarian epithelial neoplastic progression and may be potential early and sensitive markers for the evaluation of cancer risk.

▶ The objective of this study was to investigate a pattern of protein expression in patients at high risk of developing of ovarian cancer based on family history or BRCA mutational analysis. The investigators harvested the OSE, which is the tissue of origin of epithelial ovarian cancer, from women with FH-OSE and compared this tissue with that of women with NFH-OSE. The cells were grown and harvested to study the protein pattern based on 2-dimensional gel electrophoresis and mass spectrometry. The investigators found 8 proteins whose levels were significantly altered when comparing both groups. Three of these proteins were known ovarian tumor–associated proteins, while the other 5 were novel proteins. The differential expression of these genes was confirmed by Western blotting and real-time reversed transcription polymerase chain reaction. The investigators conclude that the protein alteration seen in this tissue may represent early irreversible nonmutational steps in ovarian epithelial neoplastic progression and may be potential early markers for the evaluation of ovarian cancer risk.

This is a novel and very interesting study that sheds light on our understanding of the early events and etiology of epithelial ovarian cancer. The only downside to the study was that to obtain sufficient quantities of OSE cells, the cells needed to be immortalized by transfection with the SV40 early genes. This immortalization extended the lifespan of the OSE cells in culture as they remained nontumorigenic. It is certainly possible that immortalization stimulated the expression of genes and thereby their resulting proteins that may or may not be involved in the early genesis of ovarian cancer. Nonetheless, the fact that at least 3 of the proteins identified are known ovarian tumor–associated antigens is encouraging. It should, however, be noted that the altered proteins in this study are not specific for epithelial ovarian cancer and have also been observed in other tumor types.

It is interesting that the proteins that were identified seem to be involved in protein synthesis of early response genes. Furthermore, some of the proteins identified also have antiapoptotic functions that may lead to cancer progression and drug resistance.

Overall, this study is novel and begins to unravel potential early events in ovarian carcinogenesis. Further molecular studies comparing ovarian surface epithelium from normal and high-risk individuals as well as patients with early and advance ovarian cancer will help improve our molecular understanding of this disease process.

J. A. Hurteau, MD

Prevalence of *BRCA1* and *BRCA2* Mutations in Women Diagnosed With Ductal Carcinoma in Situ

Claus EB, Petruzella S, Matloff E, et al (Yale Univ, New Haven, Conn; Brigham and Women's Hosp, Boston)
JAMA 293:964-969, 2005

39–5

Context.—The distribution of *BRCA1* and *BRCA2* mutations in women diagnosed with noninvasive breast carcinoma is unknown.

Objective.—To estimate the *BRCA1* and *BRCA2* mutation prevalence in women with ductal carcinoma in situ (DCIS), unselected for age, family history, or ethnicity.

Design, Setting, and Participants.—The data were 369 DCIS cases diagnosed among female residents aged 20 to 79 years from the state of Connecticut between September 15, 1994, and March 14, 1998. These women were participants in a large population-based case-control study of breast carcinoma in situ. Telephone interviews were used to collect risk factor information and blood or buccal specimens were collected for *BRCA1* and *BRCA2* mutation testing.

Main Outcome Measures.—Prevalence of disease-associated mutations of *BRCA1* and BRCA2 in women diagnosed with DCIS.

Results.—Three (0.8%) and 9 (2.4%) of 369 DCIS cases had disease-associated mutations in *BRCA1* or *BRCA2*, respectively. One woman had a mutation in both genes (*BRCA1* W321X and *BRCA2* 3398del5). Carriers were significantly more likely than noncarriers to report a first-degree (mother, sister, or daughter) family history of breast cancer (odds ratio [OR], 3.7; 95% confidence interval [CI], 1.1-12.4), as well as a personal history of ovarian cancer. In addition, carriers were more likely than noncarriers to be diagnosed at an early age (<50 years) (OR, 3.4; 95% CI, 1.0-11.7), as well as to report at least 1 first-degree relative diagnosed with breast cancer before 50 years (OR, 10.6; 95% CI, 3.0-37.0).

Conclusions.—Ductal carcinoma in situ is a part of the breast/ovarian cancer syndromes defined by *BRCA1* and *BRCA2*, with mutation rates similar to those found for invasive breast cancer. These findings suggest that patients with breast cancer with an appropriate personal or family history of breast and/or ovarian cancer should be screened and followed according to high-risk protocols, regardless of whether they are diagnosed with in situ or invasive breast cancer.

▶ The association of BRCA mutations with the development of breast and ovarian cancer is a well-excepted risk factor and is considered an appropriate assessment in women who are at high risk of developing breast and ovarian cancer because of personal or family history. However, controversy exists involving the roles of DCIS with respect to inherited breast and ovarian cancer syndromes associated with BRCA mutations. To this end, the authors sought to determine the contribution of BRCA mutations in early-stage breast cancer by using a population-based, case-controlled study of women diagnosed with DCIS. They found that BRCA mutation rates amongst women with DCIS were similar to those found with frankly invasive breast cancer. Accordingly, women with breast cancer with an appropriate personal or family history of breast or ovarian cancer should be screened according to high-risk protocols regardless of whether their breast cancer is diagnosed as in situ or invasive. The importance of this study is that DCIS should now be considered to be on an equal footing with regard to risk assessment to invasive breast carcinomas.

L. P. Shulman, MD

Intra-abdominal Carcinomatosis After Prophylactic Oophorectomy in Women of Hereditary Breast Ovarian Cancer Syndrome Kindreds Associated With BRCA1 and BRCA2 Mutations
Casey MJ, Synder C, Bewtra C, et al (Creighton Univ, Omaha, Neb; Ctr for Research in Women's Health, Toronto)
Gynecol Oncol 97:457-467, 2005   39–6

Objective.—Prophylactic surgical removal of the ovaries has been offered for many years as a potential preventative of ovarian cancer in women deemed to be at increased hereditary risk for this disease. Now, it is possible to test for specific mutations of the *BRCA1* and BRCA2 genes that render members of hereditary breast ovarian cancer (HBOC) syndrome families susceptible to cancer. Widespread intra-abdominal carcinomatosis, which mimics metastatic ovarian serous carcinoma, has been reported following oophorectomy in individuals at increased hereditary risk. This study was undertaken to examine and report particularly the occurrence of intra-abdominal carcinomatosis, as well as other cancers, following prophylactic oophorectomy in patients who carry cancer susceptibility mutations of *BRCA1* and *BRCA2* and to assess the cumulative risks for this disease in order to assist in developing appropriate surgical interventions, based on currently available information, and to counsel patients who choose prophylactic surgery, concerning the potential prognosis, thereafter.

Methods.—The Creighton University Hereditary Cancer Institute registry was searched for members of HBOC syndrome families who had undergone prophylactic oophorectomy. The histories and results of DNA testing for the *BRCA1* and *BRCA2* mutations carried in their families were recorded, tabulated and examined, and the aggregate data are reported along with pertinent details of those individuals who developed neoplastic diseases after prophylactic oophorectomy. All available histologic and cytologic materials of patients who were diagnosed with intra-abdominal carcinomatosis were reviewed, and life-table calculations were performed to assess cumulative risks for this disease following prophylactic oophorectomy.

Results.—From 72 HBOC syndrome families that carried either *BRCA1* or *BRCA2* cancer-associated mutations, 238 individuals who had undergone prophylactic oophorectomy were recorded in our registry between January 1985 and December 2002. During a mean follow-up of 9.3 years, cancers were diagnosed in 27 subjects, including 16 individuals with breast cancer and five patients with intra-abdominal carcinomatosis. Breast cancers were stage I in 10 of 12 proven carriers of cancer-associated mutations. All five cases of intra-abdominal carcinomatosis were serous carcinomas, and all occurred in *BRCA1* mutation carriers. Histologic review of the prophylactically removed ovaries found borderline lesions in two cases, one with possible early stromal invasion. Two of the five patients who developed intra-abdominal carcinomatosis were among 78 patients in this series who were diagnosed and treated for breast cancer before prophylactic oophorectomy. A 3.5% cumulative risk for all mutation carriers and a 3.9% cumulative risk for *BRCA1* mutation carriers were calculated through 20 years of follow-up after prophylactic oophorectomy.

Conclusions.—Intra-abdominal carcinomatosis in our series was diagnosed only in *BRCA1* mutation carriers. The calculated cumulative risks of developing intra-abdominal carcinomatosis after prophylactic oophorectomy in members of HBOC syndrome families, specifically those who carry deleterious mutations, are well below the estimated risks of ovarian cancer published in the literature for similar patients. Breast cancers, which tended to be small and localized, were the most common malignancy in *BRCA1* and *BRCA2* mutation carriers after prophylactic oophorectomy.

► Prophylactic removal of the ovaries and fallopian tubes is a very effective method for the prevention of ovarian cancer in women at increased risk. Published reports, however, have demonstrated that a small proportion of women undergoing surgical prophylaxis will subsequently develop a primary peritoneal cancer.

The study by Casey et al is one of the largest published to date detailing the subsequent outcome for women at increased risk for cancer who have undergone a prophylactic operation. Long-term follow-up in this study was more than 9 years, which is excellent. The authors have shown an approximate 3.5% cumulative risk for the development of subsequent primary peritoneal cancer in *BRCA* mutation carriers who undergo prophylactic removal of the ovaries and fallopian tubes. Strengths of the study include its large size, the presence of accurate data regarding mutation status in study subjects, and the excellent long-term follow-up.

G. Rodriguez, MD

Altered Expression and Loss of Heterozygosity of the *LOT1* Gene in Ovarian Cancer

Cvetkovic D, Pisarcik D, Lee C, et al (Fox Chase Cancer Ctr, Philadelphia)
Gynecol Oncol 95:449-455, 2004   39–7

Objectives.—Previously, we demonstrated that the *LOT1* (*PLAGL1/ZAC1*) gene encodes a zinc-finger transcription factor and has growth suppressive effects in carcinoma cell lines. The gene is localized on chromosome 6q24-25, a common site for loss of heterozygosity (LOH) in many solid tumors including ovarian cancer. In this study, we evaluated the *LOT1* gene expression and allelic deletion in the tumor tissues in order to provide additional evidence to support the gene's potential role in cancer.

Methods.—The *LOT1* gene expression was analyzed in malignant ovarian epithelium obtained from frozen human ovarian tumor tissues using laser capture microdissection (LCM) and real-time PCR techniques. Highly frequent single nucleotide polymorphic (SNP) sites within the *LOT1* gene were identified and used for PCR and direct sequencing to determine the occurrence of allelic imbalance in a series of surgically resected ovarian and breast carcinomas.

Results.—The analysis revealed that *LOT1* mRNA expression was not detectable in 12 of 31 (39%) cases of ovarian cancer and was variable between the remaining 19 tumor specimens. These findings are consistent with the previous data that showed altered expression of *LOT1* in different human ovarian carcinoma cell lines. In addition, we analyzed the occurrence of *LOT1* allelic deletion in different ovarian tumor genomic DNA samples that included papillary serous (majority), mucinous, and primary peritoneal adenocarcinomas of low- to high-grade and the corresponding normal lymphocytes. The informative samples showed 12 out of 33 or about 36.4% LOH of this gene based on allelic loss of one or more polymorphic sites within the *LOT1* genomic sequences. Similarly, primary breast carcinomas, which included invasive ductal (majority), spindle cell, mucinous, giant cell, and atypical medullary carcinomas, were examined on genomic DNA from patients for the allelic loss of *LOT1*. The informative cases showed 4 out of 10 samples or 40% LOH of this candidate tumor suppressor gene locus in breast cancer.

Conclusions.—The altered expression and LOH of the *LOT1* locus support the gene's potential role, at least in part, in the pathogenesis of ovarian cancer and possibly in other types of cancer.

▶ The association of *BRCA* mutations with the development of ovarian cancer is well known. However, most women with ovarian cancer do not carry *BRCA* mutations, making the likelihood high that other genes will have an impact on the risk of developing ovarian cancer. In this study, altered or absent expression of the *LOT1* gene occurred in all tumor specimens evaluated. Further studies of this and other genes are ongoing to identify those genes that are associated with ovarian and other organic cancer development.

L. P. Shulman, MD

Lower Cancer Incidence in Amsterdam-I Criteria Families Without Mismatch Repair Deficiency: Familial Colorectal Cancer Type X
Lindor NM, Rabe K, Petersen GM, et al (Mayo Clinic, Rochester, Minn; Univ of Southern California, Los Angeles; Cleveland Clinic, Ohio; et al)
JAMA 293:1979-1985, 2005   39–8

Context.—Approximately 60% of families that meet the Amsterdam-I criteria (AC-I) for hereditary nonpolyposis colorectal cancer (HNPCC) have a hereditary abnormality in a DNA mismatch repair (MMR) gene. Cancer incidence in AC-I families with MMR gene mutations is reported to be very high, but cancer incidence for individuals in AC-I families with no evidence of an MMR defect is unknown.

Objective.—To determine if cancer risks in AC-I families with no apparent deficiency in DNA MMR are different from cancer risks in AC-I families with DNA MMR abnormalities.

Design, Setting, and Participants.—Identification (1997-2001) of 161 AC-I pedigrees from multiple population- and clinic-based sources in North America and Germany, with families grouped into those with (group A) or without (group B) MMR deficiency by tumor testing. A total of 3422 relatives were included in the analyses.

Main Outcome Measures.—Cancer incidence in groups A and B (excluding the 3 affected members used to define each pedigree as AC-I) and computed age- and sex-adjusted standardized incidence ratios (SIRs) using Surveillance, Epidemiology, and End Results data.

Results.—Group A families from both population- and clinic-based series showed increased incidence of the HNPCC-related cancers. Group B families showed increased incidence only for colorectal cancer (SIR, 2.3; 95% confidence interval, 1.7-3.0) and to a lesser extent than group A (SIR, 6.1; 95% confidence interval, 5.2-7.2) ($P<.001$).

Conclusions.—Families who fulfill AC-I criteria but who have no evidence of a DNA MMR defect do not share the same cancer incidence as families with HNPCC-Lynch syndrome (ie, hereditary MMR deficiency). Relatives in such families have a lower incidence of colorectal cancer than those in families with HNPCC-Lynch syndrome, and incidence may not be increased for other cancers. These families should not be described or counseled as having HNPCC-Lynch syndrome. To facilitate distinguishing these entities, the designation of "familial colorectal cancer type X" is suggested to describe this type of familial aggregation of colorectal cancer.

Genetic Derangements in the Tumor Suppressor Gene PTEN in Endometrial Precancers as Prognostic Markers for Cancer Development: A Population-Based Study From Northern Norway With Long-Term Follow-up

Ørbo A, Kaino T, Arnes M, et al (Univ of Tromsø, Norway; Univ Hosp of Tromsø, Norway)

Gynecol Oncol 95:82-88, 2004   39–9

Objectives.—The purpose of the current study was to characterize the role of PTEN in malignant transformation and to evaluate the significance of mutated PTEN exons as prognostic markers in the carcinogenesis of endometrial hyperplasia. A comparison of PTEN mutations as prognostic markers with former investigated prognosticators was also intended.

Methods.—Histological material from 68 patients with endometrial hyperplasia and 10–20 years of follow-up of whom 18 later developed cancer was examined (Table 4). PCR amplification and DNA sequencing were performed, screening the most frequently mutated exons 5a-8b of the PTEN gene.

Results.—Mutations were demonstrated in 13.2% of the patients. Of the patients with cancer development, five showed to have PTEN mutations corresponding to 28%. Of the patients remaining without carcinoma, only 8% had PTEN mutations ($P = 0.04$). In total, there were three missense, three nonsense, and four frameshift mutations, and twice as many mutations leading to a truncated protein (six) than mutations altering one amino acid in the entire protein (three). Mutations were distributed in the following manner: three in exon 5a, two in exon 5b, two in exon 6, two in exon 7, and one in exon 8b. Only mutations in exons 6, 7, and 8a were connected with cancer development or coexisting cancer and six out of seven mutations within these exons were frameshift or nonsense mutations.

Conclusions.—Our results showed that mutations in the PTEN gene were statistically more frequent in cases with cancer development or coexisting

TABLE 4.—A Material of 68 Patients Was Investigated

Marker/Variable	Sensitivity	Specificity	Positive Predictive Value	Negative Predictive Value
PTEN	56	92	71	85
HMLH1	56	98	90	86
D-score < 0, > 1	100	78	100	58
PTEN mutation	27	91	56	68

A total of 18 patients developed cancer and 50 remained healthy. The morphometrical D-score, the immunomarkers for PTEN and hMLH1, and PTEN mutations are considered as tumor markers for cancer development. The sensitivity, specificity, and positive and negative predictive values are evaluated. The threshold and the D-score results correspond to the results published in former studies.

(Courtesy of Ørbo A, Kaino T, Arnes M, et al: Genetic derangements in the tumor suppressor gene PTEN in endometrial precancers as prognostic markers for cancer development: A population-based study from northern Norway with long-term follow-up. *Gynecol Oncol* 95:82-88. Copyright 2004 by Elsevier Science Inc.)

cancer. Although the specificity was acceptable, the sensitivity of PTEN mutations was too low to make it suitable as a tumor marker (sensitivity of 27% and specificity of 91%) in clinical practice.

▶ With regard to the application of genetics analyses for the delineation of risk for developing cancers, most clinicians are well aware of the association of *BRCA* mutation with the development of breast and ovarian malignancies. However, endometrial carcinoma is the most frequent gynecologic cancer in the Western world, with an incidence that continues to increase. Accordingly, clinicians should be aware that endometrial cancer is in itself associated with specific gene mutations. These 2 articles highlight 2 specific genes that, when mutated, are associated with increased rates of endometrial cancer. The article by Lindor et al reviews the risk of cancer development in families with HNPCC syndrome, an autosomal-dominant disorder characterized by a significantly increased risk for colon cancer as well as cancers of the endometrium, stomach, small intestine, kidney, and ovary. HNPCC is the result of a mutation on an MMR gene. Those individuals with MMR gene mutations have a very high risk for developing HNPCC-associated malignancies. However, certain families and individuals meet the criteria for HNPCC and yet are found to not carry detectable mutations. The goal of this study was to determine the risk of cancer development in such people and families. The authors found that those families that fulfill a criteria (Amsterdam-I criteria) for HNPCC but do have detectable mutations have a significantly lower incidence of cancers than those with MMR mutations. Accordingly, the author suggest that such families should not be described or counseled as having HNPCC (or Lynch) syndrome, but rather should be counseled concerning their risk based on another familial aggregation of colorectal and associated cancers. The second study by Ørbo et al seeks to assess the current role of the PTEN gene (localized on chromosome 10) in the risk assessment for the development of endometrial hyperplasia and carcinoma. The authors sought to characterize the role of PTEN by comparing various mutations of the PTEN gene with other gene markers in a cohort of women with endometrial hyperplasia with 10 to 20 years of follow-up, of whom 18 subsequently developed endometrial cancer. The authors found that although PTEN mutations were more frequent in cases with cancer development or coexisting cancer, the sensitivity of the PTEN mutation frequency was too low to make a suitable tumor marker for a clinical practice in this Norwegian study. Both of these studies highlight the increasing understanding of the role of germ line gene mutations and environmental factors in the development of malignancies in individuals and families.

L. P. Shulman, MD

40 Vulva and Vagina

Long-Term Survival and Disease Recurrence in Patients With Primary Squamous Cell Carcinoma of the Vulva
Bosquet JG, Magrina JF, Gaffey TA, et al (Mayo Clinic, Rochester, Minn; Mayo Clinic, Scottsdale, Ariz)
Gynecol Oncol 97:828-833, 2005   40–1

Objectives.—To assess time to failure and sites of failure with extended follow-up of patients with squamous cell carcinoma (SCC) of the vulva.

Methods.—A retrospective analysis of 330 patients with primary SCC of the vulva treated at Mayo Clinic between 1955 and 1990 was conducted. The main outcome measures were the rates of treatment failure. The Kaplan-Meier method and the log-rank test were used to estimate the rates of overall survival, disease-free survival, and recurrence. The Cox proportional hazards model was used to assess independent variables as prognostic factors for treatment failure.

Results.—All 330 patients in the cohort underwent lymphadenectomy; 113 patients (34.2%) had involvement of the inguinofemoral nodes and 88 patients (26.7%) had treatment failure. Treatment failures occurred more frequently in patients who presented with inguinal metastasis at the primary surgery and during the first 2 years of follow-up. After 2 years, both groups, with or without positive inguinal nodes, had similar treatment failure rates. Most patients with disease recurrence in the groin died within the first 2 years of follow-up. Involvement of the inguinal nodes was the main independent predictive factor for survival, disease recurrence, and metastasis.

Conclusions.—Most treatment failures occurred during the 2 years after initial surgical management. However, in 35% of patients, disease reoccurred 5 years or more after diagnosis, which demonstrates the need for long-term follow-up. Complete ipsilateral or bilateral inguinofemoral lymph node dissection ensures a thorough evaluation and treatment of the groin.

► The article reviews a retrospective study of 330 patients with squamous cell carcinoma of the vulva at the Mayo Clinic between 1955 and 1990. The objective of the study was to assess the time to failure and determine the sites of failure in these patients. The secondary objectives included long-term recurrences, survival rates, and prognostic factors for treatment failure. All patients underwent an inguinal lymphadenectomy (214 bilateral and 16 ipsilateral). The variables that correlated with outcome included comorbid condition, previous vulvar treatment, previous malignancy, type of surgery, adjuvant therapy, pathologic characteristics, and location and type of relapse. The Kaplan-Meier method was then used to estimate the rate of overall survival, disease-free survival, and recurrence. The Cox model was then used to adjust between other covariates and the events of interest. There was follow-up information available for all patients. The most life-threatening events occurred during the initial 2-year surveillance period. Also, longer follow-up is needed because 9.4% recurred more than 5 years from diagnosis. Lastly, they concluded that complete inguinofemoral dissection should be the gold standard in diagnosing nodal metastases.

Y. Collins, MD

---

p16[INK4a] and p21[Waf1/Cip1] Expression Correlates With Clinical Outcome in Vulvar Carcinomas

Knopp S, Bjørge T, Nesland JM, et al (Univ of Oslo, Norway)
Gynecol Oncol 95:37-45, 2004   40–2

Objective.—Aberrant expression of the cell cycle kinase inhibitors p16, p21, and p27 has been associated with poor prognosis in a variety of human malignancies. Little is known, however, about their clinical impact in vulvar carcinoma patients. Thus, we analyzed a larger series of vulvar squamous cell carcinomas and compared the results with clinical outcome.

Methods.—A total of 224 vulvar squamous cell carcinomas were immunohistochemically investigated for expression of p16, p21, and p27 using the biotin-streptavidin-peroxidase method and the OptiMax Plus automated cell staining system.

Results.—High p16 ($\geq 5\%$) positive nuclear immunostaining was found in 69 (31%) cases, high p21 (any staining) protein levels was detected in 95 (42%) cases, and low p27 ($\leq 50\%$ positive nuclei) staining was seen in 170 (76%) cases. High expression of p16 was related to lower patient age and low expression of p53. High expression of p16 indicated a better prognosis in the multivariate analysis (RR = 0.5, 95% CI = 0.2–1.0) and less risk of developing lymph node metastasis (OR = 0.3, 95% CI = 0.2–0.7). High level of p21 was significantly associated with shorter survival in patients staged FIGO I and II (RR = 3.4, 95% CI = 1.3–9.3). We found no significant correlation between the expression of p27 and any of the clinicopathological variables.

Conclusions.—Our study indicates a prognostic relevance for p16 and p21 immunoreactivity. Low level of p16 protein and high level of p21 protein were associated with a shorter disease-related survival. We did not find p27 protein expression to be useful as a prognostic indicator in vulvar carcinoma patients.

▶ Many human cancers have been linked to aberrant expression of genes. Cell cycle kinase inhibitors p16, p21, and p27 have been associated with a poorer prognosis in multiple human cancers. However, when related to vulvar carcinomas, the correlation isn't known. This article is an attempt to correlate these markers with clinical outcome. There were 224 vulvar squamous carcinomas diagnosed between 1977 and 1991 reviewed immunohistochemically for the expression of p16, p21, and p27. The Pearson χ^2 test was used to compare the distribution of patient characteristics by expression. The Kaplan-Meier test was then used to calculate survival rates. There was positive immunostaining for 31% with p16 and 42% with p21. p16 correlated with patient age and p53 with expression. The study found no statistically significant correlation with p27 and any clinical variables; p27 correlated only with p53. The loss of p27 expression may occur very early in the tumorigenesis process. The inconsistencies found in this study related to p16, p21, and p27 may be related to human papilloma virus involvement. The conclusions drawn from this study are that there may be some correlation with p16 and p21. Low levels of p16 and high levels of p21 were associated with shorter disease-related survival.

Y. Collins, MD

Radioguided Sentinel Lymph Node Detection in Vulvar Cancer
Merisio C, Berretta R, Gualdi M, et al (Univ of Parma, Italy; IRCCS Fondazione Salvatore Maugeri, Pavia, Italy; Policlinico San Matteo Hosp, Pavia, Italy)
Int J Gynecol Cancer 15:493-497, 2005   40–3

Abstract.—Lymph node status is the most important prognostic factor in vulvar cancer. Histologically, sentinel nodes may be representative of the status of the other regional nodes. Identification and histopathologic evaluation of sentinel nodes could then have a significant impact on clinical management and surgery. The aim of this study was to evaluate the feasibility and diagnostic accuracy of sentinel lymph node detection by preoperative lymphoscintigraphy with technetium-99 m–labeled nanocolloid, followed by radioguided intraoperative detection. Nine patients with stage T1, N0, M0, and 11 patients with stage T2, N0, M0 squamous cell carcinoma of the vulva were included in the study. Only three cases had lesions exceeding 3.5 cm in diameter. Sentinel nodes were detected in 100% of cases. A total of 30 inguinofemoral lymphadenectomies were performed, with a mean of 10 surgically removed nodes. Histological examination revealed 17 true negative sentinel nodes, 2 true positive, and 1 false negative. In our case series, sentinel lymph node detection had a 95% diagnostic accuracy, with only one false negative. Based on literature evidence, the sentinel node procedure is feasible and reliable in vulvar cancer; however, the value of sentinel node dissection in the treatment of early-stage vulvar cancer still needs to be confirmed.

▶ The single most important prognostic factor for vulvar carcinoma is lymph node involvement; however, lymphadenectomy is associated with high morbidity rates related to wound dehiscence, wound infection, and chronic lymphedema. Sentinel lymph node detection in vulvar cancer has been studied, which is confirmed in this article. This study reviewed 20 cases of vulvar carcinoma T1 to T2, clinically negative groin nodes, and no prior chemotherapy or radiotherapy. They underwent the standard radical vulvectomy with a 2-cm margin along with unilateral or bilateral inguinofemoral lymphadenectomy.

The sentinel node detection was done by lymphoscintigraphy 16 hours before surgery. The lesion was injected circumferentially and the first site detected was marked. The patient then underwent surgery where the lymphadenectomy was preceded by a radioguided sentinel node detection. The sentinel node was separated from the other nodes, and they were all sent to pathology. The nodes were studied by using immunohistochemistry and hematoxylin-eosin stains. There were 32 nodal dissections with 301 nodes removed (average, 9.4 per groin). The sentinel node was detected in all cases. Sensitivity was 80%, specificity was 100%, positive predicted value was 100%, and negative predicted value was 94%.

Only 1 patient with a medial lesion was diagnosed with bilateral sentinel nodes. The authors concluded that sentinel node detection be reserved for patients with a high operative risk. Lastly, they concluded more large multicenter trials need to be done.

Y. Collins, MD

A Prospective, Randomized Study Analyzing Sartorius Transposition Following Inguinal–Femoral Lymphadenectomy

Judson PL, Jonson AL, Paley PJ, et al (Univ of Minnesota, Minneapolis; Pacific Gynecologic Specialists, Seattle; Bellevue Surgical Associates PC, St Louis)
Gynecol Oncol 95:226-230, 2004   40–4

Objectives.—Based on the reduced morbidity seen in our retrospective study, we undertook a prospective, randomized trial to determine whether transposition of the sartorius muscle improves post-operative morbidity in women with squamous cell carcinoma of the vulva undergoing inguinal-femoral lymphadenectomy.

Methods.—Patients with squamous carcinoma of the vulva requiring inguinal-femoral lymphadenectomy were randomized to undergo sartorius transposition or not. All patients received perioperative antibiotics, DVT prophylaxis, and closed suction surgical site drainage. Outcomes assessed include wound cellulitis, wound breakdown, lymphocyst formation, lymphedema, and/or rehospitalization. Cohorts were compared using Fisher's exact test. Baseline characteristics were compared using Student's t test or Fischer's exact test as appropriate. Logistic regression was used to assess the impact of sartorius transposition, after adjusting for other factors.

Results.—From June 1996 to December 2002, 61 patients underwent 99 inguinal–femoral lymphadenectomies, 28 with sartorius transposition, and 33 without. The mean (SD) age for controls and patients undergoing sartorius transposition was 63.5 (15.2) and 73.8 (13.7) years, respectively ($P <$ 0.05). There were no statistically significant differences in BSA, tobacco use, co-morbid medical conditions, past surgical history, medication use, size of incision, duration of surgery, number of positive lymph nodes, pathologic stage, pathologic grade, pre- or postoperative hemoglobin, or length of hospitalization. There were no statistically significant differences in the incidence of wound cellulitis, wound breakdown, lymphedema, or rehospitalization. The incidence of lymphocyst formation was increased in the sartorius transposition group. After adjusting for age, however, the groups appeared similar.

Conclusions.—Sartorius transposition after inguinal–femoral lymphadenectomy does not reduce postoperative wound morbidity.

▶ This article is a prospective randomized trial of patients with invasive squamous cell carcinoma who required either a unilateral or bilateral inguinofemoral lymphadenectomy at the University of Minnesota Hospital. They were randomized to either undergo sartorius transposition or not. All patients received preoperative antibiotics, DVT prophylaxis, and drain placement. All the baseline patient characteristics were compared by using Fisher's exact test along with logistic regression to assess the impact of transposition on complication rates. There were a total of 64 patients randomized between June 1996 and December 2002; the 2 groups were very comparable in patient characteristics, comorbid conditions, and medications. There were no differences in wound cellulitis, wound breakdown, or lymphocysts with sartorius transposition.

Y. Collins, MD

Flap Algorithm in Vulvar Reconstruction After Radical, Extensive Vulvectomy
Salgarello M, Farallo E, Barone-Adesi L, et al (Catholic Univ of the Sacred Heart, Rome; Catholic Univ of the Sacred Heart, Campobasso, Italy)
Ann Plast Surg 54:184-190, 2005   40–5

Abstract.—The objective of this study was to assess the reconstructive options after radical, extensive vulvectomy; relate them to tumor characteristics; and select a choice of flaps able to correct every remaining defect. This study is a retrospective review of a 4-year experience with 31 flaps in 20 consecutive vulvar reconstructions. Three of the 31 flaps presented nonsignificant delayed healing at their tips and 3 other flaps developed a major breakdown related to an infection or an error in flap planning. According to the authors, the size of the defect is the main issue that must be taken into consideration during the establishment of reconstructive needs. Closure of vulvar defects is preferably performed using fasciocutaneous flaps, which are very reliable flaps and can be raised with different techniques to meet different needs. A flap is then chosen with the fewest potential complications. An algorithm has been thus established: Small to medium-size defects are closed with island V-Y flaps, island gluteal fold flaps, or pedicled pudendal thigh flaps. Among them, the island V-Y flap is the workhorse flap for vulvar reconstruction because of its versatility, reliability, and technical simplicity compared with its very low complication rate. If the vulvar defect is large and/or reaches the vulva–crural fold, V-Y flaps are also preferred to close these large and posteriorly extended excisions. If the vulvar defect is very large, extending both anteriorly and posteriorly, the use of a distally based, vertically oriented rectus abdominis muscle flap is recommended. Using this algorithm, immediate vulvar reconstruction with pedicled local or regional flaps can be performed easily and reliably.

▶ Most of the articles dealing with vulvar reconstruction after radical and ultraradical pelvic surgery are usually method based. They extol the virtues of this technique or that method and how that technique can be used to cover even the largest defects. Most clear-thinking, experienced surgeons readily admit that no one technique is applicable for all or even most situations. Similar surgical wisdom is revealed in this report, where a variety of techniques were used to cover vulvar defects. This included the more elaborate techniques such as vertical rectus abdominis musculocutaneous flaps or gluteal fasciocutaneous flaps as well as simpler advancement flaps. It is interesting to note that some of the biggest defects were covered by that simpler flap, the V-Y fasciocutaneous advancement flap.

D. S. Miller, MD

41 Cervix

Predictors of Outcomes for Women With Cervical Carcinoma
Leath CA III, Straughn JM Jr, Kirby TO, et al (Univ of Alabama, Birmingham)
Gynecol Oncol 99:432-436, 2005   41–1

Background.—To determine the impact of race and other factors on the management and outcomes of women treated for cervical cancer in a rural state.

Methods.—Following IRB approval, a retrospective review identified 434 eligible women treated for cervical cancer from 1994 to 2000. Collected data included: demographics, clinicopathologic data, primary and adjuvant therapy, recurrence, and survival. Statistical analyses were performed with the Chi-square test, Kaplan–Meier method, and Cox regression.

Results.—304 (70%) of the women were white and 130 (30%) were non-white. Non-whites were more likely to present with advanced stage disease [Stage IIB–IVB] (25% vs. 13%; $P < 0.01$). Whites were more likely to smoke, be married, be employed, and have private insurance. Non-whites were more likely to have medical co-morbidities such as diabetes and hypertension. Although whites with early stage disease were more likely to undergo surgery as their primary therapy than non-whites (93% vs. 84%; $P < 0.01$), survival was similar. Survival outcomes for advanced stage disease were similar between groups.

Conclusions.—Non-whites diagnosed with cervical cancer are more likely to present with advanced stage disease than whites; however, overall survival was similar between groups. Non-whites with early stage disease were more likely to receive primary radiation therapy than whites. The decision to use radiation therapy vs. surgery does not appear to have a detrimental effect on overall survival, but may impact quality of life.

▶ This study reinforces the concept that nonwhites are more likely to present with advanced-stage cervical carcinoma. In addition, it confirms previous observations that suggest whites are more likely to have cervical lesions related to tobacco use. Interestingly, nonwhites were more likely to be medically infirm. However, the most interesting observation is that patients are treated differently depending on race. However, stage for stage, race did not predict poorer outcomes for minority women with cervical cancer. Access to health care for women, especially those in rural or impoverished communities, remains paramount. Significant resources and continued research are needed to decrease health care disparities for women with cervical cancer.

B. J. Monk, MD

Preoperative Magnetic Resonance Imaging Staging of Uterine Cervical Carcinoma: Results of Prospective Study
Choi SH, Kim SH, Choi HJ, et al (Seoul Natl Univ, Korea)
J Comput Assist Tomogr 28:620-627, 2004   41–2

Objective.—To determine the accuracy of the preoperative staging of uterine cervical cancer by magnetic resonance (MR) imaging in 115 patients in a prospective study.

Methods.—A prospective study was performed in 115 patients who underwent MR imaging at 1.5 T before surgery or biopsy. Histopathologic findings were correlated with MR imaging results for all patients.

Results.—The accuracy of preoperative tumor staging by MR imaging in the 115 patients was 77%. In terms of the evaluation of parametrial status, this study had an accuracy of 94% and a sensitivity of 38%. The accuracy and sensitivity of MR imaging for vaginal invasion were 81% and 87%, respectively. In terms of lymph node metastasis, this study had an accuracy of 97% and a sensitivity of 36%.

Conclusion.—Magnetic resonance imaging has high accuracy in the preoperative staging of uterine cervical cancer.

▶ This study demonstrates that pretreatment MRI is accurate (specific) but relatively insensitive in detecting parametrial involvement. The sensitivity was only 38%, and it is unclear how this compares to clinical evaluation such as palpation, especially rectal examinations. In addition, MRI is insensitive in detecting lymphatic metastases, with PET being the preferred method once conventional imaging is negative. Although pretreatment MRI may help clarify questionable parametrial involvement, these patients are probably better treated with primary chemotherapy and radiation because postoperative chemotherapy and radiation are common and the use of all 3 modalities (radical surgery, chemotherapy, and radiation) has never been shown to be less toxic or more efficacious than 2 modalities (chemotherapy and radiation).

B. J. Monk, MD

A Comparison of Stages IB1 and IB2 Cervical Cancers Treated With Radical Hysterectomy. Is Size the Real Difference?

Rutledge TL, Kamelle SA, Tillmanns TD, et al (Univ of Oklahoma, Oklahoma City; Washington Univ, St Louis)
Gynecol Oncol 95:70-76, 2004   41–3

Objective.—To compare stages IB1 and IB2 cervical cancers treated with radical hysterectomy (RH) and to define predictors of nodal status and recurrence.

Methods.—Patients with stage IB cervical cancers undergoing RH between 1990 and 2000 were evaluated and clinicopathological variables were abstracted. The perioperative complication rate, estimated blood loss (EBL), and OR time were also tabulated. Variables were analyzed using χ^2 and t tests. Disease-free survival (DFS) was calculated by Kaplan–Meier method. Multivariate analysis was performed via stepwise logistic regression. Cox-proportional hazards were used to identify independent predictors of recurrence.

Results.—RH was performed on 109 stage IB1 and 86 stage IB2 patients. Mean age, EBL, and perioperative complication rates were similar. Overall, 38 patients (14 IB1 vs. 24 IB2) had positive nodes ($P = 0.01$) including 9 patients with positive para-aortic nodes (2 IB1 and 7 IB2). Parametrial involvement (PI) and outer 2/3 depth of invasion (DOI) were significantly more common in the IB2 tumors as well. Patients with IB2 disease received adjuvant radiation more frequently than IB1 patients (52% vs. 37%, $P = 0.04$). Univariate predictors of nodal status included lymphovascular space involvement (LVSI) ($P = 0.001$), DOI ($P = 0.011$), PI ($P = 0.001$), and stage ($P = 0.011$). Multivariate analysis identified only LVSI (OR 6.4, CI 2.4–17, $P = 0.0002$) and PI (OR 8, CI 3.1–20, $P = 0.0001$) as independent predictors of positive nodes. With a median follow-up of 35 months, estimates of DFS revealed tumor size ($P = 0.008$), nodal status ($P = 0.0004$), LVSI ($P = 0.002$), PI ($P = 0.004$), and DOI ($P = 0.0004$) as significant univariate predictors. Neoadjuvant chemotherapy, age, grade, histology, and adjuvant radiation were not associated with recurrence. The significant independent predictors of DFS were LVSI (ROR 5.7, CI 2–16, $P = 0.0064$) and outer 2/3 DOI (OR 5.8, CI 2–20, $P = 0.0029$). Neither tumor size nor nodal status was a significant predictor of DFS.

Conclusions.—The prognosis in stage IB cervical cancer seems to be most influenced by presence of LVSI and DOI and not by tumor size as the staging criteria would suggest. These factors are best determined pathologically after radical hysterectomy. This report contains the largest comparison of IB1 and IB2 patients managed by RH. Tumor size failed to predict recurrence or nodal status when stratified by LVSI, DOI, and PI. Treatment decisions based on tumor size alone should be reconsidered.

▶ This report provides provocative evidence that size is only a surrogate for lymphatic metastases. Lymphatic metastases is a stronger predictor of tumor recurrence than FIGO stage or size. In fact, lymphovascular space invasion and depth of invasion are important prognostic factors not incorporated in the FIGO system. A staging system similar to endometrial cancer should be considered where patients who undergo surgical management are staged differently than those evaluated clinically. Important surgical and pathologic factors not only help determine prognoses but are also important in determining if radiation or radiation and chemotherapy should be administered in the postoperative adjuvant setting.

B. J. Monk, MD

Laparoscopically Assisted Radical Vaginal Hysterectomy vs Radical Abdominal Hysterectomy for Cervical Cancer: A Match Controlled Study
Jackson KS, Das N, Naik R, et al (Queen Elizabeth Hosp, Gateshead, England)
Gynecol Oncol 95:655-661, 2004   41–4

Objectives.—The technical feasibility of laparoscopically assisted radical vaginal hysterectomy has been well described, but its advantages over the open technique remain largely unproven. We reviewed and compared our experiences with both approaches.

Methods.—All patients undergoing laparoscopically assisted radical vaginal hysterectomy (LARVH) between 1996 and 2003 were identified and matched for age, FIGO stage, histological subtype and nodal metastases using a control group of women who underwent radical abdominal hysterectomy (RAH) during the same time period.

Results.—Fifty-seven women were listed for LARVH, resulting in five conversions. Fifty cases were matched successfully using the criteria above. The majority of cases were FIGO stage 1B1. Statistically significant differences ($P < 0.05$) were present when the following were compared for LARVH vs. RAH: duration of surgery (median 180 vs. 120 min), blood loss (median 350 vs. 875 ml), hospital stay (median 5 days vs. 8 days) and duration of continuous bladder catheterisation (median 3 days vs. 7 days). There were no statistically significant differences with regard to nodal yield, completeness of surgical margins or perioperative complication rate. Four major complications (8%, three cystotomies and one enterotomy) occurred in the LARVH group and three in the RAH group (6%, one pulmonary embolism, one ureteric injury and one major haemorrhage). Three women in LARVH group had seen a specialist regarding postoperative bladder dysfunction, versus 12 in the RAH group ($P = 0.04$). No patients in the LARVH group reported constipation requiring regular laxatives, versus six in the RAH group ($P = 0.03$). Median follow-up was 52 months for LARVH and 49 months for RAH. There was no significant difference between recurrence rates or overall survival (94% for LARVH vs. 96% for RAH).

Conclusions.—Despite the inherent limitations of LARVH and its associated learning curve, the procedure conveys many advantages over the open technique in terms of blood loss, transfusion requirement and hospital stay. In addition, the incidence of postoperative bladder and bowel dysfunction appears low-suggesting improved quality of life-without compromising survival.

▶ This retrospective study suggest that laparoscopically assisted radical vaginal hysterectomy is a longer operation and is associated with less blood loss when compared with radical abdominal hysterectomy in the management of early invasive cervical cancer. In addition, laparoscopically assisted radical vaginal hysterectomy is associated with shorter hospital stay and less bladder dysfunction. Although complications were unusual in both surgical approaches, some investigators have suggested that more complications occur when laparoscopy is integrated into the surgical management of cervical carcinoma. Clearly, experience is critical in evaluating the rates complications and there are data to suggest a steep learning curve. Randomized trials comparing laparoscopically assisted radical surgery versus open radical surgery in cervical carcinoma are probably not feasible. Although, the Gynecologic Oncology Group is completing a study in endometrial cancer comparing these 2 diverse surgical approaches and the results of this trial are eagerly anticipated. Laparoscopically assisted radical vaginal hysterectomy should be considered in the management of small cervical carcinomas at centers where this procedure is frequently performed.

B. J. Monk, MD

A Fertility-Sparing Alternative to Radical Hysterectomy: How Many Patients May Be Eligible?
Sonoda Y, Abu-Rustum NR, Gemignani ML, et al (Mem Sloan-Kettering Cancer Ctr, New York)
Gynecol Oncol 95:534-538, 2004   41–5

Objective.—To determine the percentage of patients with early-stage cervical cancer who may be eligible for fertility preservation with laparoscopic radical vaginal trachelectomy (LRVT).

Methods.—We retrospectively reviewed the records of patients who underwent a radical hysterectomy for invasive cervical cancer at our institution from 12/85 to 8/01, before our use of LRVT at Memorial Sloan-Kettering Cancer Center. Institutional eligibility criteria for LRVT were applied. Patients ≥40 years of age were considered ineligible.

Results.—We identified 435 patients who had undergone radical hysterectomy for cervical cancer; 186 were age <40 at surgery and constituted our study population. Eighty-nine (48%) patients may have been eligible by our pathologic criteria. In 12 patients, LRVT may have been aborted or altered because of unexpected disease spread.

Conclusion.—A significant number of patients <40 with early-stage cervical cancer may be pathologically eligible for LRVT and should be counseled on this preoperatively.

▶ In 1987, Dargent et al[1] developed the radical trachelectomy as a fertility-retaining alternative to radical hysterectomy for cervical cancer. Currently, this procedure is performed in conjunction with a laparoscopic pelvic lymphadenectomy and is known as LRVT. Small studies have indicated comparable efficacy in early-stage disease. This study was a review of records of patients undergoing radical hysterectomy to determine what proportion theoretically could undergo LRVT. Patients aged 40 years and older were excluded based on age alone. The study concluded that up to 48% could potentially be candidates for the procedure. It is unclear what percentage of women who would be candidates for LRVT would desire the procedure, or the percentage of patients who would remain candidates based on surgical findings. Although many questions remain about the utility of LRVT, it appears that a considerable number of patients eligible for radical hysterectomy could potentially be candidates for this fertility-sparing alternative.

V. A. M. Givens, MD

Reference

1. Dargent D, Brun JL, Roy M, et al: Pregnancies following radical trachelectomy for invasive cervical cancer. *Gynecol Oncol* 52:105, 1994.

Vaginal Radical Trachelectomy: An Oncologically Safe Fertility-Preserving Surgery. An Updated Series of 72 Cases and Review of the Literature
Plante M, Renard M-C, François H, et al (Centre Hospitalier Universitaire de Québec; Laval Univ, Quebec)
Gynecol Oncol 94:614-623, 2004   41–6

Objective.—To review the oncological results and complication rate of our first consecutive 72 completed cases of vaginal radical trachelectomies (VRT).

Methods.—From October 1991 to October 2003, we have planned 82 VRT in patients with early-stage cervical cancer (stages IA, IB, and IIA). The VRT was preceded by a complete laparoscopic pelvic node dissection and laparoscopic parametrectomy.

Results.—The planned procedure was successfully completed in 72 cases and was abandoned in 10 cases (12%) because of either positive nodes discovered at the time of surgery (4), positive endocervical margins (5) or extensive tubal adhesions (1) (Table 3). The median age of the remaining 72 patients was 31 and most (75%) were nulliparous. The majority of the lesions were stage IA2 (32%) or IB1 (60%) and 54% were grade 1 (Table 1). In terms of histology, 58% were squamous and 42% were adenocarcinomas. Vascular space invasion was present in 20% of cases, and 90% of the lesions

TABLE 3.—Reasons for Abandoning the Planned Radical Trachelectomy (n = 10)

Reasons		Procedure Done Instead
Extensive tubal adhesions	1	ARH
Positive endocervical margins	5	Schauta in 4, ARH in 1
Positive pelvic nodes	4	PAN biopsies
		CT/RT in 3, RT alone in 1

ARH: abdominal radical hysterectomy; PAN: paraaortic node.
CT/RT: combination of chemotherapy and radiation therapy.
RT: radiation therapy.
(Courtesy of Plante M, Renard M-C, François H, et al: Vaginal radical trachelectomy: An oncologically safe fertility-preserving surgery. An updated series of 72 cases and review of the literature. *Gynecol Oncol* 94:614-623. Copyright 2004 by Elsevier Science.)

measured ≤2 cm. An average of 32 lymph nodes has been removed laparoscopically. The mean follow-up is 60 months (6–156). The intraoperative complication rate was low (6%) and the postoperative morbidity was also low mainly involving bladder hypotonia (16%) and vulvar edema (12%) (Table 2). There were no bladder or ureteral injuries. The average hospital stay was 3 days. Excluding one patient with a small cell neuroendocrine tumor who rapidly recurred and died, there were two recurrences (2.8%) and one death (1.4%). The actuarial recurrence-free survival is 95%. Tumor

TABLE 1.—Tumor Characteristics

	Total (*n* = 82)	VRT (*n* = 72)	No VRT (*n* = 10)
Stage			P = NS
IA1 with VSI	4 (5%)	4 (5%)	0 (0%)
IA2	24 (30%)	23 (32%)	1 (10%)
IB1	51 (61%)	43 (60%)	9 (90%)
IIA	3 (4%)	2 (3%)	1 (1%)
Grade			P=0.0009
1	40 (49%)	39 (54%)	1 (10%)
2	23 (28%)	21 (29%)	2 (20%)
3	16 (19%)	10 (14%)	6 (60%)
Unknown	3 (4%)	2 (3%)	1 (10%)
Histology			P = NS
Squamous	49 (60%)	42 (58%)	7 (70%)
Adenocarcinoma	29 (35%)	27 (38%)	2 (20%)
Adenosquamous	4 (5%)	3 (4%)	1 (10%)
Size			P = NS
2 cm	72 (90%)	64 (89%)	8 (80%)
>2 cm	10 (10%)	8 (11%)	2 (20%)
VSI			P = NS
No	65 (79%)	58 (80%)	6 (75%)
Yes	17 (21%)	14 (20%)	2 (25%)
Diagnosis			P = NS
Cone or LEEP	57 (70%)	53 (74%)	6 (60%)
Biopsy alone	25 (30%)	19 (26%)	4 (40%)

VSI: vascular space invasion.
(Courtesy of Plante M, Renard M-C, François H, et al: Vaginal radical trachelectomy: An oncologically safe fertility-preserving surgery. An updated series of 72 cases and review of the literature. *Gynecol Oncol* 94:614-623. Copyright 2004 by Elsevier Science.)

TABLE 2.—Surgical Complications

Intraoperative complications	5 (6.1%)
Vascular trauma to iliac vessels requiring laparotomy	2
Trauma to superficial epigastric artery	1
Parametrial bleeding requiring a laparotomy	1
Cystotomy	1
Postoperative complications	
Bladder hypotonia	13 (16%)
Urinary tract infection	2 (2%)
Vulvar edema	10 (12%)
Vulvar hematoma	6 (7%)
Suprapubic hematoma	3 (4%)
Lymphocele	9 (11%)
Lymphedema	3 (4%)
Lombalgia	2 (2%)
Femorocutaneous palsy	1 (1%)

(Courtesy of Plante M, Renard M-C, François H, et al: Vaginal radical trachelectomy: An oncologically safe fertility-preserving surgery. An updated series of 72 cases and review of the literature. *Gynecol Oncol* 94:614-623. Copyright 2004 by Elsevier Science.)

size >2 cm was statistically significantly associated with a higher risk of recurrence ($P = 0.03$). The recurrence-free survival of the nine patients who did not have the planned VRT because of more advanced disease was statistically significantly less ($P = 0.003$).

Conclusion.—VRT is an oncologically safe procedure in well-selected patients with early-stage disease. Lesion size >2 cm appears to be associated with a higher risk of recurrence. The morbidity of the procedure is low and it allows fertility preservation (Table 4).

▶ The results of this study indicate that radical trachelectomy is a valuable fertility-sparing alternative for young women with early-stage disease. The morbidity rate of the procedure is low. The recurrence and death rate of less than 5% is similar to data from radical hysterectomy. It would appear that lesions smaller than 2 cm are candidates for this procedure. Tumor between 2 and 3 cm and those with lymph vascular space invasion are at higher risk of

TABLE 4.—Recurrences and Deaths of Published Series

Author	N	Median Follow-up (Months)	Recurrences	Deaths	Abandoned Trachelectomies
Dargent et al. [19,20]	95	76 (4-176)	4 (4.2%)	3 (3.1%)[a]	13/108 (12%)
Covens [21,22]	93	30 (1-103)	7 (7.3%)	4 (4.2%)	0/93 (0%)
Plante and Roy	72	60 (6-156)	2 (2.8%)	1 (1.4%)[a]	10/82 (12%)
Shepherd et al. [23]	30	21 (1-64)	0	0	4/30 (13%)
Burnett et al. [24]	19	31 (22-44)	0	0	2/21 (10%)
Schlaerth et al. [25]	10	47 (28-84)	0	0	2/12 (17%)
Total	319	44 (1-176)	13 (4.1%)	8 (2.5%)	31/346 (9%)

[a]Excluding one case of small cell neuroendocrine tumor.

(Courtesy of Plante M, Renard M-C, François H, et al: Vaginal radical trachelectomy: An oncologically safe fertility-preserving surgery. An updated series of 72 cases and review of the literature. *Gynecol Oncol* 94:614-623. Copyright 2004 by Elsevier Science.)

occurrence. Lesions larger than 3 cm are probably not candidates for this fertility-sparing procedure. Although randomized trials in this setting are not feasible, this operation may be considered in treating small cervical lesions when future fertility is desired.

B. J. Monk, MD

The Role of Radical Parametrectomy in the Treatment of Occult Cervical Carcinoma After Extrafascial Hysterectomy
Leath CA III, Straughn JM Jr, Bhoola SM, et al (Univ of Alabama, Birmingham)
Gynecol Oncol 92:215-219, 2004   41–7

Objectives.—To assess the morbidity and efficacy of radical parametrectomy (RP) performed following extrafascial hysterectomy in patients with occult cervical carcinoma.

Methods.—An IRB approved retrospective chart review identified 23 patients that underwent RP with pelvic and/or para-aortic lymphadenectomy and upper vaginectomy. Data were collected on demographics, tumor stage, grade, histology, indication for hysterectomy, surgical findings, complications, recurrence, and survival.

Results.—Of the 23 patients, 2 patients had a stage IA_2 lesion while 21 patients had a stage IB_1 lesion. There were 5 patients with a grade 1 tumor, 10 with grade 2, 4 with grade 3, and 4 with unknown grade. Median age was 41 years (range 27–59). The most common indication (48%) for extrafascial hysterectomy was CIS of the cervix. Four patients (17%) had metastasis to pelvic nodes or evidence of tumor at the margin at the time of RP. Three of these 4 patients with a positive specimen received adjuvant radiation and all are alive (mean follow-up 66 months). One patient declined radiation and is alive at 42 months. There were 7 (30%) operative complications: Most notably 4 patients received blood transfusions. Two of 19 patients (11%) with no residual tumor in RP specimen recurred and 1 patient was salvaged with radiation (follow-up 103 months). With a median follow-up of 61 months (range 9–103), overall 5-year survival is 96%.

Conclusions.—RP is an acceptable option for patients diagnosed with an occult cervical carcinoma at the time of extrafascial hysterectomy. Careful selection of RP for patients unlikely to have residual tumor will obviate the need for radiation in most instances.

▶ This study helps define the frequency of "aborted" radical hysterectomies. This appears to occur in approximately 10% of the patients when conventional imaging studies are used preoperatively. Fortunately, these patients can be salvaged with postoperative radiation or radiation and chemotherapy. The aborted radical operation does not necessarily predict a worse prognosis, although it is clearly associated with unnecessary morbidity. However, the theoretical benefits of debulking grossly involve nodes as well as the opportunity to surgically stage the patient, with evaluation of the aortic lymph nodes possibly leading to a better prognosis among patient initially explored for a radical hysterectomy compared with those treated with chemotherapy and radiation primarily. With sophisticated imaging techniques such as MRI and PET, the incidence of aborted radical hysterectomies is expected to decline.

B. J. Monk, MD

Gene Expression Profiling of in Vitro Radiation Resistance in Cervical Carcinoma: A Feasibility Study

Tewari D, Monk BJ, Al-Ghazi MS, et al (Univ of California, Orange; Oncotech, Inc, Irvine, Calif)
Gynecol Oncol 99:84-91, 2005   41–8

Objective(s).—To determine the feasibility of integrating an in vitro chemo-radiation response assay (IVRRA) with a gene microarray system to investigate the molecular patterns of expression that contribute to radiation resistance in cervical cancer.

Methods.—Viable primary untreated cervical cancer specimens were obtained and exposed to gamma irradiation at a dose of 3 Gy in the IVRRA to determine in vitro radiation sensitivity. RNA was purified for microarray analysis with the Affymetrix Human Genome U95A Array carrying more than 12,000 gene probes. Gene expression analysis was performed, and specimen transcript patterns were correlated with radiation response using an iteration analysis model and Pearson's correlation coefficient.

Results.—A feasibility set of eight tumor specimens was studied. Tumors were classified into 4 extreme (ERR), 2 intermediate (IRR) and 2 low radiation resistance (LRR) categories. An intrinsic radiation response gene set of 54 genes transcripts with 100% accuracy for the classification of each tumor's radiation response category was identified.

Conclusion(s).—Gene sets associated with in vitro radiation response profiles in cervical cancer can be generated using the IVRRA and microarray technology. This has direct applications to the study of the biological pathways contributing to radiation resistance and may lead to the development of alternative treatment modalities. The potential of these technologies for cancers in which radiotherapy is employed warrants further investigation.

▶ Ideally, patients intrinsically resistant to irradiation therapy could be identified through the evaluation of gene expression patterns before the initiation of radiation. Such patients might be treated with alternative therapies such as radical surgery. This operation would most likely include a primary pelvic exenteration, but for selected patients with intrinsically radiation-resistant cervical cancers it might potentially be life saving.

Another approach to improving outcomes during chemoradiation is to individualize therapy by choosing the optimal radiosensitizing agent. In vitro assays such as the one described in this study might be used for this purpose. Ideally, gene expression profiles could also be found that predict which chemotherapeutic agent/radiosensitizer works best with radiation in an individual patient. This novel approach to tailoring therapy to individual patients based on tumor biology is clearly the future of oncology. Further study is needed in this area.

B. J. Monk, MD

Quality of Life Outcomes From a Randomized Phase III Trial of Cisplatin With or Without Topotecan in Advanced Carcinoma of the Cervix: A Gynecologic Oncology Group Study
Monk BJ, Huang HQ, Cella D, et al (Univ of California, Orange; Roswell Park Cancer Inst, Buffalo, NY; Northwestern Univ, Evanston, Ill; et al)
J Clin Oncol 23:4617-4625, 2005   41–9

Purpose.—To prospectively assess the impact of treatment with cisplatin alone or in combination with topotecan (CT) on quality of life (QOL) in patients with advanced or recurrent cervical cancer, and to explore the prognostic value of baseline QOL scores.

Patients and Methods.—Patients entered on Gynecologic Oncology Group (GOG) Protocol 179 were expected to complete QOL assessments at four time points using Functional Assessment of Cancer Therapy-General (FACT-G), Cervix subscale (Cx subscale), FACT/GOG-Neurotoxicity subscale (NTX subscale), Brief Pain Inventory (BPI), and UNISCALE (UNI). Adjusting for patient age, baseline scores, and effects of time, we longitudinally examined treatment effect on QOL during and after chemotherapy.

Results.—Among patients randomly allocated to receive cisplatin (n = 146) or CT (n = 147), there were no statistically significant differences in QOL up to 9 months after randomization despite more hematologic toxicity in the combination arm. QOL assessments were completed at rates of 98%, 85%, 68%, and 59%, respectively, for the four time points, with similar rates and reasons for nonparticipation between regimens. Baseline FACT-G (P = .0016) and BPI (P = 0001) scores were significantly associated with patient age; older patients had better QOL and less pain. Baseline UNI was positively correlated with FACT-G (r = 0.66; P < .001) and Cx subscale (r = 0.29; P < .001), and negatively related to BPI (r = −0.41; P < .0001). Baseline FACT-Cx (FACT-G + Cx subscale) was associated with survival.

Conclusion.—Despite increased toxicity, CT did not significantly reduce patient QOL when compared with cisplatin alone. Patient-reported QOL measures may be an important prognostic tool in advanced cervix cancer.

▶ This report quantifies the impact of QOL when topotecan is added to cisplatin in the treatment of metastatic disease on GOG 179. Importantly, the more aggressive combination did not result in a statistically significant decrease in QOL. QOL was measured using multiple sophisticated and valid questionnaires. In addition, baseline QOL as assessed by the FACT-Cx was significantly associated with overall survival. The estimated hazard of death for patients in the highest QOL quartile was 47% lower then patients in the lowest quartile (hazard ratio, 0.53; 95% confidence interval, 0.362-0.78; P = .001), 40% lower than patients in the second lowest quartile (hazard ratio, 0.60; 95%

confidence interval, 0.41-0.89; $P = .001$), 40% lower than patents in the third lowest quartile (hazard ratio, 0.60; 95% confidence interval, 0.40-0.88; $P = .001$).

This study is the first prospective evaluation of QOL to be reported by GOG in cervical cancer. It illustrates the importance of translational research end points in deciding the optimal therapy of patients with life-threatening gynecologic carcinoma.

B. J. Monk, MD

42 Uterus

Morbid Obesity and Endometrial Cancer: Surgical, Clinical, and Pathologic Outcomes in Surgically Managed Patients
Pavelka JC, Ben-Shachar I, Fowler JM, et al (Ohio State Univ, Columbus)
Gynecol Oncol 95:588-592, 2004   42–1

Background.—Surgery is a mainstay for the treatment of endometrial cancer both in removing disease and properly staging patients, a procedure that has both diagnostic and likely therapeutic benefits. One of the concerns with the treatment of women with endometrial cancer is that many are morbidly obese because of the well-recognized association of increased unopposed estrogen levels resulting from an increased body mass index (BMI). Thus, a significant concern in the treatment of women with endometrial cancer is the ability to perform proper surgery, including comprehensive staging. To examine this association, the authors examined surgical, clinical, and pathologic outcomes in women with endometrial cancer as grouped by BMI.

Methods.—A total of 356 patients with endometrial cancer who were consecutively treated served as the study population, of whom 339 were assessable and included in the final analysis. BMI was categorized into 3 groups: <30, 30 to 40, and >40.

Findings.—Definite statistically significant differences were found between the subgroups stratified by BMI. The ability to surgically stage and completely surgically stage was diminished in those patients with the greatest BMI. Positive lymph nodes were identified in 11% of the overall patient population, but this did not differ by BMI subgrouping. The majority of significant changes between groups are noted in the Table.

TABLE.

Variable	BMI <30	BMI 30-40	BMI >40
Distribution	40%	38%	22%
Underwent staging	93%	92%	81%
Staging included periaortic lymph nodes	82%	80%	59%
Grade 1 tumor	47%	51%	71%
Wound complications	4.3%	7.8%	18.7%
Mean operative time (min)	177	184	205
Estimated blood loss (mL) (staged patients)	331	576	570
Death	0.7%	1.6%	1.3%

Conclusions.—Comprehensive surgery is feasible in the majority of women with endometrial cancer, even for those with high BMIs. Those with the greatest BMI, however, do experience greater morbidity in the course of this surgical exercise.

▶ The authors present a well-written and interesting review of the experience in treating endometrial carcinoma in an academic-based gynecologic oncology service. One of the key findings was that the distribution of disease outside the uterus, such as lymph node involvement, remained similar across BMI strata. This further punctuates the need for comprehensive staging in women with the greatest BMI, despite the higher association with grade 1 tumors.

This study closely examines a number of the variables that may be expected to differ by BMI. Major morbidity and mortality did not differ for those patients who were comprehensively staged when stratified by BMI. Lymph node yield was appropriate as classified by sampling versus dissection, with a mean of 23 lymph nodes harvested for those patients who were fully staged.

One methodological concern of this study is that the authors did not control for selection bias. Some patients, even in the highest BMI subgroup, may have been more amenable to staging or were healthier at study entry versus those patients who did not undergo full staging. A second concern is the applicability of these findings to centers that perform a lower volume of endometrial cancer staging procedures. Furthermore, the number of available intraoperative assistants, such as residents and medical students, can facilitate exposure for comprehensive staging. Thus, for those centers that have fewer surgical personnel available, more difficulty may be encountered.

This article would be further strengthened by inclusion of long-term outcome data including long-term complications, progression-free and overall survival data. Despite these criticisms, this report clearly establishes the need and feasibility of attempted comprehensive staging in most patients with endometrial cancer despite increased BMI.

T. J. Herzog, MD

Hysteroscopy and Cytology in Endometrial Cancer
Bradley WH, Boente MP, Brooker D, et al (Univ of Minnesota, Minneapolis)
Obstet Gynecol 104:1030-1033, 2004   42–2

Objective.—To estimate the effect of preoperative diagnostic hysteroscopy on peritoneal cytology in patients with endometrial cancer.

Methods.—A total of 256 charts were reviewed. Two cohorts were established based on diagnosis by hysteroscopy or blind endometrial sampling via either endometrial biopsy or dilatation and curettage (D&C). Malignant or suspicious peritoneal cytology was the primary outcome. Cohorts were compared using logistic regression to correct for potential confounders of stage and grade.

Results.—A total of 204 cases were diagnosed by endometrial biopsy or D&C, whereas 52 were identified by hysteroscopy. In the endometrial biopsy or D&C arm, 14 of 204 (6.9%) patients had malignant or suspicious cytology compared with 7 of 52 (13.5%) patients in the hysteroscopy arm (*P* = .15). After logistic regression controlling for stage and grade, the odds ratio for positive cytology after hysteroscopy was 3.88 (95% confidence interval 1.11,13.6; *P* = .03). Four of the 52 (7.7%) cases diagnosed by hysteroscopy were stage IIIA due to cytology alone compared with 3 of the 204 (1.4%) cases diagnosed by endometrial biopsy or D&C (*P* = .03).

Conclusion.—Hysteroscopy appears to be associated with an increased rate of malignant cytology after controlling for confounders of stage and grade. Further, there appears to be an association between hysteroscopy and upstaging patients due to cytology alone.

▶ The potential for hysteroscopy to disseminate malignant endometrial cells into the peritoneal cavity has long been questioned. This retrospective study reviewed 254 patients who had been surgically staged. Of the 254, 52 had been diagnosed using laparoscopy as opposed to endometrial biopsy and D&C. A higher percentage of patients with positive cytology was noted in the hysteroscopy group, including 4 who were upstaged because of cytology alone. Logistic regression controlling for stage and grade of cancer showed an odds ratio of 3.88 for positive cytology if hysteroscopy was performed. Since this was a retrospective study, it was not possible to determine whether there were other confounding variables that influence the choice of hysteroscopy for diagnosis rather than simple biopsy or D&C. However, this study would seem to argue for caution in performing hysteroscopy in patients with a high likelihood of malignancy.

V. A. M. Givens, MD

Vaginal Hysterectomy and Abdominal Hysterectomy for Treatment of Endometrial Cancer in the Elderly

Susini T, Massi G, Amunni G, et al (Univ of Florence, Italy)
Gynecol Oncol 96:362-367, 2005   42–3

Objective.—The purpose of this study was to analyze the outcome of vaginal and abdominal hysterectomy for treatment of endometrial cancer in elderly patients.

Methods.—In a retrospective series of 171 patients with age ≥70 years and at stages I–III, we evaluated operative and hospitalization data, as well as morbidity, mortality, and long-term survival associated with vaginal and abdominal hysterectomy. A total of 128 patients were operated on with vaginal hysterectomy and 43 cases underwent abdominal hysterectomy.

Results.—Medically compromised patients were significantly more frequent in the vaginal surgery group (*P* = 0.01). Overall, the 10-year disease-specific survival rates after vaginal and abdominal hysterectomy were 80% and 78%, respectively (*P* = n.s.) (Fig 1). Limiting the analysis to stage I (130 patients), 10-year disease-specific survival was 83% in 95 women operated on by the vaginal route and 84% in 35 patients operated on by the abdomi-

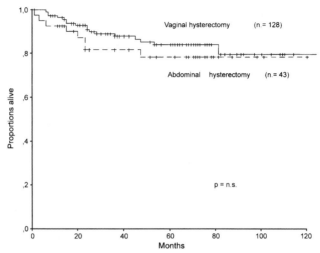

FIGURE 1.—Disease-specific 10-year survival for the overall series. Vaginal hysterectomy versus abdominal hysterectomy. n.s., Not significant. (Courtesy of Susini T, Massi G, Amunni G, et al: Vaginal hysterectomy and abdominal hysterectomy for treatment of endometrial cancer in the elderly. *Gynecol Oncol* 96:362-367. Copyright 2005 by Elsevier Science Inc.)

nal approach (P = n.s.) (Fig 2). Patients in the vaginal surgery group had a significantly shorter operative time (P = 0.01), less blood loss (P < 0.05), and were discharged earlier (P < 0.05). Severe complications occurred in 5.4% of the vaginal and in 7.0% of the abdominal procedures. Perioperative mortal-

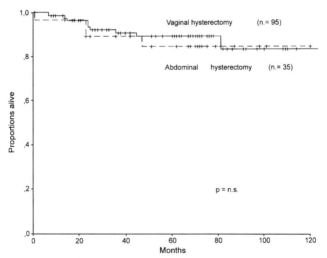

FIGURE 2.—Disease-specific 10-year survival for stage I cases. Vaginal hysterectomy versus abdominal hysterectomy. n.s., Not significant. (Courtesy of Susini T, Massi G, Amunni G, et al: Vaginal hysterectomy and abdominal hysterectomy for treatment of endometrial cancer in the elderly. *Gynecol Oncol* 96:362-367. Copyright 2005 by Elsevier Science Inc.)

ity was zero after vaginal hysterectomy and 2.3% after abdominal hysterectomy, respectively.

Conclusions.—Vaginal hysterectomy showed a high cure rate, shorter operative time, less blood loss, reduced morbidity, and no mortality and therefore may be considered the elective approach for treatment of elderly patients with endometrial cancer.

▶ The title of this study is somewhat misleading since 9% of the patients who underwent vaginal hysterectomy and 63% of those who underwent abdominal hysterectomy also had at least a pelvic lymphadenectomy. In addition, the vaginal hysterectomy done was not a typical operation in that a vaginal cuff was resected. This study adds further fuel to the ongoing debate as to what surgery is necessary and sufficient for the treatment of early endometrial cancer. Unfortunately, it also provides little clarification.

Most patients with clinical stage I endometrial cancer will be cured by hysterectomy alone. The issue is how to minimize the 15% to 20% of patients with occult lymph node metastasis or those who will recur. Many American gynecologic oncologists believe that lymphadenectomy will find most patients with occult metastasis and prevent future recurrence without the requirement for adjuvant radiation therapy.[1] Others feel that more selective use of lymphadenectomy combined with a more liberal use of adjuvant radiation therapy yields almost as good results. It was not stated in this trial how many patients did receive radiation.

Nonetheless we await the results of the MASTEC trial to provide us further information on the proper role of lymphadenectomy for early endometrial cancer. In the meantime, vaginal hysterectomy remains an option for selected patients. If we accept the assumption that a 70-year-old woman would live an average of 15 additional years or an 80-year-old will live an average of 9 more years, the greater than 78% 10-year survival seen in this group of patients leads this editor to draw several conclusions not well discussed in this report: (1) that this group of patients were not nearly as morbid as the authors contend, (2) that the diagnosis of endometrial cancer confers a survival advantage to elderly women so afflicted, or (3) that this group of elderly endometrial cancer survivors in Florence, Italy, received excellent geriatric preventive care.

D. S. Miller, MD

Reference

1. Straughn JM Jr, Huh WK, Orr JW Jr, et al: Stage IC adenocarcinoma of the endometrium: Survival comparisons of surgically staged patients with and without adjuvant radiation therapy. *Gynecol Oncol* 89:295-300, 2003. (2004 YEAR BOOK OF OBSTETRICS, GYNECOLOGY, AND WOMEN'S HEALTH, p 476-478.)

Retrospective Analysis of Selective Lymphadenectomy in Apparent Early-Stage Endometrial Cancer

Cragun JM, Havrilesky LJ, Calingaert B, et al (Duke Univ, Durham, NC)
J Clin Oncol 23:3668-3675, 2005   42–4

Purpose.—Selective lymphadenectomy is widely accepted in the management of endometrial cancer. Purported benefits are individualization of adjuvant therapy based on extent of disease and resection of occult metastases. Our goal was to assess effects of the extent of selective lymphadenectomy on outcomes in women with apparent stage I endometrial cancer at laparotomy.

Patients and Methods.—Patients with endometrial cancer who received primary surgical treatment between 1973 and 2002 were identified through an institutional tumor registry. Inclusion criteria were clinical stage I/IIA disease and procedure including hysterectomy and selective lymphadenectomy (pelvic or pelvic + aortic). Exclusion criteria included presurgical radiation, grossly positive lymph nodes, or extrauterine metastases at laparotomy. Recurrence and survival were analyzed using Kaplan-Meier analysis and Cox proportional hazards model.

Results.—Among 509 patients, the median number of lymph nodes removed was 15 (median pelvic, 11; median aortic, three). Pelvic and aortic node metastases were found in 24 (5%) of 509 patients and 11 (3%) of 373 patients, respectively. Patients with poorly differentiated cancers having more than 11 pelvic nodes removed had improved overall survival (hazard ratio [HR], 0.25; $P < .0001$) and progression-free survival (HR, 0.26; $P < .0001$) compared with patients having poorly differentiated cancers with 11 or fewer nodes removed. Number of nodes removed was not predictive of survival among patients with cancers of grade 1 to 2. Performance of aortic selective lymphadenectomy was not associated with survival. Three (27%) of 11 patients with microscopic aortic nodal metastasis are alive without recurrence.

Conclusion.—These data add to the literature documenting the possible therapeutic benefit of selective lymphadenectomy in management of patients with apparent early-stage endometrial cancer.

▶ Since the earliest studies done by the Gynecologic Oncology Group showing the prognostic significance of pelvic and periaortic lymph nodes for endometrial cancer outcome, the surgical evaluation of those lymph nodes has become more extensive.[1-3] Surgical removal of pelvic and periaortic lymph nodes became part of the FIGO staging criteria for endometrial cancer. Yet the extent of the lymphadenectomy is not defined. Several authors have reported very good results as measured by low recurrence and high survival rates in early-stage endometrial cancers treated with complete pelvic and periaortic lymphadenectomies.[4-6] The most biologically plausible hypothesis for the role of lymphadenectomy is that the more thorough the dissection, the more likely occult metastases are to be found, thus moving those patients from stage I to stage III. It is implied that these operations are not only diagnostic but also therapeutic, presumably also removing potential future reservoirs for recurrence. It is now the opinion of many gynecologic oncologists that complete pelvic and periaortic lymphadenectomy is a necessary component of endometrial cancer staging and treatment. However, others disagree.[7,8] Clearly a more extensive lymphadenectomy is more likely to detect occult lymph node metastasis. But how extensive does it need to be? Recently the Gynecologic Oncology Group defined the extent of lymphadenectomy required for its ongoing molecular staging protocol GOG 210, which specifies a minimum of 4 lymph nodes to be removed from each hemipelvic lymphadenectomy and 1 from each hemiperiaortic lymphadenectomy. But this specified criterion was not based on any data.

This study appears to confirm that requirement. The disappointments of this report are multitude. Unfortunately, it appears that only a small nugget of information was extracted from what should have been a gold mine of experience. Only the patients who had some lymph lodes removed were included in the analysis and not the more than 500 patients who had no lymph nodes done. Clearly, some of those patients who did not have lymphadenectomy, in fact, had occult metastatic disease, recurred, and died. Thus, one could have had a more meaningful comparison with patients who had lymph nodes removed. In addition, had the authors used a more powerful statistical analysis by using the number of lymph nodes as a continuous variable, receiver operator characteristic curves could have been produced that might have identified a better cutoff than 11 lymph nodes. This study leaves far too many questions unanswered.

D. S. Miller, MD

References

1. Lewis G, Mortel R, Slack N: Endometrial cancer: Therapeutic decision and the staging process in "early" disease. *Cancer* 39(2 suppl):959-966, 1977.
2. Creasman W, Morrow C, Bundy B, et al: Surgical pathologic spread patterns of endometrial cancer. A Gynecologic Oncology Group Study. *Cancer* 60(8 suppl) :2035-2041, 1987.
3. Creasman W, DeGeest K, DiSaia PJ, et al: Significance of true surgical pathologic staging: A Gynecologic Oncology Group Study. *Am J Obstet Gynecol* 181:31-34, 1999.
4. Orr J, Holimon J, Orr P: Stage I corpus cancer: Is teletherapy necessary? *Am J Obstet Gynecol* 176:777-789, 1997.
5. Straughn J, Huh W, Kelly J, et al: Conservative management of stage I endometrial carcinoma after surgical staging. *Gynecol Oncol* 84:194-200, 2002. (2003 YEAR BOOK OF OBSTETRICS, GYNECOLOGY, AND WOMEN'S HEALTH, p 467-468.)
6. Straughn J, Huh W, Orr J Jr, et al: Stage IC adenocarcinoma of the endometrium: Survival comparisons of surgically staged patients with and without adjuvant radiation therapy. *Gynecol Oncol* 89:295-300, 2003. (2004 YEAR BOOK OF OBSTETRICS, GYNECOLOGY, AND WOMEN'S HEALTH, p 476-478.)
7. Creutzberg C, van Putten W, Koper P, et al: Surgery and postoperative radiotherapy versus surgery alone for patients with stage-1 endometrial carcinoma: Multicentre randomised trial. PORTEC Study Group. *Lancet* 355:1404-1411, 2000. (2001 YEAR BOOK OF OBSTETRICS, GYNECOLOGY, AND WOMEN'S HEALTH, p 473-474.)
8. Creutzberg CL: GOG-99: Ending the controversy regarding pelvic radiotherapy for endometrial carcinoma? *Gynecol Oncol* 92:740-743, 2004.

Prospective Evaluation of FDG-PET for Detecting Pelvic and Para-aortic Lymph Node Metastasis in Uterine Corpus Cancer

Horowitz NS, Dehdashti F, Herzog TJ, et al (Washington Univ, St Louis)

Gynecol Oncol 95:546-551, 2004   42–5

Objectives.—To estimate the sensitivity and specificity of positron emission tomography (PET) with 2-[^{18}F]fluoro-2-deoxy-D-glucose (FDG) for detecting pelvic and para-aortic lymph node metastasis in patients with uterine corpus carcinoma before surgical staging.

Methods.—Patients with newly diagnosed FIGO grade 2 or 3 endometrioid, papillary serous, or clear cell adenocarcinoma or uterine corpus sarcoma scheduled for surgical staging, including bilateral pelvic and para-aortic lymphadenectomy, were eligible. PET was performed within 30 days of surgery and interpreted independently by two nuclear medicine physicians. The imaging, operative, and pathologic findings for each patient and each nodal site were compared, and the sensitivity and specificity of FDG-PET in predicting nodal metastasis were determined.

Results.—Twenty patients underwent FDG-PET before surgical staging. One patient found to have ovarian carcinoma on final pathology was excluded. Of the 19 primary intrauterine tumors, 16 (84%) exhibited increased FDG uptake (Fig 2). One patient did not undergo lymphadenectomy; her chest CT was suspicious for metastatic disease and FDG-PET

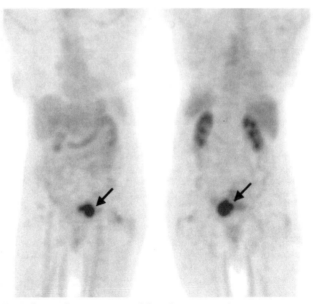

FIGURE 2.—Endometrial cancer. Anterior (**left**) and posterior (**right**) FDG-PET reprojection images demonstrate focal accumulation of FDG in the pelvis (*solid arrows*), consistent with the patient's known endometrial cancer. (Courtesy of Horowitz NS, Dehdashti F, Herzog TJ, et al: Prospective evaluation of FDG-PET for detecting pelvic and para-aortic lymph node metastasis in uterine corpus cancer. *Gynecol Oncol* 95:546-551. Copyright 2004 by Elsevier Science Inc.)

TABLE 4.—Correlation of FDG-PET Results With
Pathologic Findings in Pelvic and Para-aortic Lymph Nodes

	PET Positive	PET Negative	Total
By lymph node region			
Pathology positive	3	2	5
Pathology negative	1	68	69
Total	4	70	74
Sensitivity = 3/5 = 60%			
Specificity = 68/69 = 98%			
By patient			
Pathology positive	2	1	3
Pathology negative	1	15	16
Total	3	16	19
Sensitivity = 2/3 = 67%			
Specificity = 15/16 = 94%			

(Courtesy of Horowitz NS, Dehdashti F, Herzog TJ, et al: Prospective evaluation of FDG-PET for detecting pelvic and para-aortic lymph node metastasis in uterine corpus cancer. *Gynecol Oncol* 95:546-551. Copyright 2004 by Elsevier Science Inc.)

showed uptake in multiple nodal and pulmonary foci. Metastatic disease was confirmed by percutaneous nodal biopsy. A total of three pathologically positive nodes were found in 2 of the 18 patients (11%). FDG-PET predicted that 3 patients would have positive lymph nodes (2 true positive and 1 false positive). Analyzed by lymph node regions, FDG-PET had 60% sensitivity and 98% specificity. The sensitivity and specificity by individual patient were 67% and 94%, respectively (Table 4).

Conclusions.—FDG-PET is only moderately sensitive in predicting lymph node metastasis pre-operatively in patients with endometrial cancer. This imaging modality should not replace lymphadenectomy, but may be helpful for patients in whom lymphadenectomy cannot be, or was not, performed.

▶ Because there is significant variability in management of patients with endometrial cancer and debate about the extent to which pelvic and para-aortic lymph nodes should be removed, this prospective study was undertaken to determine the sensitivity and specificity of FDG-PET for detecting metastases to the pelvic and para-aortic lymph nodes before surgical staging for endometrial cancer. Eligible patients were those with International Federation of Gynecology and Obstetrics (FIGO) grade 2 or 3, papillary serous or clear cell carcinoma of the uterus scheduled to undergo surgical staging within 30 days of undergoing a PET scan. PET scans were scored on a 5-point system: 0 = definitely normal, 1 = probably normal, 2 = equivocal, 3 = probably abnormal, 4 = definitely abnormal. For dichotomization, scores of 0 to 2 were considered negative and scores of 3 or 4 were positive. The surgeon and radiologist were blinded to clinical information or PET results, respectively. The sensitivity and specificity of the PET scan for determining lymph node metastases were determined.

Twenty patients were enrolled into the study. One had ovarian cancer and was excluded, leaving 19 evaluable patients. A total of 3 positive nodes were found in 2 of 18 patients (11%). One patient did not undergo surgery, as she was found on PET scan to have positive supraclavicular nodes and lung nodules. Although this was not a primary outcome measure in this study, in terms of PET detection of the primary tumor, 16 of 19 patients had a positive PET, and the remaining 3 were equivocal. In terms of lymph node involvement, 2 had a true positive result, and 1 was a false positive. There was one false-negative pelvic lymph node in a carcinosarcoma patient. The sensitivity was 60% and specificity was 98%. There were a number of areas of incidental uptake in the colon and mesentery and chest wall that turned out to be a benign colonic polyp, granulomatous change in the bowel mesentery, or a rib fracture.

The benefit of PET scanning for lymph node assessment appears to be in its specificity and not sensitivity. Therefore, PET scan is only moderately sensitive in predicting lymph node metastases preoperatively and should not replace lymphadenectomy.

The advantages of this study are its prospective nature and the blinded nature of the PET scan interpretation. The small number of patients with lymph node metastases precludes making global recommendations. From a study standpoint, the dichotomization strategy for interpretation of results (scores 0-2 interpreted as negative) may not be clinically practical. For instance, an equivocal result (score = 2) would not necessarily be considered a negative result. The fact that PET-CT was not used to potentially eliminate false-positive extranodal areas of disease also may have limited the value of PET scanning in this patient population.

S. D. Yamada, MD

Vaginal Brachytherapy Alone: An Alternative to Adjuvant Whole Pelvis Radiation for Early Stage Endometrial Cancer
Jolly S, Vargas C, Kumar T, et al (William Beaumont Hosp, Royal Oak, Mich)
Gynecol Oncol 97:887-892, 2005   42–6

Objective.—Postoperative management of early stage adenocarcinoma of the endometrium remains controversial. The use of pelvic radiation therapy as shown by the Gynecologic Oncology Group (GOG)-99 trial improves the event free interval at the cost of increased toxicity. We reviewed and compared our results treating early stage endometrial adenocarcinoma using hypofractionated high dose rate (HDR) vaginal brachytherapy (VB) alone with the results of the GOG-99.

Methods.—From 1992 to 2002, 243 endometrial cancer patients were treated with TAH/BSO and selective lymph node dissection followed by adjuvant radiotherapy (RT). Of these, 50 FIGO stage I-II (occult) adenocarcinoma (no clear cell or serous papillary) of the endometrium were managed with HDR hypofractionated VB as monotherapy using Iridium-192 to a dose of 30 Gy in 6 fractions twice weekly prescribed to a depth of 5 mm and median length of 4 cm. The characteristics, toxicity rates, and outcomes of our patients were compared with the results of the GOG-99. The median fol-

TABLE 1.—Patient Characteristics Comparison to GOG-99

		GOG-99 Pelvic EBRT	VB	*P* Value	GOG-99 No EBRT
Age	≤60	77 (41%)	16 (33%)	0.5	83 (41%)
	61-70	69 (36%)	20 (41%)		75 (37%)
	>70	44 (23%)	13 (27%)		44 (22%)
FIGO	IA	NA	4 (8.2)	NA	NA
stage	IB	110 (58%)	27 (55%)	0.2	119 (59%)
	IC	62 (33%)	9 (18%)		17 (8%)
	II occult	18 (10%)	6 (12%)		19 (9%)
Tumor	1	87 (46%)	21 (43%)	0.7	79 (39%)
grade	2	74 (39%)	22 (50%)		80 (40%)
	3	29 (15%)	6 (12%)		43 (21%)

Abbreviations: GOG, Gynecologic Oncology Group; *EBRT,* external beam radiation therapy; *VB,* vaginal brachytherapy; *FIGO,* International Federation of Gynecology and Obstetrics; *NA,* not applicable.

(Courtesy of Jolly S, Vargas C, Kumar T, et al: Vaginal brachytherapy alone: An alternative to adjuvant whole pelvis radiation for early stage endometrial cancer. *Gynecol Oncol* 97:887-892. Copyright 2005 by Elsevier Science Inc.)

low up of our patients and the GOG-99 were 3.2 years and 5.8 years, respectively.

Results.—Patient characteristics including age, stage, and grade were similar in our study and the GOG-99 (Table 1). The local recurrence rate in our study, the pelvic RT arm of the GOG-99, and the no RT arm of the GOG-99 were 4% (*n* = 2), 2% (*n* = 3), and 9% (*n* = 18), respectively (Table 4). In our study, one patient failed in the vagina alone and a second patient failed in the vagina and pelvis. In the GOG-99, the vagina as a component of locoregional failure was also the most common failure site in the no RT arm 77.8% (*n* = 14) and in the RT arm 100% (*n* = 3). The 2-year cumulative recurrence rate in our study was 2%, which compares favorably with the GOG-99 pelvic RT arm (3%) and observation arm (12%). Four-year survival rates of the no RT arm of the GOG-99, the RT arm of the GOG-99, and our study with HDR VB were 86%, 92%, and 97%, respectively. Chronic grade 2 toxicity rates were reduced by the use of VB compared to pelvic RT, especially GI

TABLE 4.—Sites of Locoregional Failure

	GOG-99 Pelvic EBRT	VB	*P* Value	GOG-99 No EBRT
Locoregional	3 (2%)	2 (4%)	0.3	18 (9%)
Vagina	2 (1%)	1 (2%)	0.5	13 (6%)
Pelvis	0 (0%)	0 (0%)	NS	4 (2%)
Vagina and Pelvis	1 (0.5%)	1 (2%)	0.4	1 (0.5%)
Distant	10 (5%)	0 (0%)	0.13	13 (6%)
All failures	13 (6.8%)	2 (4%)	0.7	31 (15.3%)

Abbreviations: GOG, Gynecologic Oncology Group; *EBRT,* external beam radiation therapy; *VB,* vaginal brachytherapy; *NS,* not significant.

(Courtesy of Jolly S, Vargas C, Kumar T, et al: Vaginal brachytherapy alone: An alternative to adjuvant whole pelvis radiation for early stage endometrial cancer. *Gynecol Oncol* 97:887-892. Copyright 2005 by Elsevier Science Inc.)

toxicity 0% vs. 34% (P value < 0.001), and GI obstruction 0% vs. 7% (P value = 0.08).

Conclusion.—Stage I-II (occult) endometrial adenocarcinoma treated with postoperative HDR vaginal brachytherapy has similar overall survival, locoregional failure rates, and cumulative recurrence rates to standard fractionation external beam pelvic RT with the benefit of much lower toxicity rates and shorter overall treatment time.

▶ This article is a retrospective review of patients with stage I and II surgically staged endometrial cancer treated at William Beaumont Hospital in Michigan with adjuvant VB alone. No patients with deep myometrial invasion and grade 3 tumors or papillary serous or clear cell carcinoma were included. Patient characteristics, locoregional failure rates, and toxicity were compared between the study population and the population of patients from the prospective GOG 99, published by Keys et al,[1] in which intermediate-risk endometrial cancer patients were randomized to observation or pelvic radiation.

Fifty patients were treated with a vaginal cylinder via hypofractionated HDR brachytherapy to a dose of 30 Gy in 6 fractions twice weekly. The dose was prescribed to 5 mm from the applicator surface. In GOG 99, pelvic RT was administered to patients with "intermediate risk factors": stage IB, IC, IIA (occult), and IIB (occult). The median follow-up in this study was 3.2 years (range, 0.7-8.8 years). No significant differences existed in stage and grade distribution between the GOG 99 patients and this patient population (Table 1). The 2-year cumulative recurrence rate was 2% in the VB group and 3% in the GOG 99 group that received pelvic radiation. The overall 4-year survival was 97% versus 92%, respectively. Locoregional recurrence rates were also similar between the 2 groups. Two (4%) locoregional recurrences were noted in the VB group—one in the pelvis and another in the vagina. Vaginal failures (P = .5), vaginal and pelvic failures (P = .4), distant failures (P = .13), and overall failure (P = .7) were similar between the pelvic radiation and VB groups (Table 4). A comparison of overall failure between the GOG 99 observation group and this VB group revealed a significant difference: 15.3% in the GOG observation group and 4% in the current VB group (P = .03). No patients treated with VB experienced a toxicity grade of 2 or higher. This appeared to be significantly different than the pelvic RT arm in GOG 99 where 7% of patients experienced bowel obstructions.

This study lends support to the use of VB as sole adjuvant treatment in patients with intermediate risk factors for recurrence. The risk of recurrence appears to be similar, and the toxicity is lower. However, there are certainly some concerns when a retrospective data set of patients accrued over a 10-year period are compared with a prospective data set (GOG 99) in terms of quality of data and follow-up. In addition, the median follow-up in this study was only 36 months as opposed to 68 months for surviving patients on GOG 99. Therefore, the number of recurrences in this study may be higher with longer follow-up.

S. D. Yamada, MD

Reference

1. Keys HM, Roberts JA, Brunetto VL, et al: A phase III trial of surgery with or without adjunctive external pelvic radiation therapy in intermediate risk endometrial adenocarcinoma: A Gynecologic Oncology Group study. *Gynecol Oncol* 92: 744-751, 2004.

Whole Abdominal Radiotherapy in the Adjuvant Treatment of Patients With Stage III and IV Endometrial Cancer: A Gynecologic Oncology Group Study
Sutton G, Axelrod JH, Bundy BN, et al (St Vincent's Hosp, Indianapolis, Ind; Western Pennsylvania Hosp, Pittsburgh; Roswell Park Cancer Inst, Buffalo, NY; et al)
Gynecol Oncol 97:755-763, 2005   42–7

Objective.—To evaluate toxicity, survival, and recurrence-free interval in women with loco-regionally advanced endometrial carcinoma treated with postoperative whole abdominal radiation therapy.

Methods.—Whole abdominal irradiation with pelvic plus or minus para-aortic boost was initiated within 8 weeks of total abdominal hysterectomy, bilateral salpingo-oophorectomy, pelvic washings, and selective pelvic and para-aortic node sampling in eligible, consenting patients.

Results.—Of 180 evaluable patients entered on the study with surgically staged III and IV endometrial carcinoma maximally debulked to less than 2 cm, 77 had typical endometrial adenocarcinoma and 103 had high-risk histology, either papillary serous or clear cell carcinoma. Patients with typical endometrial adenocarcinoma were significantly younger and had significantly fewer poorly differentiated cancers. Proportionally, there were twice as many non-Whites with high-risk histologies as non-Whites with typical endometrial adenocarcinoma. Forty-five percent of patients with typical en-

---

TABLE 6.—Adverse Events

Adverse Effect	Grade (Frequency)				
	0	1	2	3	4
Hematologic	63 (36%)	35 (20%)	54 (31%)	19 (11%)	3 (2%)
Genitourinary	138 (79%)	32 (18%)	4 (2%)	0	0
Gastrointestinal	27 (15%)	42 (24%)	78 (45%)	20 (11%)	7 (4%)
Hepatic	165 (95%)	5 (3%)	0	3 (2%)	1 (1%)
Pulmonary	156 (90%)	11 (6%)	6 (3%)	1 (1%)	0
CV	159 (91%)	1 (1%)	2 (1%)	10 (6%)	2 (1%)
Neurologic	167 (96%)	3 (2%)	2 (1%)	2 (1%)	0
Cutaneous	118 (68%)	44 (25%)	10 (6%)	2 (1%)	0
Lymphatic	164 (94%)	6 (3%)	3 (2%)	1 (1%)	0
Fever	140 (85%)	26 (15%)	6 (3%)	2 (1%)	0
Other	159 (91%)	11 (6%)	2 (1%)	2 (1%)	0

Abbreviation: CV, Cardiovascular.
(Courtesy of Sutton G, Axelrod JH, Bundy BN, et al: Whole abdominal radiotherapy in the adjuvant treatment of patients with stage III and IV endometrial cancer: A Gynecologic Oncology Group study. *Gynecol Oncol* 97:755-763. Copyright 2005 by Elsevier Science Inc.)

TABLE 9.—Recurrence-Free Interval and Survival at 3 Years

Cell Type/Stage	No.	RFS (%)	Survival (%)
Typical endometrial, stage III	58	34.5	34.5
Typical endometrial, stage IV	19	10.5	21.1
Papillary serous/clear cell, stage III	75	40.1	48.1
Papillary serous/clear cell, stage IV	28	10.7	10.7

Abbreviation: RFS, Recurrence-free survival.
(Courtesy of Sutton G, Axelrod JH, Bundy BN, et al: Whole abdominal radiotherapy in the adjuvant treatment of patients with stage III and IV endometrial cancer: A Gynecologic Oncology Group study. *Gynecol Oncol* 97:755-763. Copyright 2005 by Elsevier Science Inc.)

dometrial adenocarcinomas had positive pelvic nodes compared to 51% of those with high-risk histologies. Both histologic groups had similar distribution for performance status, para-aortic node positivity, site and extent of disease, and International Federation of Gynecology and Obstetrics (FIGO) stage. The frequency of severe or life-threatening adverse effects among 174 patients evaluable for radiation toxicity included 12.6% with bone marrow depression, 15% GI, and 2.2% hepatic toxicity (Table 6). The recurrence-free survival rates were 29% and 27% (at 3 years) for the typical endometrial adenocarcinoma and high-risk histologies, respectively (Table 9). The survival rates were 31% and 35%, respectively. No patient with gross residual disease survived (Table 7).

TABLE 7.—Site of Recurrence

Sites	Typical Endometrial No. (%)	Papillary Serous/ Clear Cell No. (%)
NED	27 (35.1)	34 (33.0)
Recurred	50 (64.9)	69 (67.0)
Vagina	3	4
Pelvis	7	3
Abdomen	9	21
Retroperitoneal nodes	0	1
Lung	9	15
Other[a]	10	6
Lung and other	2	3
Abdomen and other	2	2
Pelvis and liver	1	0
Vagina and liver	0	1
Lung and pelvis	0	1
Abdomen and pelvis	1	4
Abdomen and lung	1	4
Vagina and lung	0	1
Retro. nodes and pelvis	0	1
Unknown	5	2

[a]Includes axillary, groin, and supraclavicular lymph nodes, bone, brain, spinal cord, liver, stomach, and bladder.
Abbreviation: NED, No evidence of disease.
(Courtesy of Sutton G, Axelrod JH, Bundy BN, et al: Whole abdominal radiotherapy in the adjuvant treatment of patients with stage III and IV endometrial cancer: A Gynecologic Oncology Group study. *Gynecol Oncol* 97:755-763. Copyright 2005 by Elsevier Science Inc.)

Conclusion.—Whole abdominal irradiation in maximally resected advanced endometrial carcinoma has tolerable toxicity, and it is suggested that the outcome may be improved by this adjunctive treatment in patients with completely resected disease.

▶ This is a prospective study analyzing the use of whole abdomen radiotherapy in an open field technique for surgically staged stage III and IV endometrioid, papillary serous, clear cell, and recurrent uterine carcinomas with less than 2 cm of residual disease. The purpose of the study was to evaluate toxicity, survival, and progression-free survival. A second objective was to determine differences in survival and progression-free survival between patients with endometrial adenocarcinoma and papillary serous/clear cell carcinomas. Patients with vaginal, liver parenchymal, lung, or extraperitoneal metastases were excluded.

A total of 180 patients between 1986 and 1994 were evaluable and discussed in this report. There were 77 patients with endometrioid histology and 103 with papillary serous or clear cell histology. Patients with papillary serous and clear cell cancers were significantly older than their counterparts with endometrioid cancer (median age: 68.5 years for papillary serous and 71 for clear cell vs 63 for endometrioid, $P < .01$). A larger proportion of black patients than white patients had papillary serous or clear cell cancers (78% vs 53%). Similar sites of metastatic disease distribution were present between the endometrioid and papillary serous/clear cell cancer group except that there was more diaphragmatic disease (7.8%) in the papillary serous/clear cell group than the endometrioid group (1.3%, $P < .05$).

Toxicities are listed in Table 6. Seven patients (4%) had grade 4 gastrointestinal toxicity. Three of these patients had no evidence of disease and required surgery. Two of these 3 died after surgery. A total of 22 patients (13%) had grade 3 or 4 hematologic toxicity. Patterns of recurrence are shown in Table 7. Overall, 65% of endometrioid patients and 67% of papillary serous and clear cell patients had recurrences. Recurrence-free intervals were similar for patients with endometrioid (12.6%), clear cell (22%), and papillary serous (11%) cancers at 3 years. Recurrence-free survival and overall survival at 3 years are shown in Table 9. Overall, the in-field recurrences were 40% in endometrioid cancers and 47% in papillary serous and clear cell cancers. Patients with gross residual disease and papillary serous or clear cell cancer did more poorly than those with microscopic residual disease. No patient with gross residual disease survived. Median disease-free survival (DFS) was 4.8 months (2.5-33.5 months). Median survival was 11.1 months (5.8-55.5 months). If patients had gross residual disease but was completely resected, the median DFS was 12 months (1.3-57 months) and the median survival was 27.4 months. In patients with only microscopic disease, the median survival was 65 months and the median DFS was 66 months. Although the article states the isolated recurrences in patients with endometrioid cancers with gross residual and microscopic residual, the corresponding median DFS and survival statistics are not given specifically for the endometrioid patients.

This article demonstrates that whole abdomen radiation results in 3-year survivals of 31% to 35% for patients with advanced-stage endometrioid and uterine papillary serous cancer. There is, however, a high frequency of in-field recurrences and some gastrointestinal toxicity.

S. D. Yamada, MD

A Pilot Trial of TAC (Paclitaxel, Doxorubicin, and Carboplatin) Chemotherapy With Filgrastim (r-metHuG-CSF) Support Followed by Radiotherapy in Patients With "High-Risk" Endometrial Cancer
Duska LR, for the Gynecologic Oncology Research Program of the Dana Farber/Harvard Cancer Center (Massachusetts Gen Hosp, Boston; et al)
Gynecol Oncol 96:198-203, 2005   42–8

Objectives.—To determine the toxicity, tolerability, and feasibility of delivering combination chemotherapy with subsequent radiation therapy to women with high-risk endometrial cancer and to evaluate the long-term bowel toxicity of this regimen.

Methods.—The trial was approved by the Dana Farber/Partners Cancer Care (DFPCC) Institutional Review Board (IRB). Patients with stage 3 or stage 4 endometrial cancer or patients with high-risk histology and any stage disease were prospectively entered. Complete surgical staging and a normal gated blood pool scan were required prior to entry. Patients were treated with three cycles of paclitaxel (160 mg/m^2), doxorubicin (45 mg/m^2) and carboplatin (AUC 5) (TAC) all on day 1 of a 21-day schedule as an outpatient with G-CSF support. At the conclusion of chemotherapy, patients received radiation therapy (4500 cGy to the whole pelvis) commencing within 35 days of the last cycle of chemotherapy. Paraaortic radiation and/or vaginal brachytherapy were allowed at the discretion of the treating radiation oncologist.

Results.—Twenty patients were entered into the trial from November 2000 through February 2003. Eighteen patients successfully completed the trial, and two patients came off trial during chemotherapy (both later completed planned radiation therapy). Patients were initially stage 1 ($n = 3$), stage 3 ($n = 14$), and stage 4 ($n = 3$). Papillary serous was the dominant histology with 13 patients. Chemotherapy was given on average within 32 days of surgery (range 11-63 days) and radiation was initiated on average within 14 weeks of surgery (range 10-18 weeks). Chemotherapy was well tolerated, with 57 total cycles delivered of a planned 60 cycles. Two patients required dose modification in two cycles (two patients in cycle 3 secondary to hematologic toxicity). No grade 3 or grade 4 neurotoxicity was reported. There were six episodes of grade 3 short-term toxicity with radiation therapy reported in a single patient. Late radiotherapy toxicity included bowel obstruction requiring laparotomy in two patients and grade 3 constipation in one patient. Late radiation toxicity data are still being collected as follow-up continues.

Conclusions.—The TAC chemotherapy regimen is well tolerated and three cycles were delivered successfully with G-CSF support without evidence of the neurotoxicity or cardiac toxicity reported with the cisplatin containing TAP regimen. Standard radiation was deliverable following TAC therapy without excessive toxicity. Further study of this regimen with subsequent radiation therapy is warranted in patients at risk for systemic and regional recurrence of their malignancy.

▶ This was a phase II study evaluating the use of paclitaxel, doxorubicin, and carboplatin in patients with "high-risk" endometrial cancer, defined as histologically confirmed stage III or IV endometrioid cancer or any stage papillary serous or clear cell cancer. Patients underwent surgical staging in the form of hysterectomy, bilateral salpingo-oophorectomy, pelvic washings, and selective retroperitoneal lymph node dissection. Patients with unresectable metastatic disease were not eligible. Patients received all 3 chemotherapy agents on day 1: doxorubicin 45 mg/m², paclitaxel 160 mg/m², and carboplatin at AUC 5 for 3 cycles followed by pelvic radiation. Extended field radiation and vaginal vault brachytherapy were used as needed.

Twenty patients were enrolled in the trial, and 18 completed the study. Two patients were removed from study: one who experienced intractable paclitaxel hypersensitivity, and one for recurrent ascites. Grade 3 to 4 neutropenia occurred in 50% of patients. One patient required bowel resection as a result of radiation enteritis, while another had recurrent uterine papillary serous carcinoma (UPSC). Median follow-up was 16 months (range 4-36 months). Thirteen patients have no recurrent disease, while 3 patients have died of disease and one is alive with disease. All 4 of these patients had UPSC and peritoneal but no pelvic recurrences.

This study is a prospective pilot study in a surgically staged patient population that demonstrates feasibility of this regimen. However, the follow-up to document recurrence-free survival is short. Whether this regimen could be tolerated with less toxicity if administered with intensity-modulated radiotherapy should be considered.

S. D. Yamada, MD

Adjuvant Sequential Chemotherapy and Radiotherapy in Uterine Papillary Serous Carcinoma
Low JSH, Wong EH, Khoo Tan HS, et al (Natl Cancer Centre, Singapore; KK Women and Child Hosp, Singapore)
Gynecol Oncol 97:171-177, 2005   42–9

Purpose.—To evaluate the efficacy and toxicity of adjuvant combination of sequential chemotherapy followed by radiotherapy in uterine papillary serous carcinoma (UPSC).

Methods and Materials.—From April 1994 to June 2003, 26 patients (median age 61.7 years, range 46.9-78.4) with UPSC were treated with a platinum-based chemoradiation protocol after definitive surgery. 9 patients were assigned as stage I (35%), 4 were stage II (15%), 11 were stage III (42%), and 2 were stage IV (8%) according to the FIGO staging for gynecological cancers. All patients underwent total hysterectomy, salpingo-oophorectomy, pelvic ± periaortic lymph nodes dissection/sampling, omentectomy, and peritoneal washing. The adjuvant chemoradiation protocol consists of 4 cycles of platinum-based chemotherapy followed by pelvic irradiation and vaginal vault brachytherapy. In selected stage I patients with no or minimal myometrial invasion, only vault brachytherapy was given after adjuvant chemotherapy.

Results.—After a median follow-up of 28 months (range 9-113 months), 14 (54%) patients were alive and free of disease. 12 out of these 14 patients were FIGO stage I/II. 9 patients (35%) had died (8 from distant metastases). The Kaplan-Meier 2-year and 5-year survival estimates were 69.5% and 57%, respectively. Only 4 (15%) patients had pelvic recurrence. None of the patients developed local vault recurrence. The treatment was well tolerated, only 1 patient developed congestive cardiac failure from the chemotherapy and 6 patients had grade 2 peripheral neuropathy on follow-up.

Conclusion.—In our series of UPSC patients treated with adjuvant chemotherapy followed by radiotherapy, local control can be achieved in a majority of patients. Distant failure remains the major cause of mortality. Further investigations into finding a more effective systemic therapy are required if improvement in outcome for this form of uterine cancer is to be achieved.

▶ The role of adjuvant therapy and its effectiveness in UPSC is controversial. This article is a retrospective review of 26 patients with UPSC treated with a platinum-based chemoradiation protocol. Patients underwent a total abdominal hysterectomy and bilateral salpingo-oophorectomy. The majority of patients had a pelvic lymph node dissection or sampling (24/26), and 7 of 26 had a para-aortic lymph node evaluation. All patients had an omentectomy and washings performed. The stage of patients was as follows: stage I (9 patients, 24%), stage II (4 patients, 15%), stage III (11 patients, 42%), and stage IV (2 patients, 8%). Adjuvant therapy consisted of 4 cycles of platinum-based chemotherapy followed by pelvic radiation and vaginal vault brachytherapy. In stage I patients, vaginal vault brachytherapy only was used. Chemotherapy consisted of IV cisplatin and epirubicin (19% of patients, before 1998) or paclitaxel and carboplatin (73% of patients, after 1998). The remainder received carboplatin and gemcitabine. Standard pelvic radiation (45 Gy) ± high-dose-rate brachytherapy to 10 Gy was given. Most patients (80%) were able to complete all 4 cycles of chemotherapy, and all patients completed radiation. At a median follow-up of 28 months, 14 patients (26%) were free of disease. Of the 9 patients with stage I disease, 8 had no evidence of disease (NED), and 1 was dead of disease (DOD). Of the stage II patients, all 4 had NED. Of the 11 stage III patients, 3 had NED, 5 were DOD, and 3 were alive with disease. Of the 2 stage IV patients, both were DOD. The overall Kaplan-Meier estimate of 2-year survival was 69.5%, and 5-year survival was 57%. The overall survival for stage I patients was 72.9%; for stage II, 100%; for stage III, 58.9%; and for stage IV, 0%. There were no vaginal vault recurrences. Of the stage III patients who recurred, all recurrences were distant or in the abdomen. Four patients additionally had a recurrence in the pelvis.

This article reaffirms the findings in other studies that distant and intra-abdominal sites of disease are primary sites at risk in this patient population. In addition, there was not a uniform type of chemotherapy administered. The majority of patients did not have a para-aortic node dissection, and the number of patients treated overall was small, however. Whether a para-aortic node dissection might have identified patients who would have benefited from extended-field para-aortic node radiation cannot to be determined from this study. Accurately staged stage I patients did well, but whether this was a product of surgical staging and identifying those patients with stage I disease who would have done well without adjuvant therapy, or whether this was a product of the aggressive treatment is unclear. But this study adds to the growing body of evidence that distant sites of recurrence need to continue to be a target for therapy in this patient population.

S. D. Yamada, MD

A Comparison Between Different Postoperative Treatment Modalities of Uterine Carcinosarcoma
Menczer J, Levy T, Piura B, et al (E Wolfson Med Ctr, Holon, Israel; Tel Aviv Univ, Israel; Ben-Gurion Univ of the Negev, Beer-Sheva, Israel; et al)
Gynecol Oncol 97:166-170, 2005   42–10

Objective.—Uterine carcinosarcomas are highly aggressive neoplasms with no established effective adjuvant therapy. The aim of the present study was to compare between the outcome in three medical institutions in each of which a different postoperative treatment modality was preferred, namely, chemotherapy in one, whole pelvic irradiation (WPI) in another, and sequential treatment (i.e., chemotherapy followed by WPI) in the third.

Methods.—The hospital records of all 49 uterine carcinosarcoma patients diagnosed and operated from 1995 to 2003 in the three institutions were reviewed. Non-parametric test was used to compare the median age between the treatment groups. Survival was calculated using the Kaplan-Meier method and compared by the log-rank test. Cox proportional hazard regression model was used to assess the effect of treatment type on survival after adjustment for stage.

Results.—Only about half of the patients (51%) had stage I at diagnosis and the majority of the patients (83.7%) had postoperative adjuvant treatment. The overall 5-year survival of the 41 patients that had postoperative treatment was 49.6%. The highest median survival and 5-year survival rate was observed in the sequential treatment group. Controlling for stage, this treatment modality was associated with a significant decrease in mortality of about 80% when compared to postoperative chemotherapy alone, and a non-significant decrease in mortality of about 50% when compared to WPI alone (HR = 0.20; 95% CI 0.04-0.99, $P = 0.049$ and HR = 0.50; 95% CI 0.1-2.32, $P = 0.4$, respectively).

Conclusions.—The improved outcome in patients who received postoperative sequential treatment seems to indicate that further exploration of this treatment modality is justified.

▶ This is a retrospective analysis of a series of 49 patients with stage I-IV surgically staged carcinosarcoma treated at 3 different institutions with 3 different adjuvant treatment regimens: chemotherapy alone (10 patients), WPI alone (21 patients), or sequential treatment in the form of chemotherapy followed by WPI (10 patients). The purpose of the study was to compare survival based on treatment regimen. Eight patients were excluded because they did not receive any adjuvant treatment. Approximately 50% of the patients had stage I disease, 14% stage II, 16% stage III, and 18% stage IV. WPI consisted of 4500 to 5000 cGy via a 4-field "box" technique followed by brachytherapy if radiation was the only form of adjuvant therapy. Chemotherapy consisted of ifosfamide 1500 mg/m²/d over 5 days with mesna, and cisplatin 60 mg/m² on day 1 every 21 days for 6 cycles. Sequential treatment consisted of ifosfamide 1200 mg/m²/d for 3 days with mesna, and cisplatin 80 mg/m² on day 3 every 21 days for 3 cycles followed by WPI. Side effects were reasonable for the patients who received WPI or sequential therapy. There were 3 patients with grade 3 to 4 myelotoxicity or neurotoxicity in the chemotherapy-only group. There were no differences in age or stage distribution between the 3 groups. Recurrence occurred in 16 patients (39%), with recurrence being highest in the chemotherapy-only group (7 patients, 70%). There was a significant difference in 5-year survival between the sequential therapy and chemotherapy groups (5-year survival, 75% vs 22%, $P = .05$), and a borderline significant difference between the WPI and chemotherapy groups (50% vs 22%, $P = .066$). When controlled for stage, sequential therapy was associated with a decrease in mortality compared with chemotherapy (hazard rate [HR] = 0.20, 95% confidence interval [CI] 0.04-0.99, $P = .049$), but a nonsignificant decrease in mortality when compared with WPI (HR = 0.50, 95% CI 0.1-2.32, $P = 0.4$).

This study indicates that sequential therapy may be beneficial in this patient group. Few studies have been able to show any significant survival advantages in the adjuvant treatment of uterine carcinosarcomas, and interpretation of results of earlier studies has been hampered by grouping together of uterine leiomyosarcomas and carcinosarcomas. The disadvantages of this study are that treatment assignment modality would not appear to have been a strict criteria for each institution, only that each institution had a "preferred" modality treatment. The numbers in each group are small but given the rarity of this tumor type, not unexpected. The results of this study would suggest that sequential treatment deserves to be studied in this patient population as a form of adjuvant therapy.

S. D. Yamada, MD

Phase III Trial of Doxorubicin With or Without Cisplatin in Advanced Endometrial Carcinoma: A Gynecologic Oncology Group Study

Thigpen JT, Brady MF, Homesley HD, et al (Univ of Mississippi, Jackson; Roswell Park Cancer and Data Ctr, Buffalo, NY; Albany Med Ctr, NY; et al)
J Clin Oncol 22:3902-3908, 2004   42–11

Purpose.—Doxorubicin and cisplatin have activity in endometrial carcinoma and at initiation of this study ranked as the most active agents. This trial of stage III, IV, or recurrent disease evaluated whether combining these agents increases response rate (RR) and prolongs progression-free survival (PFS) and overall survival (OS) over doxorubicin alone.

Patients and Methods.—Of 299 patients registered, 281 (94%) were eligible. Regimens were doxorubicin 60 mg/m^2 intravenously or doxorubicin 60 mg/m^2 plus cisplatin 50 mg/m^2 every 3 weeks until disease progression, unacceptable toxicity, or a total of 500 mg/m^2 doxorubicin.

Results.—There were 12 (8%) complete (CR) and 26 (17%) partial responses (PR) among 150 patients receiving doxorubicin versus 25 (19%) CRs and 30 (23%) PRs among patients receiving the combination. The overall response rate was higher among patients receiving the combination (42%) compared with patients receiving doxorubicin (25%; P = .004). Median PFS was 5.7 and 3.8 months, respectively, for the combination and single agent. The PFS hazard ratio was 0.736 (95% CI, 0.577 to 0.939; P = .014). Median OS was 9.0 and 9.2 months, respectively, for the combination and single agent. Overall death rates were similar in the two groups (hazard ratio, 0.928; 95% CI, 0.727 to 1.185). Nausea, vomiting, and hematologic toxicities were common. The combination produced more grade 3 to 4 leukopenia (62% *v* 40%), thrombocytopenia (14% *v* 2%), anemia (22% *v* 4%), and nausea/vomiting (13% *v* 3%).

Conclusion.—Adding cisplatin to doxorubicin in advanced endometrial carcinoma improves RR and PFS with a negligible impact on OS and produces increased toxicity. These results have served as a building block for subsequent phase III trials in patients with disseminated and high-risk limited endometrial carcinoma.

▶ This is a somewhat belated publication of GOG 107, the most pivotal endometrial cancer chemotherapy trial conducted by GOG to date. The study accrued patients from 1988 to 1992 and established doxorubicin and cisplatin as the standard chemotherapy for endometrial cancer during the 1990s on the basis of significantly improved response rate and progression-free survival. While overall survival was not significantly improved, one would anticipate that many of the patients who received doxorubicin only were subsequently treated with cisplatin. This combination then became the control arm for subsequent GOG phase III trials 122, 139, 163, and 177.[1-4] The last of those trials, 177, showed that the addition of paclitaxel with growth factor support to doxorubicin and cisplatin resulted in a significant improvement in response rate, progression-free survival, and overall survival.[3]

D. S. Miller, MD

References

1. Gallion HH, Brunetto VL, Cibull M, et al: Randomized phase III trial of standard timed doxorubicin plus cisplatin versus circadian timed doxorubicin plus cisplatin in stage III and IV or recurrent endometrial carcinoma: A Gynecologic Oncology Group study. *J Clin Oncol* 21:3808-3813, 2003. (2005 YEAR BOOK OF OBSTETRICS, GYNECOLOGY, AND WOMEN'S HEALTH, p 430-431.)
2. Randall ME, Brunetto G, Muss H, et al: Whole abdominal radiotherapy versus combination doxorubicin-cisplatin chemotherapy in advanced endometrial carcinoma: A randomized phase III trial of the Gynecologic Oncology Group. *Proc Am Soc Clin Oncol* 22:2, 2003.
3. Fleming GF, Brunetto VL, Cella D, et al: Phase III trial of doxorubicin plus cisplatin with or without paclitaxel plus filgrastim in advanced endometrial carcinoma: A Gynecologic Oncology Group study. *J Clin Oncol* 22:2159-2166, 2004.
4. Fleming GF, Filiaci VL, Bentley RC, et al: Phase III randomized trial of doxorubicin + cisplatin versus doxorubicin + 24-h paclitaxel + filgrastim in endometrial carcinoma: A Gynecologic Oncology Group study. *Ann Oncol* 15:1173-1178, 2004. (2005 YEAR BOOK OF OBSTETRICS, GYNECOLOGY, AND WOMEN'S HEALTH, p 431-432.)

Phase III Randomized Trial of Doxorubicin + Cisplatin Versus Doxorubicin + 24-h Paclitaxel + Filgrastim in Endometrial Carcinoma: A Gynecologic Oncology Group Study

Fleming GF, Filiaci VL, Bentley RC, et al (Univ of Chicago; Roswell Park Cancer Inst, Buffalo, NY; Duke Univ, Durham, NC; et al)
Ann Oncol 15:1173-1178, 2004   42–12

Background.—This study was performed to determine whether 24-h paclitaxel plus doxorubicin and filgrastim was superior to cisplatin plus doxorubicin in patients with endometrial cancer with respect to response, progression-free survival (PFS) and overall survival (OS).

Patients and Methods.—Eligible chemotherapy-naive patients were randomly assigned to doxorubicin 60 mg/m² intravenously (i.v.) followed by cisplatin 50 mg/m² i.v. (arm 1, $n = 157$) or doxorubicin 50 mg/m² i.v. followed 4 h later by paclitaxel 150 mg/m² i.v. over 24 h plus filgrastim 5 μg/kg on days 3–12 (arm 2, $n = 160$). Starting doses were reduced for prior pelvic radiotherapy and age >65 years. Both regimens were to be repeated every 3 weeks for a maximum of seven cycles.

Results.—There was no significant difference in response rate (40% versus 43%), PFS (median 7.2 versus 6 months) or OS (median 12.6 versus 13.6 months) for arm 1 and arm 2, respectively. Toxicities were primarily hematological, with 54% (arm 1) and 50% (arm 2) of patients experiencing grade 4 granulocytopenia. Gastrointestinal toxicities were similar in both arms.

Conclusions.—Doxorubicin and 24-h paclitaxel plus filgrastim was not superior to doxorubicin and cisplatin in terms of response, PFS or survival in advanced endometrial cancer.

▶ Paclitaxel is one of the few drugs tested by the Gynecologic Oncology Group (GOG) that has both frontline and second-line activity against endometrial cancer.[1,2] But doublet of doxorubicin and paclitaxel was not superior to doxorubicin and cisplatin. While this study did not produce a winner it does provide useful information. A subsequent GOG trial, #177, showed that the addition of paclitaxel to doxorubicin and cisplatin produced an improvement in response rate, PFS, and OS.[3] The results of all these studies taken together lead one to conclude that the most active 2-drug combinations against endometrial cancer might be cisplatin and paclitaxel. That combination can be toxic and many have suggested carboplatin and paclitaxel as a less toxic and more convenient alternative. Thus the design of the present open GOG trial #209, which compares the combination of paclitaxel, doxorubicin, and cisplatin with carboplatin and paclitaxel.

D. S. Miller, MD

References

1. Ball HG, Blessing JA, Lentz SS, et al: A phase II trial of paclitaxel in patients with advanced or recurrent adenocarcinoma of the endometrium: A Gynecologic Oncology Group study. *Gynecol Oncol* 62:278-281, 1996.
2. Lincoln S, Blessing JA, Lee RB, et al: Activity of paclitaxel as second-line chemotherapy in endometrial carcinoma: A Gynecologic Oncology Group study. *Gynecol Oncol* 88:277-281, 2003. (2004 YEAR BOOK OF OBSTETRICS, GYNECOLOGY, AND WOMEN'S HEALTH, p 480-481.)
3. Fleming GF, Brunetto VL, Cella D, et al: Phase III trial of doxorubicin plus cisplatin with or without paclitaxel plus filgrastim in advanced endometrial carcinoma: A Gynecologic Oncology Group study. *J Clin Oncol* 22:2159-2166, 2004. (2005 YEAR BOOK OF OBSTETRICS, GYNECOLOGY, AND WOMEN'S HEALTH, p 431-432.)

Randomized Phase III Trial of Cisplatin With or Without Topotecan in Carcinoma of the Uterine Cervix: A Gynecologic Oncology Group Study

Long HJ III, Bundy BN, Grendys EC Jr, et al (Mayo Clinic, Rochester, Minn; Roswell Park Cancer Inst, Buffalo, NY; Northwestern Univ, Chicago; et al)
J Clin Oncol 23:4626-4633, 2005   42–13

Purpose.—On the basis of reported activity of methotrexate, vinblastine, doxorubicin, and cisplatin (MVAC) or topotecan plus cisplatin in advanced cervix cancer, we undertook a randomized trial comparing these combinations versus cisplatin alone, to determine whether survival is improved with either combination compared with cisplatin alone, and to compare toxicities and quality of life (QOL) among the regimens.

Patients and Methods.—Eligible patients were randomly allocated to receive cisplatin 50 mg/m² every 3 weeks (CPT); cisplatin 50 mg/m² day 1 plus topotecan 0.75 mg/m² days 1 to 3 every 3 weeks (CT); or methotrexate 30 mg/m² days 1, 15, and 22, vinblastine 3 mg/m² days 2, 15, and 22, doxorubicin 30 mg/m² day 2, and cisplatin 70 mg/m² day 2 every 4 weeks (MVAC). Survival was the primary end point; response rate and progression-free survival (PFS) were secondary end points. QOL data are reported separately.

Results.—The MVAC arm was closed by the Data Safety Monitoring Board after four treatment-related deaths occurred among 63 patients, and is not included in this analysis. Two hundred ninety-four patients enrolled onto the remaining regimens: 146 to CPT and 147 to CT. Grade 3 to 4 hematologic toxicity was more common with CT. Patients receiving CT had statistically superior outcomes to those receiving CPT, with median overall survival of 9.4 and 6.5 months ($P = .017$), median PFS of 4.6 and 2.9 months ($P = .014$), and response rates of 27% and 13%, respectively.

Conclusion.—This is the first randomized phase III trial to demonstrate a survival advantage for combination chemotherapy over cisplatin alone in advanced cervix cancer.

▶ This study is a randomized phase III trial analyzing use of cisplatin alone or cisplatin with topotecan in patients with advanced (stage IVB), recurrent, or persistent carcinoma (squamous, adenosquamous, or adenocarcinoma) of the uterine cervix. The study was originally designed as a 3-arm trial to include (1) cisplatin 50 mg/m² IV every 21 days; (2) topotecan 0.75 mg/m² IV on days 1,2, and 3 followed by cisplatin 50 mg/m² on day 1; or (3) MVAC every 28 days. A total of 364 women were entered onto the trial of which 356 were eligible. Because of 4 treatment-associated deaths in the MVAC arm, this arm was closed after 63 patients were accrued. Hematologic toxicity was more severe in the CT arm as compared with the CPT arm. Grade 3 and 4 neutropenia, febrile neutropenia, infection, and thrombocytopenia occurred significantly more often in the CT patients than in the CPT patients. One patient who received CT died of hemorrhagic complications of disease possibly complicated by thrombocytopenia, while 2 others in the CT arm died of pulmonary emboli.

There was a statistically significant improvement in PFS and median survival in the group that received CT. The median PFS was 2.9 months for CPT and 4.6 months for CT. The adjusted relative risk (RR) estimate for the CT arm was 0.738 (95% confidence interval [CI], 0.578-0.942, $P = .0075$, one tailed). Median survival was also significantly improved for the CT arm: 6.5 months for CPT versus 9.4 months for CT. The adjusted RR estimate for survival was 0.77 (95% CI, 0.600-0.992, $P = .021$, one tailed) favoring the CT arm. Overall response rate was 13% for CPT and 27% for CT (95% CI, 0.194-0.350, $P = 004$) (Table 2 in the original article). The CT arm demonstrated an improvement in PFS and overall survival even when prior cisplatin therapy use was taken into account.

The impact of this study is that it is the first randomized trial to demonstrate a survival advantage for a chemotherapy arm in advanced or recurrent cervical cancer. This 2.9-month improvement in median survival does come at the cost of increased toxicity, however.

S. D. Yamada, MD

▶ This pivotal study known as GOG 179 is the first randomized clinical trial to show a survival advantage to any therapeutic program among women with FIGO stage IVB or recurrent cervical carcinoma. Although the combination of cisplatin and topotecan is associated with more myelosuppression, it produces a 2.9-month prolongation in survival. This is particularly significant since many patients with recurrent and/or advanced cervical cancer are young, making any prolongation in survival clinically significant. This clinical trial also makes 2 important observations relevant to the treatment of patients with recurrent or advanced cervical carcinoma.

First, the study shows the effect of prior treatment with cisplatin-based chemoradiation therapy on overall survival for the 2 treatment regimens. This was significant by univariate and Cox regression analysis with patients who had not received prior radiosensitizing chemotherapy and did receive topotecan in addition to cisplatin at the time of recurrence having a prolonged survival.

The second observation made by GOG 179 is the prognostic significance of the time from diagnosis to treatment of recurrent disease among patients with recurrent metastatic cancer. This strong prognostic factor was significant even after accounting for performance, status, and age. For example, among patients with recurrent disease, every 6-month increment from the time of diagnosis to the beginning of treatment of disease was associated with a decrease in risk expressed as a relative risk of 0.81 (ie, 19% risk reduction), with a plateau at 30 months and a relative risk of 0.35. Figure 4 illustrates the effect of time from initial diagnosis to study entry of patients with recurrent disease.

The combination of cisplatin and topotecan is being compared with other cisplatin-containing doublets in a current GOG trial, protocol 204. This study compares cisplatin plus topotecan to cisplatin plus gemcitabine, cisplatin plus paclitaxel, and cisplatin plus vinorelbine.

B. J. Monk, MD

43 Fallopian Tube and Ovary

Additional Salpingectomy After Previous Prophylactic Oophorectomy in High-Risk Women: Sense or Nonsense

Olivier RI, Lubsen-Brandsma LAC, van Boven H, et al (The Netherlands Cancer Inst, Amsterdam; Academic Med Ctr, Amsterdam)

Gynecol Oncol 96:439-443, 2005   43–1

Objectives.—Since BRCA1/2 germ line mutation carriers are also at a higher risk of developing fallopian tube carcinoma, resection of the fallopian tubes is currently included at the time of risk reducing surgery. In this study,

TABLE 1.—Patient Characteristics of the Group Studied

	Additonal BPS After BPO (N = 15)	BPO (N = 27)
DNA results		
BRCA1 mutation	10	17
BRCA2 mutation	1	3
BRCA1 and 2 mutation	1	—
Non-informative test results	3	2
Not tested	—	3
Non-carrier BRCA1	—	2
Mean age at oophorectomy	42.7 (32-60)	48.7 (32-65)
(year, range)		
Mean follow-up	80 (64-112)	66 (1-109)
(months, range)		
Mean age at salpingectomy	47 (37-65)	NA
(year, range)		
Salpingectomy		
Laparoscopic	13	NA
Laparotomic	2	NA
Interval between BPO and BPS	65 (6-101)	NA
(months, range)		
Post-oophorectomy peritoneal	0	3
papillary serous cancer (N)		
Age at diagnosis (year, range)	NA	57 (53-64)
Follow-up time to diagnosis	NA	60 (33-77)
(months, range)		

NA = not applicable.
(Courtesy of Olivier RI, Lubsen-Brandsma LAC, van Boven H, et al: Additional salpingectomy after previous prophylactic oophorectomy in high-risk women: Sense or nonsense. *Gynecol Oncol* 96:439-443. Copyright 2005 by Elsevier Science Inc.)

we comment on the need of additional bilateral prophylactic salpingectomy (BPS) following previous bilateral prophylactic oophorectomy (BPO) in women at high risk of ovarian cancer.

Methods.—Retrospectively, the medical files of 42 high-risk women, who had undergone BPO only, were reviewed (Table 1).

Results.—In our center, risk-reducing surgery consisted of BPO only for 42 women. Twenty-seven women received an informative letter in which counseling for additional BPS was offered. In total, 15 women opted for additional BPS. Surgery was performed with a mean interval of 65 months (range 6–101) in 10 BRCA1 carriers, one BRCA2 carrier, one BRCA1 and 2 carrier, and three women with non-informative test results. The procedure was readily done by laparoscopy in 13 women and two needed a laparotomy. No post-operative complications had occurred. Histopathological examination revealed no malignancy.

Conclusions.—We believe that additional risk reduction of cancer necessitates BPS in BRCA1/2 carriers after previous BPO. BPS after previous BPO was easily performed. Today, physicians should include resection of the fallopian tube at prophylactic surgery in high-risk women and should consider additional BPS in women who have undergone BPO only.

▶ Women who are carriers of *BRCA1* or *BRCA2* germ line mutations are at a considerably increased risk for developing ovarian and fallopian tube carcinomas compared with the general population. The detection of *BRCA1* or *BRCA2* mutations commonly leads to a frank discussion of prophylactic oophorectomy to reduce the woman's risk for developing ovarian cancer. However, the removal of ovaries from women who carry *BRCA* mutations does not result in an absolute prevention against peritoneal carcinomatosis. This study by Olivier et al from The Netherlands Cancer Institute in Amsterdam shows that there can be considerable benefit for women who carry *BRCA* mutations to be offered not only bilateral oophorectomy but bilateral salpingectomy at the time of surgery. As removal of the entire adnexa does not result in an increased risk of adverse surgical outcomes, such interventions should be offered routinely to all women who seek to reduce their risk of developing ovarian and fallopian tube carcinomas as a result of inheriting *BRCA* mutations. In addition, those women who have previously undergone bilateral oophorectomy to reduce their risk for ovarian cancer should be offered prophylactic bilateral salpingectomy to further reduce their risk for fallopian tube carcinoma and peritoneal carcinomatosis. The authors report that performing bilateral salpingectomy in women who have previously undergone bilateral oophorectomy is usually not a difficult procedure, and the benefits may be profound.

L. P. Shulman, MD

The Utility of Hand-Assisted Laparoscopy in Ovarian Cancer

Krivak TC, Elkas JC, Rose GS, et al (Daivid Grant Med Ctr, Vacaville, Calif; Walter Reed Army Med Ctr, Washington, DC; Brooke Army Med Ctr, Fort Sam Houston, Tex; et al)

Gynecol Oncol 96:72-76, 2005   43–2

Background.—Traditionally, patients with ovarian cancer are subjected to midline vertical incision to facilitate cytoreductive surgery and comprehensive surgical staging. With the growing interest in minimally invasive techniques, alternative methods to accomplish the goals of surgical care in patients with ovarian cancer are being explored.

Methods.—The authors examined the feasibility of using hand-assisted laparoscopy in 25 patients with ovarian cancer who underwent staging or cytoreduction.

Findings.—Of the 25 patients, 6 patients had apparent advanced-stage cancer with gross spread of disease and thus were candidates for cytoreduction, while 19 had apparent early-stage disease and thus were candidates for comprehensive surgical staging. Of these 19 patients, 5 were found to have positive retroperitoneal lymph node involvement, 3 had other disease confined to the pelvis, and 2 had microscopic omental disease. Twenty-two of the 25 patients had their intended surgery completed by the hand-assisted technique, and the other 3 patients required conversion to a laparotomy to complete their debulking surgery. The complication rate was low, with 3 patients requiring either reoperation or hospitalization. The mean operative time was 201 minutes (range, 81-365 minutes), and the mean estimated blood loss was 271 mL. The median hospital stay was 2 days.

Conclusion.—Laparoscopy with the use of the hand-assisted technique is feasible in comprehensively staging patients with apparent early-stage ovarian cancer. Furthermore, the majority of patients with advanced disease are able to be cytoreduced with this technique as well.

▶ This article highlights the growing interest in utilizing minimally invasive techniques to facilitate equal surgical outcomes in terms of efficacy, while offering the significant advantages of minimally invasive surgery such as reduced length of stay, decreased pain and recovery time, and earlier return to employment. Laparoscopy has been widely used in the management of pelvic masses and, more recently, for staging patients with gynecologic malignancies, most commonly endometrial cancers. The addition of the hand-assisted technique allows for the surgeon to have greater exposure to the peritoneal cavity while still utilizing a small incision.

These authors used a 6- to 7-cm periumbilical or suprapubic incision to place the hand port. This intervention allows for greater tactile sensation, the ability to palpate intraperitoneal structures, and the opportunity to deliver structures extracorporally for possible resection.

The concerns raised by review of this retrospective analysis include the applicability of the technique to less experienced surgeons and the assessment of true benefit. For example, hospital stay may not be greatly reduced in that many patients. With a staging procedure performed via a laparotomy, patients will be hospitalized for 2 to 4 days, which overlaps with the average length of stay in this study. Furthermore, there is no evidence that the adequacy of the procedure was equal to what would be achieved with an open procedure in terms of thoroughness, although the mean lymph node count of 18 appeared reasonable, but not conclusive of equivalent efficacy. There were no recurrence or survival data reported. Another significant concern is the 14% complication rate. It is unclear if this rate would be reduced via a laparotomy. Despite past reports, there were no instances of port site recurrences in this series.

In summary, this proof-of-principle study has shown that the hand-assisted technique warrants further exploration in well-controlled trials in comparison with not only open laparotomy, but also with laparoscopy alone. Only then will one be able to understand the relative benefits of this interesting surgical access option.

T. J. Herzog, MD

Improved Optimal Cytoreduction Rates for Stages IIIC and IV Epithelial Ovarian, Fallopian Tube, and Primary Peritoneal Cancer: A Change in Surgical Approach

Chi DS, Franklin CC, Levine DA, et al (Mem Sloan-Kettering Cancer Ctr, New York; Harvard Univ, Boston; Nassau County Med Ctr, Long Island, NY)
Gynecol Oncol 94:650-654, 2004   43–3

Objective.—To determine the impact of the incorporation of extensive upper abdominal debulking procedures on the rates of optimal primary cytoreduction and complications in stages IIIC and IV epithelial ovarian, fallopian tube, and primary peritoneal carcinomas.

Methods.—Two groups of patients were identified for comparison. Group 1, the control group, consisted of 70 consecutive patients who underwent "standard" primary cytoreductive surgery before May 2000. Group 2, the study group, was composed of 70 consecutive patients who underwent surgery after January 2001, during which time, a more comprehensive debulking of upper abdominal disease was used, including diaphragm stripping/resection, splenectomy, distal pancreatectomy, liver resection, resection of porta hepatis tumor, and cholecystectomy.

Results.—The median age of the entire cohort was 60 years (range, 36-88 years). The majority had stage IIIC disease (86%) and serous histology (76%). Optimal cytoreduction (residual disease ≤ 1 cm) rates were 50% for group 1 and 76% for group 2 ($P < 0.01$). Patients in group 2 were more likely to have undergone extensive procedure(s) (27% versus 3%; $P < 0.001$). Operative time and estimated blood loss were greater in group 2 than group 1 (264 versus 174 min, 880 versus 460 cc, respectively; $P < 0.001$ for both). Complication rates and length of hospitalization were not significantly different between the two groups.

Conclusion.—The use of extensive upper abdominal surgical procedures significantly increased the rate of optimal primary cytoreduction. Although operative time and estimated blood loss were increased, the rate of major complications and length of hospitalization remained the same.

▶ Since the original work published by Griffiths in 1975, numerous studies have demonstrated a strong inverse correlation between amount of residual disease after primary cytoreductive surgery for ovarian cancer and overall survival. Five-year survival rates approach 50% in women with advanced-stage disease who undergo optimal cytoreduction (no residual disease greater than 1 cm in size). The outcome is significantly poorer in cases where residual tumor is greater than 1 cm in size, supporting the importance of reducing the bulky disease to minimal residual in women with ovarian cancer. The failure to achieve optimal cytoreductive status is often related to an ability to optimally debulk disease in the upper abdomen. In this study, the authors instituted a multidisciplinary surgical approach that included surgeons with sufficient expertise to perform procedures such as a distal pancreatectomy, partial liver resections, resection of tumor from the porta hepatis, as well as a diaphragmatic resections as needed to achieve optimal cytoreduction of ovarian cancer. The surgical team was able to increase the optimal cytoreductive rates significantly by 50%. Overall morbidity was not significantly enhanced in women who required advanced radical procedures to achieve optimal cytoreductions. The strengths of the study include the large number of cases and that all cases were all accrued at 1 institution. It is likely that the enhanced cytoreductive rate that has been achieved will lead to improved outcomes. The authors demonstrate the feasibility of optimal cytoreductive surgery with acceptable morbidity when implementing radical resection procedures in the upper abdomen.

G. Rodriguez, MD

Factors Associated With Cytoreducibility Among Women With Ovarian Carcinoma
Eltabbakh GH, Mount SL, Beatty B, et al (Univ of Vermont, Burlington)
Gynecol Oncol 95:377-383, 2004   43–4

Objectives.—The aim of the current study is to investigate the clinical and molecular factors associated with cytoreduction among women with advanced stage epithelial ovarian carcinoma EOC.

Methods.—Seventy-two women with FIGO stage III and IV EOC or primary peritoneal carcinoma (PPC) underwent similar attempt at surgical cytoreduction, mostly by the same surgeon. The histologic material of these patients was reviewed and the histologic subtype and grade were assigned. Immunohistochemical tests were performed for expression of molecular regulators of apoptosis (p53, p21, Bcl_2, Bcl_x, Bax) and chemoresistance (PGP, MRP, LRP, GST). The following factors were assessed for their association with complete (no residual tumor) and optimal (residual tumor < 1 cm) cytoreduction: type of carcinoma (EOC versus PPC), stage, CA-125 val-

TABLE 2.—Clinical Factors Associated With Complete Cytoreduction Among Women With Advanced Stage Ovarian or Primary Peritoneal Carcinoma ($n = 72$)

Factor	Number With Complete Cytoreduction/ Total Number (%)	P Value	Odds Ratio	95% Confidence Interval
Type:				
Ovarian carcinoma	21/63 (33.3%)	0.50	1.8	0.3, 9.2
Primary peritoneal carcinoma	2/9 (22.2%)			
Stage				
IIA + IIIB	10/15 (66.7%)	<0.001	6.8	2.0, 23.4
IIIC + IV	13/57 (22.8%)			
CA-125 values				
≤500 IU/ml	17/30 (56.7%)	<0.001	7.9	2.5, 24.2
>500 IU/ml	6/42 (14.3%)			
Ascites				
≤1 1	20/43 (46.5%)	<0.001	7.5	2.0, 28.7
>1 1	3/29 (10.3%)			
Histology				
Non serous	12/20 (60.0%)	<0.001	5.6	1.8, 17.0
Serous	11/52 (21.2%)			
Grade				
1 + 2	14/38 (36.8%)	0.35	1.6	0.6, 4.4
3	9/34 (26.5%)			

(Courtesy of Eltabbakh GH, Mount SL, Beatty B, et al: Factors associated with cytoreducibility among women with ovarian carcinoma. *Gynecol Oncol* 95:377-383. Copyright 2004 by Elsevier Science Inc.)

ues, ascites, histology, tumor grade, and p53, p21, Bcl_2, Bcl_x, Bax, PGP, MRP, LRP, GST expression using the odds ratio and associated 95% confidence intervals. Significant univariate odds ratios were assessed jointly in a multivariate logistic regression model. Receiver operating characteristic curve analysis was performed to determine the CA-125 level with the maximal cytoreduction prognostic power.

Results.—Twenty-three (31.9%) women had no residual tumor, 35 (48.6%) had ≤1 cm residual tumor and 14 (19.4%) had residual tumor >1 cm. Factors with significant univariate associations with complete cytoreduction included stage, CA-125 level, ascites, histology, and p53 (Tables 2 and 3). p53 expression was the only factor which remained significant in the multivariate analysis (odds ratio 7.2, 95% CI 1.5, 34.9). A preoperative CA-125 value of ≤500 IU/ml best determined complete cytoreducibility.

Conclusions.—Innate tumor characteristics determine cytoreducibility of women with ovarian carcinoma. Preoperative evaluation of p53 expression may be of value in predicting the outcome of cytoreductive surgery in women with advanced stage EOC.

TABLE 3.—Molecular Factors Associated With Complete Cytoreduction Among Women With Advanced Stage Ovarian or Primary Peritoneal Carcinoma ($n = 63$)

Factor	Number With Complete Cytoreductoin/ Total Number (%)	P Value	Odds Ratio	95% Confidence Interval
p53 expression				
Mild or moderate	14/28 (50.0%)	0.003	5.6	1.7, 18.7
Strong	5/33 (15.2%)			
p21 expression				
Mild or moderate	17/57 (29.8%)	0.40	0.4	0.1, 3.3
Strong	2/4 (50.0%)			
Bcl₂ expression				
Mild or moderate	13/50 (26.0%)	0.06	0.3	0.1, 1.1
Strong	6/11 (54.6%)			
Bclₓ expression				
Mild or moderate	0/3	0.23	0.3	0.0, 5.9
Strong	19/58 (32.8%)			
Bax expression				
Mild or moderate	2/6 (33.3%)	0.90	1.1	0.2, 6.7
Strong	17/55 (30.9%)			
PGP expression				
Mild or moderate	10/32 (31.3%)	0.99	1.0	0.3, 3.0
Strong	9/29 (31.0%)			
MRP expression				
Mild or moderate	12/38 (31.6%)	0.93	1.1	0.3, 3.2
Strong	7/23 (30.4%)			
LRP expression				
Mild or moderate	12/44 (27.3%)	0.29	0.5	0.2, 1.7
Strong	7/17 (41.2%)			
GST expression				
Mild or moderate	5/12 (41.7%)	0.38	1.8	0.5, 6.6
Strong	14/49 (28.6%)			

(Courtesy of Eltabbakh GH, Mount SL, Beatty B, et al: Factors associated with cytoreducibility among women with ovarian carcinoma. *Gynecol Oncol* 95:377-383. Copyright 2004 by Elsevier Science Inc.)

▶ The objective of this study was to investigate the clinical and molecular factors associated with cytoreduction among women with FIGO stage 3 and 4 EOC or PPC. This is a retrospective study evaluating 72 women with advanced-stage EOC who underwent similar attempts of surgical cytoreduction. The authors studied a number of clinical characteristics, including residual tumor, type of carcinoma, stage, CA-125 value, ascites, histology, and tumor grade to determine the association with complete (no residual tumor) and optimal (residual tumor less than 1 cm) cytoreduction. Furthermore, the authors performed immunohistochemical analysis of tissue blocks to assess expression of molecular regulators of apoptosis and chemoresistance. By odds ratio and associated 95% confidence intervals, significant univariate odds ratios were assessed jointly in a multivariate logistic regression model. The authors found that factors with significant univariate association for complete cytoreduction included stage, CA-125 level (less than 500 IU/mL), ascites, histology, and p53 expression. In a multivariate analysis, p53 expression was the only factor that remained significant. The authors concluded that tumor biology may be a determinant of cytoreducibility in women with advanced ovarian cancer.

This is a very interesting study in light of the current standard of care in EOC. The cornerstone of therapy includes an attempt at aggressive cytoreductive surgery that may include small and large bowel resections as well as block resection of the pancreas, spleen, and diaphragm. Proponents of this aggressive surgical approach believe that it is the main factor involved in improving survival. Others believe that the survival benefit achieved in patients who are completely cytoreduced is not entirely related to the surgical procedure itself but to the biology of the tumor.[1-3] Undoubtedly, the truth lies between both philosophies. With the advent of biologic serum markers that reflect tumor characteristics such as aggressiveness, angiogenic potential, and chemoresistance, we hope that in the future we are able to better define a patient population whose tumor biology may not lend itself to optimal surgical cytoreduction. It may be that a subgroup of these patients would be better served by neoadjuvant chemotherapy up front. Currently, we are selecting a patient population for neoadjuvant treatment that is founded solely on clinical impression as opposed to molecular data. We look forward to additional studies that will allow us to further characterize the molecular biology of the tumor to help guide our clinical management.

J. A. Hurteau, MD

References

1. Covens AL: A critique of surgical cytoreduction in advanced ovarian cancer. *Gynecol Oncol* 78:269-374, 2000.
2. Hoskins WJ, Bundy BN, Thigpen JT, et al: The influence of cytoreductive surgery on recurrence-free interval and survival in small-volume stage III epithelial ovarian cancer: A Gynecologic Oncology Group Study. *Gynecol Oncol* 47:159-166, 1992.
3. Potter ME, Partridge EE, Hatch KD, et al: Primary surgical therapy for ovarian cancer: How much and when. *Gynecol Oncol* 40:195-200, 1992.

Secondary Surgical Cytoreduction for Advanced Ovarian Carcinoma
Rose PG, Nerenstone S, Brady MF, et al (Case Western Reserve Univ, Cleveland, Ohio; Univ of Connecticut, Hartford; Roswell Park Cancer Inst, Buffalo, NY; et al)
N Engl J Med 351:2489-2497, 2004   43–5

Background.—We evaluated the effect of adding secondary cytoreductive surgery to postoperative chemotherapy on progression-free survival and overall survival among patients who had advanced ovarian cancer and residual tumor exceeding 1 cm in diameter after primary surgery.

Methods.—Women were enrolled within six weeks after primary surgery. If, after three cycles of postoperative paclitaxel plus cisplatin, a patient had no evidence of progressive disease, she was randomly assigned to undergo

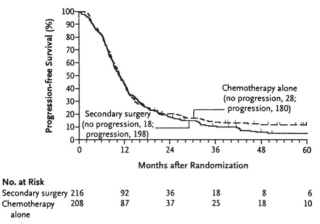

FIGURE 2.—Progression-free survival. (Courtesy of Rose PG, Nerenstone S, Brady MF, et al: Secondary surgical cytoreduction for advanced ovarian carcinoma. *N Engl J Med* 351:2489-2497, 2004. Copyright Massachusetts Medical Society. All rights reserved.)

secondary cytoreductive surgery followed by three more cycles of chemotherapy or three more cycles of chemotherapy alone.

Results.—We enrolled 550 women. After completing three cycles of postoperative chemotherapy, 216 eligible patients were randomly assigned to receive secondary surgical cytoreduction followed by chemotherapy and 208 to receive chemotherapy alone. Surgery was declined by or medically contraindicated in 15 patients who were assigned to secondary surgery (7 percent). As of March 2003, 296 patients had died and 82 had progressive disease. The likelihood of progression-free survival in the group assigned to secondary surgery plus chemotherapy, as compared with the chemotherapy-alone group, was 1.07 (95 percent confidence interval, 0.87 to 1.31; P=0.54) (Fig 2), and the relative risk of death was 0.99 (95 percent confidence interval, 0.79 to 1.24; P=0.92).

Conclusions.—For patients with advanced ovarian carcinoma in whom primary cytoreductive surgery was considered to be maximal, the addition of secondary cytoreductive surgery to postoperative chemotherapy with paclitaxel plus cisplatin does not improve progression-free survival or overall survival.

▶ Over the past 3 decades, a large number of retrospective studies have shown an inverse correlation between the size of residual tumor remaining after primary surgical debulking and both progression-free and overall survival in women with ovarian cancer. Notably, superior outcomes have been demonstrated in the setting where no residual tumor deposit is greater than 1 cm. Thus, the 1-cm residual threshold has been accepted as defining optimal cytoreductive surgery. Unfortunately, optimal debulking is not feasible in all women with advanced ovarian cancer. Factors that would limit optimal resection have included medical comorbidities that would increase the risks associated with radical tumor debulking, or technical limitations related to the extent or location of metastasis that would preclude optimal debulking.

In women in whom optimal cytoreductive surgery is not feasible, a secondary attempt at optimal cytoreductive surgery after induction chemotherapy has emerged as a potential strategy to both reduce tumor burden and improve survival. A prior randomized study conducted by the EORTC demonstrated significant improvement in median progression-free and overall survival in women who had suboptimal debulking of their ovarian cancer at their primary operation, but who demonstrated evidence of a response to several cycles of platinum-based chemotherapy, and then had optimal cytoreduction of their disease followed by completion of their chemotherapy.

The goal of this Gynecologic Oncology Group study by Peter Rose et al was to determine whether a secondary attempt at optimal cytoreduction of ovarian cancer would improve survival in women with advanced ovarian cancer who received a chemotherapy regimen comprised of a platinum agent and Taxol. Eligible patients for the study were those with advanced-stage ovarian cancer who had undergone a maximal attempt at optimal debulking surgery and in whom the residual intraperitoneal tumor burden exceeded 1 cm in diameter at any location. Women who responded to 3 cycles of chemotherapy with cisplatin and Taxol were randomized to either undergo secondary surgical cytoreduction followed by 3 more cycles of chemotherapy vs. 3 more cycles of chemotherapy alone.

Results of the study suggest no difference in overall outcome in those women who underwent an interval secondary cytoreductive procedure. The strengths of the study include the large sample size and the uniform attempt in all cases to perform a maximal surgical effort to optimally cytoreduce the tumor. The results of this study contrast with those of the prior EORTC trial. Both studies involve similar patients with advanced ovarian cancer. However, the EORTC study did not contain a chemotherapy regimen comprising Taxol. The differences in outcome may have been related both to differences in the 2 studies with regard to the degree of surgical effort to maximally cytoreduce ovarian cancer at the primary operation as well as differences in the chemotherapeutic regimens used, in that the GOG study included use of a taxane. It is possible that a more effective platinum/Taxol regimen administered in the GOG study may have abrogated any potential benefits associated with a secondary cytoreductive effort. Overall, the study calls into question the merit of a secondary debulking when a maximal attempt at tumor debulking has occurred at the primary operation.

G. Rodriguez, MD

Subject Index

A

Abortion
  breast cancer risk and, 273
  fetal pain in, multidisciplinary review of the evidence, 265
  mifepristone for, safety and efficacy in routine clinical use, 266
  misoprostol for
    6 vs. 12 hour vaginal administration in second trimester, 262
    alone in early abortion, comparison of 7 potential regimens, 264
    residents' attitudes toward participation in, 261
  risk factors for complications in Nigeria, 267
Adnexal cysts
  in postmenopausal women, prevalence and histologic diagnosis, 378
Adolescents
  age at first sexual intercourse and sexually transmitted infections in, 219
  cervical dysplasia in, 224
  combined estrogen and progestin transdermal contraceptive use in, 229
  DMPA contraception use and discontinuation, changes in bone mineral density with, 231
  fertility and parental consent for contraceptives for, 225
  high-dose estrogen treatment for reduction of adult height of tall girls, long-term effects on fertility, 177
  oral vs. vaginal sex among, 222
  positive experience of teenage motherhood, 228
  prescription contraception use and reactions to mandated parental notification for, 226
  virginity pledges and sexual behavior in, 220
Advanced maternal age
  blastocyst transfer with or without preimplantation diagnosis for aneuploidy screening in, 207
AGC (atypical glandular cells)
  utility of human papillomavirus triage in management of, 314
Airway management
  initiation for preterm newborn in delivery room, 166

Alcohol use
  breast cancer risk and, 276
Amnioinfusion
  for prevention of meconium aspiration syndrome, 169
Amniotic fluid
  proteomic profiling and novel biomarkers for diagnosis of intra-amniotic infection, 78
Anal sphincter
  risk of injury with occiput posterior fetal head position in forceps-assisted vaginal deliveries, 133
Androgens
  circulating levels in women
    correlates of, 238
    sexual function and, 240
  testosterone patch for low sexual desire in surgically menopausal women, 242
Aneuploidy
  anaphase lagging in blastocysts and, 211
  blastocyst transfer with and without preimplantation diagnosis for screening in advanced maternal age, 207
  post-zygotic chromosome loss in, 211
  preimplantation genetic diagnosis for screening in patients with unexplained recurrent miscarriages, 205
Angiotensin II type I (AT_1) receptors in preeclampsia, 75
Anorectal function
  effect of vaginal distention on, 368
Anovulation
  metformin for, in normoandrogenic women, 180
Anticoagulants
  pregnancy in women using, 108
Antiphospholipid syndrome
  heparin for prevention of pregnancy loss in, mechanisms of action, 188
Antiretroviral drugs
  maternal toxicity and pregnancy complications, 99, 100
  during pregnancy, birth defects risk associated with, 98
Aortic stenosis
  fetal, intrauterine balloon dilation for, 130
Apgar score
  cut-off point for identifying at-risk newborns, 165

Author Index

A

Abbà C, 385
Abd Essamad HM, 108
Abdel-Fattah M, 353
Abrao MS, 347
Abu-Rustum NR, 394, 429
Addis IB, 244
Aguirre O, 242
Ailawadi M, 291
Alborzi S, 346
Alexandre PK, 148
Al-Ghazi MS, 434
Allahdin S, 352
Allen GO, 259, 344
Allouche C, 144
Almeida PA, 193
Alonso AM, 338
Alvero R, 11
Aly H, 166
Ambroggio S, 385
Amini SB, 6
Amundsen CL, 358
Amunni G, 439
An H, 28
Andersen W, 314
Andrews WW, 81
Aparecida do Carmo Rego M, 85
Appleby PN, 388
Armstrong A, 11
Arnes M, 416
Arroyo C, 351
Arunkalaivanan AS, 353
Aschkenazi-Steinberg SO, 332
Avgidou K, 41
Avis N, 13
Awad R, 319
Axelrod JH, 449

B

Bajo-Arenas J, 191
Bakker PCAM, 148
Baksu A, 134
Ballow D, 15
Barak S, 286
Barnhart KT, 283, 291
Barone-Adesi L, 423
Barrington JW, 353
Barron J, 154
Baskett TF, 61
Beatty B, 467
Beckerman K, 98
Belinson JL, 333

Belkin A, 113
Benavides L, 133
Benet J, 210
Ben-Shachar I, 437
Benson CB, 45
Benson LJ, 163
Bentley RC, 458
Bernstein DI, 316
Berntrop K, 50
Berretta R, 421
Bersamin MM, 220
Bewtra C, 412
Beyene J, 63
Bhoola SM, 433
Bindra R, 41
Birgisdottir BE, 128
Bixby S, 284
Bjørge T, 420
Black S, 187
Blanchard K, 264
Blanchard MH, 6
Blank SV, 406
Blom GP, 378
Boente MP, 438
Bonney A, 233
Borkowski A, 359
Bose P, 187
Bosquet JG, 419
Boyer KM, 90
Bradley WH, 438
Brady MF, 457, 470
Brass LM, 374
Breborowicz G, 115
Bretelle F, 356
Brinton LA, 381
Broder MS, 308
Bromberger JT, 13
Brooker D, 438
Brown MB, 148
Brown ZA, 79, 80
Browning A, 362
Bruinsma F, 177
Brumfield CG, 57
Bryman I, 50
Bueno-de-Mesquita HB, 278
Bufin L, 137
Buhimschi CS, 72
Bujold E, 281
Bulterys M, 97
Bundy BN, 449, 459
Burger H, 237
Burkman RT, 252
Buster JE, 242
Butsashvili M, 93
Butte NF, 25
Buttin BM, 393

C

Cai J, 14
Calingaert B, 376, 442
Campagnoli C, 385
Cannon T, 355
Card TR, 106
Carmina E, 180
Cartar L, 64
Casey MJ, 412
Castrillon DH, 403
Caughey AB, 47
Cella D, 435
Centofanti P, 107
Chakravarty EF, 104
Chan AMY, 114
Chandna P, 400
Chanrachakul B, 262
Chaoui R, 119
Chauhan SP, 111, 137
Chavkin W, 53
Cheema R, 115
Cherpes TL, 316
Chervenak FA, 43
Chi DS, 394, 466
Chichester P, 20
Chien EK, 34
Childs AJ, 10
Chim SSC, 26
Chiu RWK, 26
Choi HJ, 426
Choi SH, 426
Chong DSY, 165
Christensen EE, 111
Chwalisz K, 340
Claeys P, 328
Claus EB, 411
Cleves MA, 32
Clifton VL, 73
Cohen L, 406
Colenbrander GJ, 148
Collins LL, 17
Colón I, 104
Condous G, 287
Connell K, 245
Constantinides C, 364
Coonen E, 211
Cooper GS, 14
Cooper JM, 337
Cornell JL, 222
Costa RLR, 327
Cottier JP, 338
Coutifaris C, 185
Covington DL, 98
Coyaji K, 264
Cragun JM, 442
Crawford A, 246